Behavior Problems in Preschool Children

Clinical and Developmental Issues

Second Edition

SUSAN B. CAMPBELL

THE GUILFORD PRESS
New York   London

KH

© 2002 The Guilford Press
A Division of Guilford Publications, Inc.
72 Spring Street, New York, NY 10012
www.guilford.com

Paperback edition 2006

Printed in the United States of America

This book is printed on acid-free paper.

Last digit is print number: 9   8   7   6   5   4   3

Library of Congress Cataloging-in-Publication Data

Campbell, Susan B.
  Behavior problems in preschool children : clinical and developmental
  issues / Susan B. Campbell.— 2nd ed.
      p. cm.
  Includes bibliographical references and index.
  ISBN-10: 1-57230-784-6   ISBN-13: 978-1-57230-784-1 (hardcover: alk. paper)
  ISBN-10: 1-59385-377-7   ISBN-13: 978-1-59385-377-8 (paperback)
  1. Behavior disorders in children.   2. Child development.   3. Preschool
children—Mental health. I. Title.
RJ506 .B44 C36 2002
618.92′89—dc21
                                                                2002008925

10/28/13

In memory of my mother, Estelle Goodman,
who was a career woman long before it was considered
acceptable for women with young children
to work outside the home;
she was a role model and inspiration.

About the Author

Susan B. Campbell, PhD, is Professor of Psychology at the University of Pittsburgh, where she has served as Chair of both the Clinical and Developmental Programs. She was the editor of the *Journal of Abnormal Child Psychology* from 1999 to 2005, and she has served on numerous editorial boards and review committees. Dr. Campbell is currently the principal investigator at the Pittsburgh site of the 10-site National Institute of Child Health and Human Development Study of Early Child Care and Youth Development. She is coauthor (with E. Mark Cummings and Patrick T. Davies) of *Developmental Psychopathology and Family Process*, published by The Guilford Press in 2000.

Preface

Three-year-old Jamie L. was expelled from preschool after frequent fights with other children. He seemed to have a "chip on his shoulder," and the rough-and-tumble play and toy struggles so common in preschool classrooms tended to escalate and become serious fights whenever Jamie was involved. Jamie seemed to lose control with other children; he was able to share toys and play quietly for only a few minutes at a time. If Jamie and some other boys were playing with trucks, Jamie was always the one to start the crashes, which got wilder and wilder. In the sandbox, it was always Jamie who threw sand in someone's face or grabbed the shovel from another child. Jamie got into fights almost daily, and at times he would get angry enough to bite, kick, and hit anyone—including the teacher—who wouldn't let him have his way. After a month in school, the teacher became worried that Jamie might seriously harm another child, and she asked Jamie's mother to keep him at home.

Jamie's mother was shocked and dismayed by this request. She knew that Jamie was a difficult child—hard to discipline, explosive, and prone to temper tantrums. He'd been hard to handle since early infancy. But she wanted to believe her pediatrician's reassurances that Jamie was just going through a difficult period of development and that she needn't worry. Mrs. L. and her husband agreed that Jamie was a handful, but they wavered between seeing his difficult behavior as "just a phase" and as a sign of more serious problems to come. There were many possible explanations for Jamie's unruly behavior in preschool. Maybe the preschool teacher didn't understand how to handle him. Maybe she was too strict. Maybe she didn't intervene soon enough when he was beginning to get wound up and overexcited. Maybe a school with more structure would be better for him. Or maybe at age 3, he just wasn't ready for a preschool program.

By contrast, 3-year-old Annie adapted well to preschool and loved it. Her teacher saw her as bright and sociable, though somewhat dependent and anxious. But she followed the school routines well and got along fine with other children. Annie's mother, however, was at her wits' end. She found Annie virtually impossible to manage, and the daily temper tantrums and constant battles were getting her down. She had enrolled Annie in preschool to give herself a break and was quite surprised at the teacher's report of Annie's good adjustment. Annie seemed to store up all her anger and defiance for her mother. She seemed a different child with other adults and was "Daddy's girl," putting additional stress on an already fragile marriage.

These vignettes describe typical problems encountered in the preschool period and raise a number of questions that developmentalists and parents alike must confront. It is obvious why parents would be upset by behavior such as this in their preschooler, but it is less clear whether they need to worry about its long-term implications. Is it important for the pediatrician, developmental specialist, or mental health professional to intervene with children like Jamie or Annie? Are they just going through a difficult period, or does their angry and uncontrolled behavior presage later, more serious problems? Even if the current problems are outgrown, what about the toll such children can take on parental self-esteem and marital harmony? Or are the problems themselves reflections of marital dysfunction, family distress, or inappropriate approaches to childrearing? Are Jamie's problems more likely to persist than Annie's, or vice versa? Or are they each likely to develop persistent problems, but of a different type? For example, will Jamie be likely to develop into an aggressive and/or hyperactive child? Will Annie develop problems with relationships or become a depressed or withdrawn adolescent?

In this book an attempt is made to address these issues, drawing on theoretical viewpoints and evidence from the fields of child development, developmental psychopathology, clinical child psychology, and child psychiatry. The focus is on late toddlerhood and the preschool period, with a particular emphasis on distinguishing those problems of early childhood that may be typical and transient from those that may be signs of a more persistent disorder. I explore problem behaviors in young children such as Jamie and Annie (roughly ages 2½–5) who may be going through a difficult and explosive, albeit temporary, developmental transition, or who may be showing early signs of more serious psychopathology with the potential to impede developmental progress. These are the children who confront parents, preschool teachers, pediatricians, and mental health professionals with particularly complex diagnostic and treatment decisions. However, prognostic predictions about the developmental course of problems in individual children are especially difficult to make with certainty, despite the growing empirical data on the emergence of problems in young children and their likely outcome at the group level.

It is widely accepted that the period between 2 and 5 is one of extremely rapid developmental change and that there are wide individual differences in the rates at which such change occurs. When the first edition of this book was written in 1989, it was generally assumed that early problems would be outgrown. Thus difficult toddlers were routinely seen as just going through the "terrible 2's," and aggressive 3-year-olds were viewed as learning how to operate in the peer group. However, a growing body of work calls these conclusions into question to some degree. It is now accepted that a small proportion of children with problems in the preschool period will continue to have significant difficulties later on. Persistent problems usually reflect some complex combination of child characteristics (including biological and genetically determined predispositions), parenting, and family dysfunction that may vary for different children; conversely, early problems that are transient may indicate merely a perturbation in development and/or the influence of developmentally appropriate and effective parenting that helps a particularly difficult toddler cope with developmental challenges and transitions. Therefore, it is important to determine which child characteristics in combination with which family factors are associated with the amelioration of early difficulties and which appear to be associated with the development of more long-standing psychological disorders. There were almost no data on this question when the first edition of this book was written, but over the past 12 years or so, numerous studies have provided information on which children are truly at risk and which are likely to be going through a more temporary problem with a developmental transition. Many of these studies are synthesized in this book.

It should also be emphasized that the recognition of early-emerging behavior problems over the past decade has also led to a tendency not to ignore problems, as was the case when the first edition of this book was written, but to seriously overpathologize and overgeneralize from short-lived or age-related difficulties. There is an increasing tendency to make predictions about serious and long-term difficulties from age-appropriate expressions of aggression, noncompliance, or irritability. This is particularly evident in writings about delinquency and violence. Although it is true that *most* violent adults had very troubled childhoods, the reverse is *not* true. Most aggressive toddlers and noncompliant preschoolers will *not* end up delinquent, antisocial, or even poorly adjusted. Only a small proportion of aggressive and defiant toddlers develop into seriously impaired children and adolescents. This prediction fallacy is too often forgotten, and it is evident in many studies that justify examining behavior problems in relatively small normative samples of young children and in the media's focus on issues such as child care and aggression, in which the meaning of small associations has been overblown.

Theoretical debates within developmental psychology and developmental psychopathology have focused on issues of continuity and change over time. Some developmentalists believe that early experiences in the first 3 years determine the course of social and cognitive development thereafter; others emphasize the plasticity of young children's behavior; still others assume that both continuity and change occur but that certain key experiences can influence developmental outcome. Within the developmental psychopathology field, the debate hinges on issues of risk and resilience. Which factors place children at risk for problems, and what determines whether children exposed to one or more risk factors will be resilient enough to overcome negative early experiences? What balance among risk and protective factors predicts outcome? These are extremely important questions for professionals concerned with the development of young children to consider, as the answers will ultimately influence the nature of prevention programs and the types of advice it is reasonable to give to parents.

Some of these theoretical and conceptual issues are examined in Chapter 1. One particular conceptual approach, the transactional model of development, is explored as it relates to the onset and course of problem behavior in young children. The transactional model, which emphasizes the interaction over time between children and parents, is integrated with a discussion of the child's social context, bringing in other

BEHAVIOR PROBLEMS IN PRESCHOOL CHILDREN

Second Edition

aspects of relations in the family, peer group, and wider social network. Questions of continuity and change are considered, because they are among the central issues that developmental psychopathologists must address. Important determinants of individual differences are also discussed, including infant temperament and the quality of early parent–infant relationships. In Chapter 2 the development of toddlers and preschoolers is discussed, with a focus on the major developmental tasks of this age period: exploration and environmental mastery; the development of autonomy and a sense of self; perspective taking and pretend play; the establishment of internalized standards of control; and advances in cognitive functioning, including language and memory. The establishment of autonomy, self-awareness, and self-regulation are viewed as normal, but critical, developmental transitions that children must negotiate. If they are dealt with successfully, the children are likely to develop into competent and psychologically healthy youngsters; difficulties coping with one or more of these tasks may set the stage for the onset of problems.

Chapter 3 explores clinical issues relevant to an understanding of symptomatic behavior in young children, including the epidemiology of behavior disorders, factors influencing referral, and diagnostic issues. Several prototypic children are described to illustrate the nature of behavior problems in early childhood. These examples are composites derived from a longitudinal study of hard-to-manage toddlers and preschoolers who have been followed through elementary school and to early adolescence. The importance of childrearing and other family factors, sibling relationships, and friendships and peer relations are addressed in Chapters, 4, 5, and 6 and illustrated with specific examples. Prevention and treatment of problems in young children are considered in Chapter 7; course, outcome, and prognostic indicators are discussed in Chapter 8, with specific examples used to highlight salient findings. Finally, Chapter 9 summarizes the major points and addresses social policy implications.

Although this second edition follows the same structure and organization as the first, many chapters have been entirely rewritten, and others have been substantially updated to incorporate more sophisticated conceptual models and new findings, especially concerning family and peer influences on development, and to highlight recent longitudinal studies exploring differing developmental pathways from early childhood to adolescence and young adulthood. This volume also places a greater emphasis on prevention and treatment, exploring what we know about evidence-based interventions for young children. Social policy issues are also given more attention, especially as they pertain to the increased use of child care and the implications of this social change for the socioemotional and cognitive development of young children.

Acknowledgments

Thanks are due to the many graduate students and staff who worked with me over the years on my preschool studies, funded by the National Institute of Mental Health. In particular, I want to acknowledge Dr. Linda J. Ewing, Dr. Elizabeth Pierce, and Dr. Susan Marakovitz, whose dedication and hard work made it possible for us to continue to follow up the children, adolescents, and parents who participated in these studies after my funding ended. Other former students who deserve special mention for their participation in various phases of these studies include Dr. Anna Marie Breaux, Dr. Cynthia March, and Dr. Emily Szumowski. Ms. Sarah McAuliffe was a dedicated project coordinator during the final phases of the data collection.

The families who participated in this research over the years deserve special recognition and heartfelt thanks. They provided helpful insights into the way that young children, some with early signs of problems, developed over the crucial years from preschool age through the transition to school and then through middle childhood and beyond. Sincere appreciation and gratitude is expressed to the parents and children who let us into their homes and schools, and were willing to share their experiences with us. The case studies described in this book are based on these families, but with circumstances altered, names changed, and some compositing across families to protect the identities of participants.

Drs. John Bates and Stephen Hinshaw provided helpful feedback on an earlier draft of this second edition, and many of their comments have been incorporated into this version. They certainly made this a better book by forcing me to confront some difficult issues head on.

However, I did not take heed of all their criticisms, so they cannot be blamed for my failure to cover material that others may see as missing or handled too briefly.

Thanks are also due to my current graduate students and the staff of the Pittsburgh site of the National Institute of Child Health and Human Development Study of Early Child Care and Youth Development. They had to put up with my moodiness, preoccupation, and unavailability, as I worked feverishly last year to complete the revisions to this book.

My sincere appreciation is also expressed to my husband for his support and patience while I was struggling to finish this book, and neglecting family, friends, and pets. My dogs have made it clear to me that they now expect me to join them in hikes in the woods and jaunts to the park.

Finally, thanks go to Seymour Weingarten and his colleagues at The Guilford Press for their patience and support.

Contents

CHAPTER 1

Theoretical and Conceptual Issues

A DEVELOPMENTAL PSYCHOPATHOLOGY PERSPECTIVE

In this book, I argue that in order to understand the different developmental pathways that young children follow, from early signs of difficulties or even good adjustment to later functioning, it is necessary to begin with a detailed knowledge of normal development. Normal development then serves as the backdrop from which to study individual differences in processes and outcomes that may be associated with the early emergence and stabilization of behavior problems in some children. Thus the focus is on universal processes in development (e.g., the development of an attachment relationship, the emergence of relationships with peers) as a context for understanding individual differences that can sometimes be markers of emerging problems in early childhood (e.g., the development of an insecure attachment; being rejected or victimized by peers). This "developmental psychopathology" perspective (Cicchetti & Cohen, 1995; Cummings, Davies, & Campbell, 2000; Rutter & Sroufe, 2000; Sroufe & Rutter, 1984) represents a theoretically and empirically grounded attempt to understand why development "goes awry" in some children but not in others who have ostensibly similar histories and experiences.

Because developmental psychopathology focuses primarily on determinants of individual differences in development, it has necessarily been dominated by complex transactional or biopsychosocial models

1

that take into account a range of biological, psychological, and social factors that converge to influence behavior and adaptation at one point in time and that also may account for changes in functioning over the course of development (Cummings et al., 2000; Sameroff, 2000; Sroufe, 1997). A transactional model underscores the multiplicity of factors that influence the course of development and also provides a framework for thinking about the different pathways that young children may follow from infancy to adulthood. This framework also suggests why it is difficult, if not impossible, to predict outcome in the individual case. The reason is that predictions are at best probabilistic, not deterministic. That is, children may follow a variety of different pathways, depending on how particular factors converge at important developmental transition points. This fact gives rise to the concepts of *equifinality* and *multifinality* in development (Cicchetti & Rogosch, 1996; Cummings et al., 2000). That is, children may reach the same end point (e.g., a diagnosis of oppositional defiant disorder) by different routes, and, conversely, children with apparently similar developmental histories and risk factors may have different outcomes (e.g., oppositional defiant disorder, depression, or even good adjustment). These issues are illustrated throughout this book.

When children have problems or are likely to develop problems, outcomes will be determined, in part, by the relative balance of risk and protective factors (e.g., Masten & Coatsworth, 1998; Rutter, 1994). Thus children who experience many adverse circumstances, such as premature birth, neglectful or harsh parenting, poor nutrition, and low quality child care, will be at higher risk for negative outcomes than children who have fewer adverse experiences. This multiple or cumulative risk model (e.g., Greenberg, Lengua, Coie, & Pinderhughes, 1999; Sameroff, Seifer, Baldwin, & Baldwin, 1993) is based on the premise that the more risk factors that are present, the worse the outcome will be. It is unclear, however, whether the relationship between risk factors and poor outcomes is linear or whether there is a threshold above which outcomes will be poor but below which risk factors will not necessarily have a long-term negative impact (Shaw & Vondra, 1993). Theoretical models must also take into account the particular risk factors apparent in any one child's life and how they may exacerbate each other. This necessity underscores the importance of understanding the synergy among risk factors or the cascading processes that may be unleashed when negative factors converge (e.g., birth complications, infant irritability, and maternal depression may set off a cascade of negative mother–infant interactions that result in an insecure attachment and harsh parenting; these also may be exacerbated by marital conflict). In addition to the number and types of risk factors and their interactions, consideration must be given to whether protective factors are also present in the child or the child's environment and whether they are potent enough to help the child overcome risk. Thus, for example, a child growing up in poverty in a dangerous neighborhood may evidence adaptive development if a strong parent–child relationship serves to keep the child off the streets and instills feelings of self-worth. Sroufe (1997) has used the metaphor of the branching tree to illustrate the diverse pathways that different children will follow based on the complex interplay of child, parent, family, and contextual factors over the course of early development.

In addition to risk and protective factors in development, certain key theoretical issues must also be addressed, because they also have important implications for the conceptualization of developmental change in both "normal" and disturbed populations, as well as for etiological formulations of childhood problems. One major debate within both developmental psychology and child psychopathology revolves around issues of continuity and change: How well does earlier behavior predict later behavior? What changes as development proceeds, and what remains stable?

It is now well established that developmental stability reflects more than a link between a particular behavior that is evident in early infancy and that same behavior later on. Rather, the focus has shifted to more general questions, such as whether earlier behavior predicts later behavior at all and whether qualitative or stylistic aspects of an individual's behavior show evidence of stability. Some theorists argue that one can predict at least certain aspects of a child's development from knowledge of earlier behavior and social influences (Carlson & Sroufe, 1995; Sroufe, 1979). Other theorists disagree and assert that developmental change is both so irregular and so profound that developmental course is not predictable (Lewis, 2000; Sameroff, 2000). The question of predictability is a central one for developmental psychopathology because the early identification of children with problems and the delineation of prognostic factors rests on the assumption that development is at least partially predictable from knowledge of earlier behavior and of the caretaking environment.

Before proceeding with this discussion, I must define several terms. *Continuity* is used to refer to general similarities in behavior or personality over time, whereas *discontinuity* refers to a lack of demonstrated stability in behavior or personality characteristics. *Predictability* is used to indicate a theoretically meaningful relationship between earlier and later behavior, whether or not the behaviors themselves are similar. Knowledge of earlier behavior may allow one to predict later behavior, despite developmental changes in the manifestations of the behavior itself; or earlier behavior may lead, in predictable ways, to the appearance of a quite different behavior. Finally, the terms *qualitative* and *quantitative* characterize the nature of developmental change. Quantitative change indicates an increase in capacity with development, although the behavior remains the same in terms of underlying processes and overt manifestations. Qualitative change refers to the reorganization and modification of behavior with development, which leads to major alterations in underlying processes.

In addition to the debate about whether or not developmental course can be predicted, a related debate on the nature of developmental change exists. What things change with development? Some would argue that developmental change reflects a quantitative increase in certain skills or processes such as memory capacity or sociability; that is, the capacity to remember facts or events increases such that older children remember more of them. Others would argue that developmental change is qualitative. Children may remember more with development, but their increased capacity reflects a reorganization of memory processes and a change in the nature of memory strategies rather than an increase in the number of stimuli that can be remembered. Similarly, in the area of social development, children's increased capacity to play cooperatively with peers may be conceptualized as a quantitative increase in the acquisition of social skills, such as a larger repertoire of social approach behaviors, or, alternatively, as a reorganization of the cognitive structures that are thought to underlie the ability to cooperate with others, such as perspective taking and means–end thinking. At a logical level, continuity positions might be seen as allied with notions of quantitative change, whereas a discontinuity view would appear to fit with the idea that change reflects complex reorganizations. This is more or less the case, although the debates over these two related issues are both heated and complex. (See, e.g., Brim & Kagan, 1980; Cummings et al., 2000; Kagan, 1984; Overton & Reese, 1981; Sroufe, 1979.)

A third theoretical issue revolves around the nature–nurture question. Although either/or formulations of this issue are no longer accepted, the question of how biological and environmental factors interact to produce either normal or pathological development remains a central issue in the field. In most theoretical models of abnormal development, some attempt is made to address this issue (Rutter et al., 1997; Rutter & Sroufe, 2000). In particular, diathesis–stress models of adult psychopathology implicate both biological vulnerabilities and psychosocial stressors as central to the development of both schizophrenia and depression (e.g., Zubin & Spring, 1977). Similarly, transactional models of development focus on the interaction among biological and environmental determinants, while allowing for qualitative changes in biological, behavioral, and social factors as a function of development. These changes in turn may alter the nature of the organism–environment interaction (Sameroff, 2000; Sameroff & Chandler, 1975). Moreover, concepts of gene–environment correlation and gene–environment interaction (Rutter et al., 1997) underscore the complexities of these issues and the fact that it is not really meaningful to try to determine the relative degree of genetic and environmental influences. Rather, questions of process are the focus, that is, how do biological and environmental influences combine to predict outcome? How does a child's genetic makeup influence the quality of parenting that is elicited (e.g., more noncompliant children elicit more negative parenting, something that presumably partly reflects the child's genetic predispositions)? How much of the quality of parent–child interaction reflects gene–environment correlation related to similarities in personality and behavioral style (e.g., high-strung parents have high-strung children, and they are more likely to enter into conflict because of their similar personality styles)? How do differences in children's genetic predispositions, presumably partly reflected in their temperamental characteristics, lead not only to differences in parenting but also to differences in the degree of influence parents may have—for example, susceptibility to parenting or willingness to be socialized (Belsky, Hsieh, & Crnic, 1998; Kochanska, 1997)? This is an example of gene–environment interaction; that is, some children elicit certain types of parental responses but also respond differentially to childrearing attempts because of their genetically determined personality characteristics. (See Collins, Maccoby, Steinberg, Hetherington, & Bornstein, 2000, and Rutter et al., 1997, for a discussion of this topic, which is beyond the scope of this book.)

In this chapter, some of these theoretical issues are discussed, and the implications of one or another position for the development of behavior disorders in young children are addressed. A discussion of transactional and ecological models as they apply to developmental psychopathology follows. In illustrating the implications of these various issues and models, the roles of infant temperament and infant attachment security are examined as well, because both are seen as sources of individual differences in young children and as possible early precursors of childhood problems, according to some theoretical models of developmental psychopathology (Carlson & Sroufe, 1995; Rothbart, Posner, & Hershey, 1995).

CONTINUITY–DISCONTINUITY AND THE NATURE OF DEVELOPMENTAL CHANGE

Decades of research in child development have been devoted to investigating continuity in behavior over time. For example, much early research attempted to predict later IQ from measures of infant functioning or to find personality traits, such as dominance or shyness, that were stable over time (e.g., Bayley & Schaefer, 1964; Kagan & Moss, 1962). It was assumed that simple knowledge of early behaviors would allow one to predict later functioning. As stage theories of development that emphasized qualitative change and reorganization (such as the work of Piaget) came to dominate the field, the notion that one could find continuities in development became suspect (e.g., Overton & Reese, 1981; Sameroff & Chandler, 1975). Thus Overton and Reese (1981) argued that the profound transformations in cognitive structures and in behavior that characterize development make it unrealistic to expect to find consistencies over time, a view that was echoed by Kagan and his colleagues (Kagan, Kearsley, & Zelazo, 1978). That is, most developmental theorists see qualitative change as synonymous with development and argue that the role of the developmentalist is to describe and attempt to explain the nature of developmental transitions rather than to search for elusive developmental continuities. Indeed, it is nearly impossible to discuss developmental continuity or discontinuity without also addressing the question of quantitative or qualitative change.

The discontinuity view arose partly because of the difficulties in predicting from infant behavior to later functioning. For example, early studies of IQ or of social behavior did not suggest clear links between early behavior and later functioning (e.g., Kagan & Moss, 1962). In addition, a number of studies failed to find the predicted link between pregnancy and/or delivery complications ("reproductive risk") and deviant development (see Sameroff & Chandler, 1975, for a review). These findings led some theorists to question whether the importance accorded to early experience was exaggerated and to argue that developmental course is both less continuous and less predictable than was once supposed (e.g., Kagan, 1984; Lewis, Feiring, & Rosenthal, 2000; Sameroff, 1975, 2000).

Other researchers and theorists have assumed that development shows predictability not in terms of the continuity of specific behaviors (see Kagan, 1971) but more generally in terms of certain attributes that cut across the domains of both cognitive and social functioning (e.g., Sroufe, 1979; Thomas, Chess, & Birch, 1968) or reflect similar underlying cognitive (Bornstein & Sigman, 1986) or social (Bowlby, 1969) schemas. These authors argue that within some general and broad parameters, knowledge of early behavior and the caretaking environment allows one to predict certain outcomes. Sroufe (1979) has termed this the "coherence" of development. Thus the issue becomes one of predictability rather than behavioral continuity. Furthermore, predictability can be demonstrated despite developmental transformations that reflect the qualitative reorganization of developmental processes. For example, some work suggests that a secure infant–mother attachment predicts competence in problem solving in toddlerhood and in the peer group in preschool (Sroufe, 1983). Sroufe argues that these data illustrate the fact that the organization of behavior changes to meet developmental challenges but that the general approach to new developmental tasks remains consistent or coherent across development (see also Cicchetti, Cummings, Greenberg, & Marvin, 1990). Infants who are competent in one domain, partly because of the responsiveness of their primary caretakers, move on to face new developmental challenges with age-appropriate strategies. From this perspective, specific behaviors would not logically be expected to show consistency. Temperament researchers likewise hypothesize that certain enduring personality characteristics can be identified in early infancy and that they shape, to some extent, the course of later development (e.g., Rothbart & Bates, 1998; Thomas et al., 1968).

One complication in the study of change and continuity revolves around how one defines consistency in behavior and what denotes transformation and reorganization (Lewis, 2000). If one behavior is a necessary precursor of a later behavior, does that imply continuity, even if the later behavior differs considerably from the earlier one, as, for example, in the shift from babbling to language? This is a particularly thorny problem when one attempts to relate infant behavior to later functioning because qualitative aspects of many behaviors show dramatic change. How does one define behavior at vastly different developmental levels in order to investigate continuity? For example, how would one look for continuity in a disposition such as sociability over time? Which behaviors would define it at three months? Three years? Which behaviors in infancy might logically be considered early precursors of social engagement at school entry? Lewis (2000) argues that an understanding of continuity or discontinuity depends on interpretation and level of analysis. Conclusions will vary according to which constructs are selected for study, how they are defined in terms of specific behaviors at different ages, how the chosen behaviors are measured, the time intervals between measurements, and how the data are interpreted.

Others agree that the interpretation of the data will reflect a pre-existing stance or worldview (e.g., Cummings et al., 2000; Kagan, 1984; Overton & Reese, 1981). In fact, Kagan suggests that a continuity perspective is one that we ourselves bring to the data to provide some order and meaning to experience. The babbling-to-language example illustrates this issue well. If it were demonstrated that frequency of babbling in infancy were correlated moderately, but significantly, with some measure of language development obtained at age 3, would that finding be interpreted as evidence for continuity or for change? The continuity theorist would argue that it showed consistency in the use of vocalization as a means of communication and that the early babbling laid the groundwork for later verbal development. On the other hand, the discontinuity theorist would argue that the vocalizations and babbling of infancy had been so transformed and reorganized over the course of the ensuing months that it would be meaningless to talk of continuity between the babbling of an infant and the communicative and syntactically correct speech of a preschooler. From this perspective, the apparent continuity (i.e., as reflected in a measure of statistical association) would not lie in the child's behavior but would probably best be explained as an example of environmental continuity. That is, an evaluation of the caregiving environment over time would probably reveal consistencies related to the encouragement of differing types of age-appropriate vocal communication. Continuity might be found in the fact that maternal behavior encouraged vocalization, but the specifics of maternal behavior would change with the child's development—for example, from contingent responses to babbling and cooing in infancy to facilitating labeling in toddlerhood to reframing sentences and asking questions during the preschool period.

The continuity–discontinuity debate is further complicated by the fact that examples of continuity, transformation, and coherence abound in development. No one would expect continuity in certain behaviors, for example, smiling or crying, because it is obvious that they change their meaning with development and that other behaviors (e.g., separation distress at maternal departure) drop out of the typical repertoire completely. For instance, smiling or crying in a 3-month-old is interpreted very differently from smiling or crying in a toddler, despite the consistency in the topography of the behavior. One would not necessarily expect frequency of smiling at 3 months to predict frequency of smiling or even more general sociability at 2 years. Similarly, one would not expect the intensity of separation protest at 8 months to predict shyness at preschool age. These are examples of social behaviors that are highly age-determined and in which transformation and reorganization are the rule.

On the other hand, although transformation and reorganization characterize most aspects of social and cognitive development, and although predictability from infancy to later functioning is generally poor, there is some suggestive evidence for stability in a few behavioral dispositions. For example, evidence exists that activity level in early infancy predicts activity level in the preschool period (Korner et al., 1985) and that activity level in preschoolers predicts activity level at school entry (Buss, Block, & Block, 1980; Campbell, Pierce, March, Ewing, & Szumowski, 1994). Even for this apparently circumscribed aspect of behavior, the focus is not on continuity in specific behaviors, because activity is measured differently in infants and preschoolers. Rather, the continuity lies in the finding that children who are in the higher ranges on some measures of infant activity are somewhat more likely than less active infants to score at higher levels on measures of activity obtained in preschool as well.

Three issues are embedded in this statement. First, these studies show only moderate stability in individual differences (McCall, 1977).

Children maintain some similarity in rank order over time, but the behavior itself may or may not be stable. Developmental changes mean that behaviors are manifested differently (e.g., from the restlessness of an infant to the running and jumping of a preschooler) and, therefore, are measured differently. Thus whatever continuity is implied is really consistency in behavioral style or intensity of response. Second, because studies find only low to moderate correlations between earlier and later behaviors, interpretations depend on the theoretical stance of the researcher. That is, these correlations may be interpreted as demonstrating continuity because there is some relationship between activity in infancy and activity later; or they may be interpreted as reflecting discontinuity because the relationship is only moderate. Third, as McCall (1977) argues, even when we can demonstrate stability of individual differences, we are not shedding light on the processes underlying development. Studies that examine the stability of individual differences do not clarify *how* a child develops from a squirmy infant to an active and energetic preschooler.

Studies also suggest coherence in other general aspects of personality and social relations. This coherence probably reflects a combination of consistency in certain genetic predispositions and overt behaviors within children and certain stable characteristics of the caregiving environment. For example, studies suggest that fussy and difficult behavior in infancy may translate into defiance and confrontation in toddlerhood, particularly when mothers use relatively intrusive and angry methods of discipline (Belsky et al., 1998; Lee & Bates, 1985). However, this association between temperamental characteristics and childrearing may also change with development. Bates and colleagues (Bates, Pettit, Dodge, & Ridge, 1998) found that difficult and resistant toddlers had fewer problems in the early elementary school years when their mothers employed restrictive disciplinary control, but children high in resistance showed more continuing problems in the absence of maternal intervention. Other studies indicate that hard-to-manage preschool children are more likely than more subdued and tractable preschool children to continue to have difficulties in early childhood and in elementary school, especially when the quality of the mother–child relationship is negative and conflicted (Campbell, Pierce, Moore, Marakovitz, & Newby, 1996; Shaw, Keenan, & Vondra, 1994; Shaw et al., 1998). Work by Sroufe and his colleagues suggests that when mothers are responsive to their infants' communications and facilitate exploration of the environment, their infants are more independent and invested in problem solving in toddlerhood, suggesting coherence at the positive end of the spectrum as well (Matas, Arend, & Sroufe, 1978). These findings have been supported in a number of recent studies that link maternal warmth, positive approaches to discipline, and positive engagement with more cooperative behavior and better self-regulation in early childhood (e.g. Belsky et al., 1998; Feldman, Greenbaum, & Yirimiya, 1999; Kochanska, 1995, 1997; National Institute of Child Health and Development [NICHD] Early Child Care Research Network, 1998; Shaw et al., 1994).

Taken together, these studies and theoretical perspectives suggest that the issue is not one of behavioral continuity per se but of consistency along some general dimensions of social and cognitive functioning and that consistency in behavior may well be partly a function of environmental continuity (Waters, Weinfeld, & Hamilton, 2000). Said differently, these studies document (Thomas, Chess, & Korn, 1982), some consistency in personality development, despite marked change as a function of both development and caregiving; consistency is mediated in part by certain stable aspects of the environment. Furthermore, studies of problem children suggest that predictability may be better for behavioral extremes than for behaviors in the moderate range (Campbell et al., 1994; Campbell, Shaw, & Gilliom, 2000; Moffitt, Caspi, Dickson, Silva, & Stanton, 1996; Nagin & Tremblay, 1999). Children who are extremely active or irritable or noncompliant or aggressive may be more likely to continue to respond maladaptively than children who are only average or slightly above average in their early levels of noncompliance, aggression, or negative affect. Children at the extremes of irritability or noncompliance may also be more sensitive to stable, but negative, environmental influences or more disorganized by environmental instability (e.g., Belsky, Woodworth, & Crnic, 1996; Belsky et al., 1998; Crockenberg, 1981). Similarly, at the positive end of the distribution, children who are more easygoing and compliant may be more likely to show consistency on these dimensions of behavior, particularly in the context of supportive parenting (Belsky et al., 1998; Crockenberg & Litman, 1990; Lee & Bates, 1985), and they may be less disorganized by environmental instability (Belsky, Woodworth, & Crnic, 1996). However, there is also evidence that irritability and lack of manageability in early childhood are linked directly to later adjustment problems, suggesting that prediction may be possible across the spectrum of child difficulty, not just at the extreme ends of the continuum (see Rothbart & Bates, 1998, for an extended discussion of the processes by which irritability and other aspects of difficult temperament may be transformed over the course of early development).

These issues have obvious implications for the study of psychological disorder in young children and for approaches to intervention. Early identification of children at risk for disorder is predicated on the idea that behavior is predictable. Preventive and therapeutic interventions are based on the assumption that problems may persist in the absence of treatment, that is, that maladaptive behavior is often stable but that, in the face of appropriate environmental interventions, change and transformation are possible. An extreme continuity view might lead to the conclusion that early behavior is unchanging and that interventions are fruitless. At the other extreme, a strongly held discontinuity view might lead to the conclusion that problems are likely to be outgrown in the absence of treatment, as part of a normal developmental transition. Whereas some behaviors such as aggression appear to be relatively resistant to treatment, providing support for a continuity position (Coie & Dodge, 1998), some children at high risk for psychopathology appear to develop normally (Masten & Coatsworth, 1998), providing support for the competing discontinuity view. Extreme adherence to either position, however, is probably an oversimplification: It seems clear that a more complex view that highlights the interaction among child characteristics and environmental factors, some stable and some changing, will be necessary to identify children at risk and to pinpoint directions for intervention.

TRANSACTIONAL MODELS OF DEVELOPMENT

Most etiological models of adult psychopathology are considered "interactionist" because they incorporate both genetic–biological and environmental factors (e.g., Zubin & Spring, 1977). That is, both a biological diathesis or vulnerability and environmental stress are necessary to precipitate the onset of disorder. Thus a genetically vulnerable individual might not break down if the environment is generally supportive and free from strain; similarly, even in the face of severe stress, some individuals continue to function well, presumably because they are biologically "resilient." The combined effects of biological vulnerability and an adverse environment are seen as necessary to produce the disturbed behavior. Although this model has much appeal and successfully accounts for much of the data on schizophrenia and manic–depressive disorder, disorders with well-documented genetic loadings, it is basically static and fails to allow for developmental change.

On the other hand, the transactional view, as outlined by Sameroff (1975, 1995, 2000), incorporates both organismic and environmental determinants in continual and mutually interactive flux over time. Several basic premises underlie this systems perspective. First, development is assumed to be discontinuous and characterized by qualitative change and reorganization. Second, the young child is seen as an active organizer of experience, participating in his or her own development. Third, interactions between young children and caretakers are viewed as bidirectional (Bell, 1968); that is, both children's responses to stimulation from adults and their influences on the behavior of adults are important. Fourth, neither child characteristics nor the environment are considered static. Both are changing over time in a mutually regulated and reciprocal fashion. Fifth, strong, biologically based self-righting tendencies are assumed to be present in all but the most severely damaged infants; that is, movement is inherently toward normal development, and this movement is under strong genetic control.

Taken together, then, the process of development is seen as an active and dynamic one in which the infant moves toward more complex functioning as cognitive and social processes reorganize with each new phase of development. Maturation plays a central role in this process, especially early on (McCall, 1981; Ramey & Ramey, 1998); but the role of the environment is likewise central, and it takes on added importance with development (Ramey & Ramey, 1998; Sameroff, 1975, 2000; Shonkoff & Phillips, 2000; Thompson & Nelson, 2001), particularly a responsive and appropriate caretaking environment that changes over time to meet the infant's developmental needs. For example, responsive caretaking in the early weeks would involve accurately reading the infant's cues regarding hunger, fatigue, and the need for cuddling or soothing. By 8 months, the infant's needs expand dramatically to include a variety of requirements for social and cognitive stimulation and the availability of a safe environment that facilitates the exploration of objects. From a transactional view, the infant's requirements and the responses of the caregiver change over time in a mutually regulated and reciprocal fashion. Stress and strain at one point in development may give way to more adaptive functioning as the infant overcomes a difficult developmental hurdle (e.g., weaning, colic) or the mother learns to anticipate the infant's needs and to read social communications more accurately (e.g., by not letting him or her become overtired or overly hungry). Thus changes in either member of the dyad feed back to influence the relationship in a dynamic and adaptively regulated system.

Therefore, given a reasonably responsive and adequate caretaking environment in which mutual adaptations can occur, the odds favor good outcomes. Thus an infant who is only moderately developmentally delayed is likely to overcome early deficits if the primary caretakers are generally responsive and stimulating, thereby facilitating development. On the other hand, a moderately delayed infant born into an unresponsive or neglecting family is less likely to overcome early problems. In the absence of environmental supports for development, one might predict continuing decline in cognitive functioning, as well as the onset of signs of emotional distress. Similarly, an irritable and unconsolable infant need not develop into a toddler with behavior problems unless his or her primary caregivers are unable to accommodate to his or her needs. Exceptional outcomes are due only rarely to deficits solely in the infant, but they usually derive from "some continuous malfunction in the organism–environment transaction across time which prevents the child from organizing his world adaptively" (Sameroff, 1975, p. 282). One potentially traumatic experience, such as anoxia at birth or the death of a parent, is not expected to lead inexorably to a poor outcome. Rather, chronically negative or inconsistent and confusing parenting, particularly of a vulnerable infant, might be expected to predict continuing problems. Knowledge of infant characteristics alone or of the caregiving environment alone is not sufficient to predict outcome except in the most extreme cases; furthermore, a longer term view is needed, as only more chronic maladaptation is likely to be associated with long-term negative consequences. Thus the focus is on multiple determinants of development and the complexity of their interactions over time. Both child characteristics and factors in the caregiving environment, what Sameroff and Chandler (1975) have termed the "continuum of caretaking casualty," need to be entered into the equation predicting outcome.

Recent reports from the English–Romanian Adoptees (ERA) Study Team (Rutter & the ERA Study Team, 1998) underscore some of these issues, most notably resilience, the need for at least adequate caretaking, and the importance of the timing of experiences. Despite extreme deprivation in Romanian orphanages, infants adopted into homes in Great Britain showed amazing "catch-up" in social-emotional and cognitive development, but the timing of the adoptions was important as well. Infants adopted by 6 months of age did not differ from British-born adoptees, despite marked differences in early experience, whereas children adopted from Romanian orphanages later than 6 months, and especially after their first birthdays, fared much more poorly. Despite dramatic gains in cognitive and social functioning, they continued to lag behind comparison groups of early-adopted children, and they were much more likely to evidence attachment disturbances. These data highlight the marked ability of young infants to overcome early deprivation when placed into more stimulating and responsive environments, as well as the importance of the time in development at which particular experiences occur. Prolonged deprivation and the lack of important experiences with stimulating and responsive caregivers during the early months of life could not be overcome totally. This finding suggests that particular early experiences are necessary during sensitive periods of development, despite the marked resilience that these children also demonstrated. These findings make it clear that early experience is important but that infants are also able to adapt to a wide range of circumstances and can show marked improvement with positive changes in the affective and physical environment.

The transactional model presents a reasonably optimistic view, because it suggests that most children, especially in the absence of extreme early deprivation or serious biological insult, are able to overcome early problems and that interventions focusing on the child or the primary caretaker or, better still, on their interaction over time may be sufficient to reverse a trend toward deviant development. Because this model provides a systems framework for understanding developmental change, it also suggests that one can intervene at multiple points to perturb or reorganize the system, thereby leading to improved functioning. Furthermore, multiple risk factor models (Sameroff et al., 1993) suggest that it is possible to identify those infants or young children most at risk for disorder and that the caregiving environment should be the major focus of preventive and therapeutic efforts (Shonkoff & Phillips, 2000). In addition, especially in the context of severe deprivation, neglect, or environmental adversity, the timing of intervention appears to be important as well (Ramey & Ramey, 1998; Shonkoff & Phillips, 2000).

ECOLOGICAL MODELS OF DEVELOPMENT

A strong consensus now exists among child development researchers and developmental psychopathologists that children's development is influenced by a range of factors beyond the parent–child relationship. The child must be viewed in a broader social context, that is, as a member of a family, peer group, wider social network, community, and culture. Thus the focus has been broadened to consider a range of direct and indirect influences on the developing child and on the family in which he or she lives (Belsky, 1984; Bronfenbrenner, 1986; McLoyd, 1998; Parke & Buriel, 1998; Shonkoff & Phillips, 2000). As with the transactional model, the metaphor is that of mutually regulated and interacting systems but at varying contextual levels (e.g., those that directly impinge on the child, such as the family and peer group, and those that indirectly influence behavior, such as prevailing cultural beliefs about childrearing).

An ecological perspective is based on the assumption that multiple factors have a direct impact on the child and that these and other factors also influence the quality of caregiving the child receives from parents. For instance, within the family it is necessary to consider the quality of both father–child and mother–child relationships. In addition, the quality of the marital relationship is likely to influence the child (Belsky, 1984; Cowan, 1997; Cummings et al., 2000; Davies & Cummings, 1994). Furthermore, these effects should be both direct and indirect. The overall climate of the home (e.g., whether it is generally warm and supportive or fraught with tension) would be expected to have a direct effect on the child's mood, as well as his or her sense of security and comfort (Davies & Cummings, 1994). In addition, marital stress is likely to impinge on the child indirectly through its effects on parents, who, because they are upset or preoccupied, may be less available to their children. The complexities of these interacting relationships become even more complicated when a second child is born. The availability of extended family or close friends, for example, would also be expected to have both direct and indirect effects on the child by providing additional adult attention and stimulation to the child and by providing social support to parents.

Cochran and Brassard (1979) suggest that all people outside the household who engage in regular social exchange with family members have the potential to influence a child's development. Direct influences include the opportunity to interact with different individuals and thus learn about new roles, styles of interaction, or activities. Children develop close relationships with network members such as regular babysitters or close friends of the family. Network members also have an indirect impact on children through their relationship with parents. For example, they may provide them with emotional, material, or informational support that has a positive effect on the family; they also may model more appropriate childrearing behaviors. Of course, members of the wider network might also have a negative effect on the children if, for example, they took parental attention away from them or served as negative role models.

Community and cultural influences are also seen as relevant (Bronfenbrenner, 1986; McLoyd, 1998; Parke & Buriel, 1998; Shonkoff & Phillips, 2000). For example, physical aspects of the community, such as the availability of playgrounds and the safety of the neighborhood; community resources, such as the availability and quality of preschool or day care settings; the nature and availability of work for parents and of educational and medical institutions have all been hypothesized to influence the quality of the child's environment and hence development, as have the availability of less formal social structures such as clubs, parent groups, church groups, and so on. In addition, different cultural groups have different perspectives on childrearing, and the cultural network in which a child is raised is another important determinant of values and attitudes (Parke & Buriel, 1998). In other words, a range of factors is seen as influencing the quality of family life, and these factors should converge to affect the child's development and overall well-being. Moreover, other formulations based on this model suggest that children, by virtue of their biological–genetic predispositions and the experiences provided to them by parents, will seek certain environmental niches and that the fit between the child and environmental supports and challenges will be another important influence on adaptation and adjustment (Scarr & McCartney, 1983).

Of course an ecological perspective is generally inherent in most clinical approaches. Clinicians, regardless of theoretical orientation, almost always obtain information about a child's family environment and the resources available to the family, as well as those in the wider community, that are needed to support the child's growth and development. Differences obtain in the use to which such information is put in clinical practice and how it is utilized in treatment. However, developmental psychologists are now trying to systematize and evaluate empirically influences that clinicians routinely attend to in assessing a child and family and that often play a role in their case formulations.

INDIVIDUAL DIFFERENCES IN TEMPERAMENT

The concept of infant temperament has been the focus of much recent research and conceptual development (e.g., Rothbart & Bates, 1998). The issue of temperament and the role of temperament in the development of behavioral disturbance was first addressed by Thomas, Chess, and Birch (1968). These authors developed one of the first truly interactive models of development, in which they stressed the combined contributions of individual differences in infant behavior and in the behavior of caretakers in determining social development. This work represented an early reaction to the strict environmental determinism and unidirectional (mother-blaming) view inherent in psychoanalytic formulations of childhood problems, and it has stimulated much recent research and theory within a transactional developmental model.

Thomas et al. (1968) conducted an early descriptive, longitudinal study within this framework. They concluded that individual differences in infant characteristics interacted with childrearing style to determine outcome. In particular, they stressed the importance of the "goodness of fit" between infant and caretakers, as well as the active role the infant played in eliciting caretaking behavior from adults (see also Bell, 1968). Thomas et al. (1968) proposed that particular individual-difference dimensions of infant behavior were, at least in part, constitutionally based and reflected stylistic aspects of infant behavior that were central to an understanding of early social development. These dimensions included regularity in biological functioning, threshold of response, intensity of reaction, quality of mood, adaptability, and activity level. Based on their typical patterns of behavior, some infants could be characterized as "difficult," that is, intense, negative, irregular, and slow to adapt to change. The combination of a difficult infant and an insensitive parent was seen as a risk factor for later deviant development, although Thomas et al. (1968) also noted that these interaction patterns were not fixed and that infant behavioral style could change as a function of environmental support. Thus this theory directly raised issues of nature–nurture and continuity–discontinuity.

More recent debates have focused on the definition of temperament, its stability over time, the relative importance of constitutional and environmental influences on the expression of temperament, and whether infant difficultness is a risk factor for or precursor of later behavior problems (for a comprehensive review, see Rothbart & Bates, 1998). Thomas et al. (1968) defined temperament in terms of the "how" of behavior, or stylistic aspects of social and cognitive functioning, but did not take a position on its determinants except to assume that both genetic and environmental factors interacted to produce a child's characteristic response style. Thus they argued that temperamental style was not necessarily immutable and unchanging because environmental events and parental caretaking styles would be expected to modify a child's inborn tendencies to behave in one way or another. Others suggested, however, that the very construct of temperament implies both constitutional–genetic determinants and stability over time (e.g., Buss & Plomin, 1975; Sroufe, 1985), a position that has been modified in the light of recent evidence (see Rothbart & Bates, 1998).

Goldsmith and Campos (1982) synthesized a number of views of infant temperament and defined temperament as an individual-differences construct that refers to stable personality dispositions, although the degree and nature of the stability may vary both across individuals and over time. In contrast to Thomas et al. (1968), who emphasized the stylistic aspects of temperament, Goldsmith and Campos (1982) stressed the affective and motivational aspects. Thus individual differences in intensity or threshold of affect expression may be reactive or may serve to initiate behavior. For example, infants differ in the speed and intensity of their response to annoying or aversive stimuli: Some infants react slowly or fuss quietly, whereas others are quick to protest and may do so with great intensity. Infants also initiate social encounters that vary as a function of the nature, intensity, and timing of their expressions of affect, be they positive, playful, and exuberant or negative and demanding. Thus these authors consider temperament to reflect individual differences in the intensity and timing of emotional expressions. As such, temperamental characteristics are not different from personality dispositions.

In their extensive review of the literature, Rothbart and Bates (1998) conclude that temperament can be conceptualized as part of personality, "constituting the affective, activational, and attentional core of personality" (p. 108), with biological–genetic roots reflected in *some stability* in underlying processes *despite changes* in the manifestations of temperamental characteristics as a function of maturation and experience. Rothbart and Bates (1998) also emphasize reactivity and regulation as core features of temperament, reflected in the onset, intensity, and duration of emotional reactions, as well as the ability to control arousal and affect. In addition to the dimensions of negative and positive emotion noted by others (Buss & Plomin, 1975; Goldsmith & Campos, 1982), Rothbart emphasizes attentional control and task persistence as temperamental traits (Rothbart et al., 1995).

Thus, regardless of definition, a general consensus exists that it is meaningful to talk about endogenous individual differences in infant behavior that are evident very early (i.e., before differences in caretaking styles would be expected to have a profound effect on behavior) and that influence the nature of parent–infant interaction in a bidirectional fashion. For example, Bates (1987) suggests that infant temperament is a useful construct because it highlights the role that infant characteristics play in socialization. Focusing attention on individual differences in infants helps to elucidate the processes by which different infants elicit different responses from primary caregivers in their social environment. Bates (1987) emphasizes fussiness, irritability, and negative mood in his conceptualization of the difficult infant, aspects of behavior that are more easily operationalized in observational studies of infant behavior and maternal caretaking (e.g., Crockenberg, 1981). Thus infants who are fussy, demanding, and difficult to console may elicit anxiety, feelings of incompetence, and/or anger in their mothers, especially if their mothers are themselves preoccupied with other problems or are impatient or depressed. This initial clash of needs and feelings may abate as early feeding difficulties such as colic are overcome or as infants develop ways of soothing themselves; further, initially stressed and anxious mothers may relax as they adapt to their infants' characteristics and learn to read their social signals, gain confidence, or make better use of alternative caregivers to help them weather a difficult early developmental phase.

On the other hand, early mother–infant conflict may set the stage for more persistent problems in the relationship. For example, some mothers with irritable and demanding babies may become less responsive over time. The study by Crockenberg (1981) suggests that this occurs in cases in which fussy infants are born to stressed and overwhelmed mothers with low levels of social support. Lack of maternal responsiveness may lead, in turn, to increased demandingness on the part of an infant whose needs for social stimulation are not being met (Bates, 1987). Data from a longitudinal study by Bates (Bates, 1987; Bates & Bayles, 1988) suggest that difficult temperament, paired with a lack of affectionate and playful interaction with mothers in infancy, may fuel a cycle of demanding and coercive interaction. This pattern of interaction may become particularly problematic in toddlerhood, as young children's strivings for autonomy conflict with parental expectations for compliance, as well as with their own ambivalence and need for structure and security.

Whereas there is wide agreement that it is meaningful to think about individual characteristics of infants, the stability versus modifiability of these individual-difference parameters has been the subject of some debate. Within the context of developmental psychopathology, one question focuses on whether infants who show "difficult" behavior over time can be identified and whether they are or are not at increased risk to develop behavior problems. A second question addresses whether irritable infants will become less difficult to care for as a function of more sensitive and responsive care, as some studies suggest (van den Boom, 1994). Findings from several longitudinal studies do suggest that such children may indeed be at greater risk for developing problems but that parenting does make a difference, especially by toddlerhood. For example, Bates and his colleagues (Bates & Bayles, 1988; Bates, Maslin, & Frankel, 1985) found that infant difficultness was predictive of behavior problems at ages 3 and 5. Low levels of maternal play and positive interaction were also independent predictors of problem behavior. Several more recent studies reveal statistical interactions between child characteristics and parenting behavior. Irritable, negative infants (Belsky et al., 1998) and inhibited infants (Kochanska, 1997) appear to respond differently from more easygoing or less fearful infants to various aspects of parenting, consistent with a "goodness-of-fit" model. Belsky and colleagues (1998) found that irritable infants who experienced more positive parenting were not especially problematic in toddlerhood, whereas irritable infants with negative, intrusive parents were more likely to be noncompliant and difficult at ages 2 and 3. Kochanska (1997) found that inhibited infants were more responsive to gentle guidance than to emotionally charged interactions. Consistent with a transactional view, it appears that responsive, involved, consistent and positive parenting may support an irritable and distressed infant as he or she learns to regulate negative emotions more effectively, whereas harsh parenting may exacerbate early difficulties with the control of negative feelings. It is also clear that, over and above the affective aspects of parenting, limit setting is important, and this may be especially true in early childhood. Bates et al. (1998) found that toddlers high on resistance to control were more likely to have continuing difficulties in middle childhood if their mothers were low on measures of control and child management.

A difficult temperament in infancy may or may not be considered a "risk factor," depending on one's view of the continuity–discontinuity issue. From the continuity perspective, it would be concluded that difficult infants are more likely to continue to have problems in adaptation, especially in the context of an unsupportive environment. From a discontinuity stance, early infant difficultness would be viewed as a developmental phase with few necessary implications for later maladaptive behavior. However, advocates of both positions would probably agree that an extremely difficult infant living in a chaotic and rejecting family would be at high risk for behavior problems. Interpretations differ in terms of the relative emphasis placed on child characteristics and family background factors in contributing to the persistence of difficulties.

INSECURE ATTACHMENT AND LATER ADJUSTMENT

The early parent–infant relationship has been conceptualized primarily within the framework of attachment theory (Ainsworth, Blehar, Waters, & Wall, 1978; Bowlby, 1969; Thompson, 1998), an integration of psychoanalytic, cognitive, systems, and ethological views on the nature of the child's affective bond with its parents. Briefly, attachment theorists argue that infants have a biologically based propensity to become attached to one or two primary caregivers and that adults, likewise, have a biologically based tendency to care for and nurture helpless and dependent members of the species. Within this framework, inborn infant behaviors such as crying and clinging are assumed to promote and maintain proximity to caretakers, thereby protecting the infant from exposure or harm and also ensuring sustenance. Attachment develops over the course of the first year, progressing from indiscriminant responsiveness to any adult in very early infancy to a highly specific and goal-directed emotional bond with the primary caregivers, usually the parents. Once a focused attachment to the mother develops, the infant's behavior becomes organized toward the goal of maintaining proximity to her when in unfamiliar surroundings or when tired or upset. She thus serves as the major source of comfort, protection, and support in times of stress. The attachment figure also serves as a secure base for exploration of the environment, facilitating the infant's mastery of the physical and social world.

According to attachment theory, the attachment figure plays a central role in the infant's cognitive and social development, as well as in the development of a sense of self. It is argued that when the attachment figure is available and responsive, the infant will be more likely to develop a sense of security and trust. Because the world appears predictable, the infant learns that he or she will be protected and cared for. Expectancies about self-efficacy and worthiness and about the availability of others are thought to derive from early experiences with responsive attachment figures (see Bretherton, 1985; Thompson, 1998). On the other hand, unavailability and/or unresponsiveness on the part of attachment figures are seen as resulting in heightened anxiety as the infant learns that the world is unpredictable, threatening, or rejecting and that basic needs for nurturance and emotional support will not be met consistently. Within this framework, then, unresponsive, rejecting, or capricious caregiving may lead to insecurity and lack of basic trust; the infant, preoccupied with maintaining proximity to a caregiver who is unavailable or available only inconsistently, may develop into an anxious, clingy infant who is easily distressed and difficult to calm (resistant or ambivalent attachment); and infants whose mothers are rejecting, intrusive, or overstimulating may learn to avoid emotional and physical contact and become sober and withdrawn or angry and explosive (Ainsworth et al., 1978; Belsky, Rovine, & Taylor, 1984; Bowlby, 1969, 1973; Bretherton, 1985; Carlson & Sroufe, 1995). In addition to these avoidant and resistant patterns, other infants become totally disorganized by separation and do not appear to have a coherent strategy when reunited with their mothers (Main & Solomon, 1990). Instead, disorganized infants may freeze, look frightened, or show other atypical behaviors in response to their mothers' return.

Attachment theorists see the quality of the attachment relationship as laying the groundwork for much subsequent socioemotional development, especially in close relationships, and they argue that coherence in development partially emerges from the way an infant's behavior is organized vis-à-vis the attachment figure (Carlson & Sroufe, 1995; Sroufe, 1979). Individual differences in attachment derive primarily from maternal behavior, especially the mother's responsiveness to infant cues and communications and her availability as a source of comfort during the first year of life. Individual differences in infant characteristics, for example, in irritability or consolability, play a role in some formulations of attachment (e.g., Campos, Barrett, Lamb, Goldsmith, & Stenberg, 1983), but a less central one in others (Sroufe, 1985). However, researchers generally agree that both infant characteristics and the responsiveness of caregivers combine to determine the specific nature of the attachment relationship in infancy and that the attachment relationship influences later social and emotional development in both direct and indirect ways (Thompson, 1998).

A large number of research studies demonstrate that individual differences in maternal behavior in early infancy predict the quality of the infant–mother attachment relationship that develops during the first year. In a recent meta-analysis, De Wolff and van IJzendoorn (1997) concluded that there was a modest relation between maternal sensitivity and responsiveness and secure attachment, although other aspects of the mother–infant relationship and other factors in the family system need to be examined as well (Cowan, 1997; Thompson, 1998). In addition, knowledge of whether the infant is securely or insecurely attached may have implications for social and cognitive development across contexts and over the life span, although this issue is also the subject of debate (e.g., Carlson & Sroufe, 1995; Lamb, 1987a; Lewis et al, 2000; Thompson, 1998; Waters et al., 2000). Some longitudinal studies have found that infants who were insecurely attached at 1 year are less competent in problem solving, less compliant with maternal requests, less sociable in the peer group, and more disorganized and deviant in their play with peers in toddlerhood and the preschool years (see Thompson, 1998, for a review). Other studies suggest even longer term implications of insecurity, especially in the context of family disruption or major stressful life events (Weinfield, Sroufe, & Egeland, 2000; Waters et al., 2000). Bowlby (1969), for example, has suggested that the attachment relationship is the prototype for later intimate relationships; others (Sroufe & Fleeson, 1986; van IJzendoorn, Juffer, & Duyvesteyn, 1995) have suggested that parents who were themselves rejected as infants will in turn be unresponsive to their infants, establishing an intergenerational pattern of insecure attachment in some dysfunctional families. However, the empirical data on the consequences of early insecurity have been quite inconsistent, with some studies suggesting links between early insecurity and later functioning (Waters et al., 2000) and others not finding attachment security to be a robust predictor even of child outcomes at 36 months, such as compliance or self-regulation (e.g., NICHD Early Child Care Research Network, 1998).

The specific relationship between insecure attachment in infancy and toddlerhood and later behavior problems has also been the subject of research and debate. Some studies suggest such a link, with resistant and avoidant infants showing patterns of anger, aggression, and noncompliance or of social withdrawal and depression in the preschool and early elementary school years (Lewis, Feiring, McGuffog, & Jaskir, 1984; Sroufe, 1983). In other studies, no relationship between insecure attachment and later behavior problems has been found (Bates & Bayles, 1988; Lewis et al., 2000; NICHD Early Child Care Research Network, 1998). More recent studies suggest clearer links between disorganized attachment patterns, reflecting a lack of coherently organized behavior toward the mother, and later behavior problems, especially in children living in highly dysfunctional families (e.g., Lyons-Ruth, 1996). Moreover, preschool children with behavior problems are more likely to be insecure than nonreferred children (Speltz, DeKlyen, & Greenberg,1999), but security does not necessarily predict subsequent symptom levels or later diagnoses. This finding suggests that some of the behaviors that are thought to reflect insecurity in preschool children (e.g., coercive behavior toward mother) may be a manifestation of the behavior problems themselves.

The links between early attachment security and later behavior should partly be accounted for by characteristics of the infant, as well as social context, for example, aspects of the mother's social network and her life circumstances. In one study, the combination of infant irritability and low social support was associated with the development of an insecure attachment relationship, presumably because mothers under stress had fewer resources to allow them to cope responsively and sensitively with a difficult infant (Crockenberg, 1981). However, infant irritability in the context of adequate support was not associated with insecure attachment (see also Bates, Maslin, & Frankel, 1985). This fact may suggest that unmeasured features of maternal behavior, possibly maternal affective engagement and limit-setting, that are modified by stress and depression (e.g., Campbell et al., 2001; NICHD Early Child Care Research Network, 1999a) really explain why family stress is linked to attachment security. Other studies suggest that environmental disruption is associated with changes in the quality of the attachment relationship in early childhood (Vaughn, Egeland, Sroufe, & Waters, 1979) and beyond (Weinfield, Sroufe, & Egeland, 2000). In the Vaughn et al. (1979) study, securely attached infants became insecure as their environments became less stable and their mothers less available to meet their needs. However two recent studies do not support these findings (Belsky, Campbell, Cohn, & Moore, 1996; NICHD Early Child Care Research Network, 2001a). In neither of these studies could changes in attachment security be meaningfully explained by changes in family functioning or the in quality of mother–child interaction. Finally, Lewis et al. (1984) have found that environmental stress interacts with early mother–infant attachment to predict good versus poor outcome at age 6. Although insecure attachment was associated with higher ratings of symptomatology, this held true only for insecure children experiencing stressful life circumstances. A further follow-up of this same sample (Lewis et al., 2000), however, found no link between early attachment and adolescent outcomes, although later stressful events such as parental divorce did predict adjustment in adolescence. These data highlight the importance of changing experiences and circumstances in predicting outcome and indicate that the effect of early experiences is modified by ongoing and contemporaneous life events (Lewis et al., 2000; Waters et al., 2000).

Based on the extant evidence, Thompson (1998), in his thorough review of the literature, concludes that the evidence for long-term predictions from attachment security in infancy are weak at best and that when links between early attachment and later functioning are found, the specific mechanisms accounting for them are unclear. One possibility is that stable aspects of parental behavior and the parent–child relationship are implicated; another possibility is that children's internal representations of relationships and their expectations of others, derived in part from early parent–infant interaction and feelings of security, are carried forward to interactions with peers and other adults. Still a third possibility is that the way children learn to regulate emotions and behavior in the context of the early parent–child relationship accounts for later behavior in other situations and with other people. For a thorough discussion of this issue, the reader is referred to Thompson

(1998). Clearly, however, the picture is still more complex than this, and several mechanisms are likely to be involved; only a combined transactional and ecological model that takes into account changes over time in dyadic and wider systems will begin to explain the complex links between attachment security and later functioning.

As an infant's needs change, the nature of maternal responsiveness and of the attachment relationship may change in predictable ways; furthermore, ecological variables such as the availability of support for the mother and maternal adjustment appear to have an effect on child outcome, presumably indirectly through their impact on the mother and her ability to respond appropriately to meet her child's needs for support and nurturance. On the basis of available evidence, it appears that a poor mother–infant relationship is sometimes reflected in early insecure attachment but that this is only *one* risk factor among many that may be associated with later problems in socioemotional development. However, insecure attachment is likely to confer risk only in the absence of alternative attachment figures or in the context of chronic family instability or disruption. Insecure attachment in infancy by itself is not likely to predict difficulties in later adjustment. As noted by Rutter (1994), in addition to characteristics of individuals and relationships, particular life events over the course of development set off causal chains of other events that in turn determine what developmental pathway a particular individual will follow. The quality of the parent–child relationship, broadly construed, is undoubtedly an important ingredient in this dynamic process, but the quality of infant–mother attachment is only a small, albeit developmentally important, piece of the puzzle.

A FINAL COMMON PATHWAY MODEL OF INTERACTING FACTORS

The theoretical issues discussed in this chapter highlight questions about the determinants of problem behaviors in young children, the predictability of a good versus poor outcome, the nature of developmental change, and the way biological and environmental factors interact to predict the onset of deviant behavior, as well as changes in behavior with development. Although none of these theoretical debates can yet be resolved unequivocally, either because they are basically philosophical questions without definite answers or because the empirical data do not provide overwhelming support for one view over another, it is possible to draw together a "working model" of interactive factors. That is, it is possible to synthesize a large body of empirical data and theoretical ideas that implicate a range of child, parent, family, and social context effects in the development and/or maintenance of behavior problems. Furthermore, empirical studies suggest that some factors are more important than others. Moreover, it does not appear logical to suppose that the same factors are operative for all children. Rather, there are undoubtedly multiple pathways to the development of disordered behavior in young children. That is, although within-child factors (both genetically determined and constitutional factors, such as biological vulnerability and difficult temperament) and parenting factors (such as childrearing practices and the affective quality of the parent–child relationship) are both implicated, different combinations of factors are likely to converge to produce good adjustment or disorder in each individual case and to determine whether or not a problem, once apparent, persists. Thus the common problems of early childhood, such as temper tantrums, defiance, separation distress, and sleep disturbances, may result from a variety of environmental stressors or developmental challenges both in biologically vulnerable children and in those without specific biological risk factors for psychopathology. The intensity of the disturbance and its ultimate outcome also will vary as a function of multiple factors in the child and the family environment.

Table 1 lists a number of factors that have been associated with the onset and/or persistence of problem behaviors in young children. This list is far from exhaustive. Furthermore, it is not clear in some instances whether the factor in question is a cause, a correlate, or a reaction to a problem. For example, problems may emerge from early irritability and unconsolability ("difficult" temperament); the difficult temperament may be an early indicator or marker of a problem; or the behaviors labeled "difficult temperament" may be a response to inconsistent and/or insensitive caregiving. Similarly, harsh disciplinary practices may be of etiological significance, a symptom of a disturbed parent–child relationship that developed initially for other reasons, or a parental reaction to a child's lack of response to more low-key attempts at behavioral control. Although it is not possible to delineate specific factors that *cause* disorder and to differentiate them from concomitants of behavior problems in young children, a sufficiently large and robust database exists to allow us to speculate on factors that are likely to be significant in some cases, but not all.

TABLE 1. Some Factors Associated with the Development of Behavior Problems in Preschool-Age Children

Child characteristics	Family composition and interaction
Biological/risk vulnerability	Single-parent family
Temperamental "difficultness"	Marital discord
High reactivity	Parental psychological disorder
High negative affect	Parental disagreements over childrearing
Limited ability to regulate arousal	
and negative affect	*Family environment/social context*
Insecure attachment	Low educational level
Uneven or delayed cognitive	Unemployment or underemployment
development	Limited financial/material resources
Deficits in social skills	Low social support
	Inadequate institutional support
Parenting behavior	Inadequate child care facilities
Insensitivity/unresponsiveness	Family stress
Unavailability	Neighborhood disadvantage
Lack of warmth and engagement	
Limited social and/or cognitive	
stimulation	
Harsh, inflexible control strategies	
Strict physical punishment	
Overly lax control strategies	
Inappropriate developmental	
expectations	

Table 1 highlights biological vulnerabilities that may underlie children's problems, as well as personality or temperamental factors, and developmental and behavioral competencies that may be associated with deviant development. These interact with childrearing practices, the affective quality of parental behavior, and parental attitudes and expectations to produce an ongoing parent–child relationship that may or may not facilitate the child's optimal development. Other factors in the family environment also are seen as significant, including family structure (e.g., single- vs. two-parent; family size), the quality of the marital relationship in a two-parent family, the postdivorce arrangements and the role of the father in single-parent families, and parents' general personality characteristics and overall psychological adjustment. Finally, as noted earlier, social context effects also have an impact on the child.

Figure 1 illustrates the nature of the relationships among child characteristics, parental childrearing strategies and behaviors, family interaction patterns, and social context effects. First, child characteristics and childrearing behaviors influence each other, as illustrated by the bidirectional arrows, reflecting both genetic and environmental influences. Similarly, patterns of interaction in the family influence and are influenced by parenting behaviors and child characteristics. For example, marital distress, as reflected in frequent arguments, may be caused, in part, by disagreements over childrearing that are fueled by a child's temper tantrums and disobedience. Family interaction patterns may also have indirect effects on the child, mediated by their effect on the parents and their childrearing strategies. These indirect effects are depicted by the dotted lines. For example, marital discord may create tension in parents that spills over into harsh or inconsistent discipline. Finally, limited resources likewise have both direct and indirect effects on children by constraining their options and experiences and by influencing parental behavior. Models such as these are presented in more specific detail in several recent publications on parent–child relations and child development (Cummings et al., 2000; Greenberg, Speltz, & DeKlyen, 1993; Greenberg, Speltz, DeKlyen, & Jones, 2001; McLoyd, 1990). In the model proposed here, some combination of child characteristics and parenting behavior is seen as the primary determinant of problems, with family and social context effects exacerbating and/or maintaining them. Family factors and social context effects may also lead to the onset of transient disturbances, as exemplified by children's reactions to divorce (e.g., Hetherington, 1989), but they are not likely

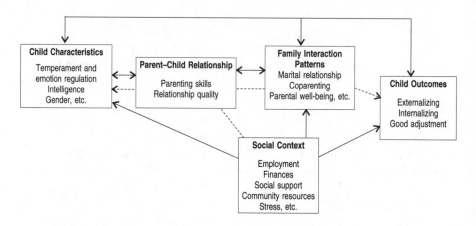

FIGURE 1. Model of interactive factors in the development of childhood problems.

to cause serious and long-term difficulties in the absence of vulnerabilities in the child and/or problems (ongoing or newly created) in the parent–child relationship. These issues are addressed in subsequent chapters.

SUMMARY

In summary, several theoretical issues have been outlined that appear relevant to an understanding of the early development of young children and to conceptualizations of problem behavior. General issues that influence theoretical perspectives on development were addressed first. Questions of interest include continuity in behavior over time and the predictability of later behavior from knowledge of earlier behavior, the nature of developmental change, and the combined contributions of hereditary and environmental influences to developmental outcomes. These complex theoretical issues cannot be unequivocally resolved, but the approach taken to them influences one's view of development. The adoption of a transactional perspective on development implies the acceptance of both discontinuity and overall developmental coherence or meaningful change, change that is primarily qualitative in nature and that is influenced by complex organism–environment interactions that themselves change over time in reciprocal fashion. The addition of ecological variables to a transactional model increases the complexities even further by including bidirectional and indirect pathways of influence from sources beyond the nuclear family and by considering factors other than those that operate directly within the parent–child relationship.

Such a theoretical perspective underlines the complexities inherent in development and highlights the myriad influences that impinge on individual children. Predictions about which developmental pathways particular children will follow and about probable outcomes at different points in development are obviously difficult to make in the face of so many interacting factors, most of which are changing over time. This dynamic perspective enhances our understanding of the general principles of developmental change, but it also makes clinical prediction more risky. Knowledge, even of a well-documented risk factor, may contribute little to prediction in the individual case. However, our increasing sophistication in conceptualizing the nature of development, in identi-

fying and tracing different developmental trajectories, and in understanding the relative importance of various influences on development,
both typical and atypical, suggests that examination of multiple risk factors may be a more fruitful approach. Furthermore, it is evident that
children with similar histories will have different outcomes and that
children with similar outcomes may reach them by different developmental pathways, some more direct than others. An appreciation of this
complexity is a necessary first step in describing and understanding the
nature of development in young children with behavior problems and,
ultimately, in devising effective treatments and predicting outcomes.

CHAPTER 2

Developmental Issues

Wenar (1982) has suggested that problems in children can best be conceptualized as "normal development gone awry" (p. 198). Thus it seems appropriate to examine the major developmental challenges of toddlerhood and the preschool years in order to suggest junctures at which development may proceed normally or may set the stage for the onset of problems. First, several aspects of infant development are described briefly, followed by an overview of some of the main developmental achievements that occur from roughly 18 months to 5 years. This discussion sets the stage for the material in the following chapters.

Among the major goals of early infancy are the development of state control and self-soothing ability, the establishment of routines, the modulation and coordination of motor activity, and the ability to focus attention on and to begin to derive meaning from environmental events (Kagan, 1984; Kopp, 1982, 1989; Sroufe, 1979). It is generally agreed that these early acquisitions are under strong biological/maturational control (Kagan, 1984; Ramey & Ramey, 1998; Thompson & Nelson, 2001), but the role of the caretaking environment is also seen as central to the successful negotiation of these developmental challenges (Kopp, 1982, 1989; Sroufe, 1979; Thompson, 1998). As noted in the previous chapter, it is assumed that the sensitivity and responsiveness of caretakers will influence how well the infant is able to cope with environmental demands and the degree to which the infant will develop feelings of self-efficacy and competence. For example, the ability of infants to wait and to soothe themselves when hungry is thought to derive, in part, from parental responsiveness, as the baby's expectation that hunger and other needs will be met promptly will be determined by past experi-

33

ences with predictable caretakers. Similarly, infants derive meaning from the repetition of environmental events and the predictability of outcomes, both of which are features of many adult–infant games. Kagan (1971, 1984) has written about the development of cognitive schemas for environmental events and the anxiety and distress attendant on the violation of expectancies. At roughly between 6 and 8 months, infants develop a focused attachment to primary caregivers and begin to recognize that people and objects exist even when they are out of sight. At about this time they not only protest parental departures but may also show wariness or outright fear at the approach of strangers. These changes in behavior signal advances in cognitive and social development that set the stage for numerous other developmental attainments, as infants reach their first birthdays.

By the end of the first year or the beginning of the second, most children begin to walk and to use rudimentary language skills to communicate. These advances in motor coordination and symbolic processing usher in a period of rapid cognitive, affective, and social development. The hallmarks of this period include exploration and mastery of the environment and the development of autonomy and independence. By toddlerhood and the early preschool period, the focus of parent–child interaction broadens to include demands for greater self-control, including compliance with parental requests and the ability to share and play cooperatively with other children. The development of independence, self-control, and satisfactory peer relations occurs in tandem with marked advances in cognitive abilities. Children begin to make sense out of their physical and social worlds and are able to convey their rudimentary understanding of the events in their environment in increasingly complex language. Brownell (1986, 1988) suggests that advances in self–other understanding and the ability to combine and sequence behavioral elements may underlie the profound cognitive and social changes that are evident during the second year. At this time children not only begin to sequence words into short sentences but also to engage in smooth and reciprocal interactions with peers that involve complementary roles, to evidence role taking in early pretend play, and to modify their behavior in accordance with the behavior of their partners.

Throughout the preschool period, children continue to demonstrate advances in cognitive and social development that are reflected in more complex reasoning and language skills, an emerging self-awareness and understanding of the feelings and thoughts of others, improved ability to balance one's own needs with the needs of partners during social interaction, and increased knowledge of the physical world. Overall, children's development, across domains, moves from a focus on the concrete and physical to an appreciation of more abstract and symbolic representations of experience. At the same time, as children become increasingly aware of the self as an autonomous agent, behavior becomes more organized and under the control of internal, rather than external, processes. In this chapter, some of the major developmental accomplishments that occur during the period from roughly 18 months to 5 years are discussed. These include language and memory development, mastery motivation, pretend play, self-awareness and a sense of self, self-regulation, and social understanding and perspective taking. The development of peer relationships, another major achievement of the preschool period, is discussed in detail in Chapter 6.

All intact infants who experience normal, expectable caretaking that meets both basic physical and psychological needs will show changes in behavior that signal the achievement of these developmental accomplishments that appear to be invariant features of psychological growth. Thus all normal and biologically intact toddlers explore the environment and begin to engage in pretend play; they develop some degree of autonomy and a sense of self that eventually includes an emerging awareness of their own inner states; they begin to use language to communicate; and they show gains in memory capacity and attentional control. All normal preschoolers show major advances in social-cognitive processing that reflect awareness of social conventions and the fact that others can have feelings and experiences that are different from their own. Preschoolers demonstrate major advances in self-control, including the regulation of emotion, and they develop the ability to play cooperatively with other children. Individual differences in the ease or difficulty young children have coping with these milestones and transitions will be influenced by the child's biological predispositions (including individual differences in intelligence) and by subtle aspects of parenting and the quality of the parent–child relationship. Indeed, young children's cognitive, social, and emotional development are thought to derive in part from early parental responsiveness and availability and from the infant's quality of attachment security (Thompson, 1998). Individual differences also derive from variations in infant abilities and temperamental characteristics, for example, in such attributes as activity level, sociability, attentional control, affect regulation, and mood. In keeping with a transactional model of development, it is assumed that reciprocal influences between children's biological predispositions and personality and caregiver responsiveness and sensitivity to developmental needs will contribute to the child's competence in each of these domains.

In keeping with current conventions, the term *cognitive development* is used to refer primarily to knowledge of and reasoning about objects and abstract events that are not interpersonal, whereas the term *social cognition* is used to refer to thoughts about social relationships and events (e.g., Bjorklund, 2000). Much of the thinking about young children's cognitive and social-cognitive development has been shaped by the theorizing of Jean Piaget (e.g., Piaget, 1926, 1928; Flavell, 1963). Although Piaget's theory per se no longer dominates current thinking in cognitive development, various features of his theory continue to have a major influence on contemporary theories and to frame debates about the nature of children's cognitive development (Bjorklund, 2000). In particular, Piaget's views of the child as an active contributor to his or her own development, his emphasis on exploration and experience, and his arguments about intrinsic motivation are generally accepted. Moreover, many of his descriptions about the nature of young children's concrete and egocentric thinking, as well as the transition from the concrete to the symbolic, are widely accepted, even if theorists reject other aspects of the theory (Bjorklund, 2000).

Piaget proposed a stage theory of cognitive development in which children's logical reasoning progressed from the sensorimotor stage of infancy and toddlerhood (roughly to age 2) through the preoperational stage of the preschooler (roughly from ages 2 to 7) to the more advanced concrete operational stage of the school-age child. Various modifications of Piaget's stage theory have been proposed, but there is general agreement among stage theorists that children go through a series of cognitive reorganizations, reflecting qualitative changes in knowledge structures and mental operations, and that these occur in the same sequence in all children who have normal expected experiences (Bjorklund, 2000), despite some individual differences in the rate at which development proceeds. There is less agreement currently among stage theorists, or cognitive developmentalists generally, about the degree to which children's reasoning about and understanding of a range of topics develops in an integrated fashion, reflecting some general underlying cognitive competence, or whether development is more differentiated and domain specific.

However, at some level, many, if not most, cognitive developmental theorists would agree that early cognitive and social-cognitive development are interrelated and that biological constraints on attention, memory, and representation and interpretation of experience, as well as coordination across modalities (e.g., visual and motor systems) limit the cognitive capacities of the infant. The rapid development of the brain during infancy and toddlerhood underlies cognitive and social-cognitive advances, but these also rely on appropriate cognitive and social stimulation (Bjorklund, 2000; Shonkoff & Phillips, 2000; Thompson & Nelson, 2001). With brain maturation, appropriately timed experiences, and support from caretakers, preverbal and reasonably helpless infants become verbal preschoolers, capable of symbolic thinking, reciprocal conversation, problem solving, and a rudimentary awareness of their own and others' inner states. Given the rapidity of development during these early years and the interrelationships among these various social and cognitive advances, problems in one area (e.g., self-control) may spill over to affect development in other areas (e.g., peer relations). Many children with problems that become more serious or resistant to treatment begin to show adjustment difficulties early on, for example, in a lack of interest in exploration or in delayed language or social development.

LANGUAGE DEVELOPMENT

It has often been argued that the main characteristic that differentiates the human from other primates is the capacity to use spoken language to communicate. Over the course of the first 36 months of life, children move from being preverbal and unable to comprehend spoken language to being able to communicate using complex and syntactically correct sentences (Bjorklund, 2000; Clark, 1983; Shatz, 1983; Sroufe, Cooper, & De Hart, 1992). The major transitions in cognitive functioning that occur over the first 3 years are dramatized by a consideration of the accomplishments made in language development. Language development is intricately tied to conceptual and memory development and to the more general capacity to represent reality with symbols (Bjorklund, 2000; Clark, 1983; Kagan, 1981; Nelson, 1996) required for pretend play and other social-cognitive advances.

The specific ways that cognitive and language development interact, with one supporting advances in the other, has been the subject of some debate. For example, Nelson (1996) argues that language underlies cognitive and memory development, as the emergence of language allows children to organize and interpret their experiences. In contrast, Clark (1983) argues that there are cognitive constraints on language development. She suggests that children learn words that map onto conceptual categories that they have already mastered at a representational level. Furthermore, the ability to think symbolically, that is, to recognize that something (such as a word) can stand for something else, would appear to be a cognitive prerequisite for language. Although this debate is beyond the scope of this book, it highlights the interdependence among conceptual, language, and memory development in early childhood.

Language develops in a highly predictable sequence that is invariant across children regardless of their linguistic and cultural background, suggesting that early language development is under strong maturational control and dependent on the growth of brain structures (Clark, 1983). Furthermore, this sequence is clearly consistent with the view that cognitive developmental advances either precede or emerge simultaneously with early linguistic competence, rather than that language precedes cognitive transitions. For example, the child's ability to link two objects in thought and to sequence two events in pretend play appear at about the same time that toddlers begin to put two words together, somewhere around 24 months (Brownell, 1988; Kagan, 1981).

Young infants vocalize to express distress and pleasure, and they respond to the sound of the human voice, localizing sounds in the early weeks of life. In the early months, infants play with sounds and are able to discriminate between differing consonant–vowel combinations. The cooing of the young infant gives way to babbling as infants practice making various sound combinations. By the latter half of the first year, infant babbling takes on the cadence of the child's own language, and by about 8 to 10 months, children are able to understand some simple commands and names for familiar people and objects. By 12 months, most infants have a vocabulary of a few simple words, though they may only be recognizable to those familiar with their idiosyncratic use of a particular speech sound to designate a particular object, person, or category of objects or people (e.g., "Da" for Daddy or for all men). Infants' first words are almost universally object words that signify familiar people and things in their immediate environment (e.g., *mama, ball, doggie, bottle*), although some properties of objects are also learned early (e.g., *hot*). At this early stage, infants can recognize many more words than they produce, and, in general, receptive language is superior to expressive language over the course of the preschool period (Bjorklund, 2000). By 18 months, children tend to have words for people, common animals, vehicles, toys, food, body parts, and household objects. In addition to nouns, children also begin to acquire vocabulary to describe situations and states (Clark, 1983). For example, they begin to use verbs such as *go*, *eat*, and *sleep*, as well as words that describe other aspects of situations or states, such as *broken, up, little*. These words all describe ongoing experiences, as well as familiar objects and events in concrete terms (Clark, 1983). At about 18 months, toddlers also use one-word utterances to imply an entire sentence. For example, "allgone" may mean that the milk, ice cream, and so forth is all finished.

Once children begin to use words to communicate, they show a rapid increase in vocabulary, primarily an increase in the acquisition of object words. This language spurt, at about 18 months, has been called the naming explosion, because children may triple their functional vocabulary in just a few weeks (Gopnik & Meltzoff, 1988). Children going through this stage of language acquisition may go around the house asking constantly, "What's that?" in an active attempt at vocabulary building. Another feature of early language is the use of what has been termed overextensions (Clark, 1983). That is, a word may be used to refer to a range of objects that are perceptually similar or that belong to a larger class of things. The word is being used in a more inclusive manner than it would be in adult speech, but the errors are usually logical. For example, a toddler may refer to dogs, horses, cows, and sheep as "doggie" until more differentiated terms are learned. Clark (1983) notes that overextensions may account for up to 30% of vocabulary usage during the period from 12 to 30 months but that overextensions systematically drop out of the vocabulary as word knowledge increases. She interprets these as approximations that young children use when vocabulary is not yet adequate, but they still wish to communicate. As they learn the appropriate word (e.g., *horsey*), they do not need to rely on the inappropriate and more generic use of the word *doggie*. Underextensions are also apparent, although less well documented. Thus children may use a word such as *kitty* to refer to a specific cat rather than to the class of animals that adults call cats.

Roughly at the time of their second birthdays, toddlers begin to put words together into two-word sentences. This is a major transition in language development and ushers in a new period of language complexity. At this time children begin to create sentences on their own. Shortly after the appearance of two-word sentences, sentence length increases. At this time, too, children increase their use of self-referent statements, including descriptions of their own internal states. These advances in language development underline the reciprocal relationships among self-awareness, self-regulation, and language competence (Kagan, 1981). By the third birthday, children are speaking in increasingly complex sentences that may include clauses and connectives, as well as statements of causality, descriptions of past events, and planning for the future. Thus, whereas early vocabulary is focused almost exclusively on concrete objects or ongoing events in the here and now, by 36 months, children are able to use language to convey information about internal states, relationships, and other abstractions.

It is generally agreed that, like the motivation to explore, the motivation to become verbal is intrinsic, a given of development. Furthermore, the capacity to develop language appears to be inherent in brain structure, although exposure to the language of the culture is an obvious prerequisite for its development (Clark, 1983). However, children are not taught language as such. Rather, the combination of physical maturation and environmental exposure combine to lead first to the recognition of speech sounds, then to comprehension, and finally to the production of language. Thus children spontaneously learn the phonemics, as well as the syntax and semantics, of their native language without direct instruction. They also learn the cadence and can mimic the prosody of their native language before they can produce a comprehensible sentence. In addition, children learn the basic rules of grammar and apply them diligently. This is evident in the logical errors that young children make, for example, in forming plurals or past tenses (e.g., feets, mans, bringed, goed; see Bjorklund, 2000). Finally, it is worth emphasizing the point that children construct new sentences all the time by putting together, in logical and appropriate sequence, series of words that they have heard in other contexts. It is this creative aspect of language that has fascinated students of child development.

Although early language appears to develop relatively predictably, given a wide range of normal experiences with caretakers, the language environment also plays an important role, and this probably becomes more important as young children use speech to communicate (Shatz, 1983). Early adult–infant interaction often involves reciprocal vocalization and turn taking, and this appears to set the stage for later language. There is no doubt that children must hear language if they are to learn to speak appropriately and at the expected time. Observations of adult–infant interaction also indicate that adults automatically adapt their speech to that of their young child. Thus, Snow (1972) described "motherese" or "child-directed speech," the tendency of adults, but particularly mothers, to use simple, well-formed sentences, more exaggerated voice inflections, and repetition when speaking to toddlers. In fact, there is evidence that children as young as 4 modify their speech when talking to younger children, producing shorter and less complex sentences than they do when talking to adults or peers (Shatz & Gelman, 1973). Mothers also correct young children's speech, for example, by supplying the correct word ("That's not a doggie, it's a horse") and elaborating on a child's utterance. They also keep conversations going by adding new information. During the course of early language learning, adults spontaneously encourage children's language competence by expanding, explaining, questioning, and rephrasing (Weizman & Snow, 2001). There is strong evidence that communicative competence is associated with the amount of conversation in the household and that conversations, even with prelinguistic infants, are important. However, the specific relationships between parental language input and children's later language competence are far from clear, as there is likely to be a large genetic influence on language competence.

There are several clinical implications of marked delays in language development in young children. Whereas language delays are most obviously associated with more general delays in cognitive development, they are also frequently associated with behavior problems in children with normal abilities. Children referred to speech clinics because of language delays are very likely to experience a range of behavior problems as well (Cantwell, Baker, & Mattison, 1979) and, conversely, children referred to child psychiatry clinics often have unsuspected language immaturities or disorders that may be overshadowed by their behavior problems (Cohen, Davine, & Meloche-Kelly, 1989). Both of these studies reported an overlap between language delays and behavior problems of roughly 50%. Furthermore, Richman, Stevenson, and Graham (1982) found an association between delayed language development and behavior problems in an epidemiological study of London 3-year-olds, and language delays were associated with reading and learning problems at age 8.

At the level of process, a language delay may be a sign of a difficulty in expressive language that can have an impact on social development by influencing peer relationships, parent–child relationships, or teacher–child interaction. For example, children may tease, reject, or isolate a child with less developed speech or speech that is hard to understand. Such youngsters may have difficulty participating in social games that involve dramatic roles and conversation. Parents may become impatient with children who misunderstand instructions or who do not easily communicate their wishes or thoughts. Parents and teachers may underestimate the abilities of children with language delays or in other ways communicate to them that they are not competent. Children's impaired language abilities may also be one manifestation of an unstimulating or otherwise unsupportive environment. The specific relationships among language development, general cognitive development, social development in the peer group, and parent–child relationships are complex and poorly understood. Research is only beginning to delineate associations among these different facets of cognitive and social development. These associations are a first step that will naturally lead to the more interesting questions about developmental process.

MEMORY DEVELOPMENT

The ability to learn language and to profit from experience is obviously intertwined with the development of memory. Memory development in young children shows both qualitative and quantitative change over the period from infancy through preschool. Changes in memory, as in other domains of functioning, are partly due to brain maturation and occur in relation to major advances in language and conceptual development. Theorists propose that memory depends on information processing at different levels of analysis and organization (Ornstein, 1978). Thus it has been suggested that at least a three-step process ensues: Stimuli are first attended to and perceived, then they are encoded in short-term working memory, and then they are integrated into long-term memory. In addition, distinctions are made between recognition and recall; among semantic, episodic, and autobiographical memory; and between explicit and implicit memory.

Over the first few months of life, infants begin to derive meaning from environmental stimuli, and by between 2 and 3 months they begin to recognize the familiar. This is evident from studies that rely on infants' innate preferences for novelty and use looking time as an index of interest in unfamiliar, as compared with familiar, stimuli. Recent research by Rovee-Collier and colleagues (as cited in Bjorklund, 2000) indicates that infants as young as 2 months can recognize familiar visual displays after a 2-week period. Six-month-olds can also recognize visual stimuli after various delay intervals, although changes in context (e.g., place of testing, background stimuli) can interfere with retention. It is not surprising that 6-month-olds can remember complex visual stimuli, because they are able to recognize familiar people or favorite toys that they do not see daily. Bjorklund points out that the visual memory capacities of infants reflect recognition (not active recall) and implicit memory; that is, the infants did not consciously try to remember, nor are they aware of their memory processes.

Olson and Sherman (1983), in an extensive review of infant memory development, note the rapid changes in infant memory capacity over the first year of life, as infants become better able to organize information about the world. They are able to rely on a growing knowledge base to help them make sense of new experiences, and this organizational capacity facilitates the retention of information about familiar objects, people, and events. Diary studies provide evidence for fairly complex memory ability, as evidenced by expectancies, surprise, and recognition in young infants. Thus, by 12 months, infants give clear evidence of remembering both routine events and past experiences, such as visits to the pediatrician. More controlled research also demonstrates that 1-year-olds can recognize pictures shown only briefly in a large array. Furthermore, object permanence clearly relies on memory both for the hidden object and for its location.

Memory in young children also tends to be very context specific (Daehler & Greco, 1985). It has been suggested that the improvements noted in memory between ages 2 and 5 can be accounted for by conceptual development and an increase in the knowledge base, rather than by a change in the strategies children use (Daehler & Greco, 1985; Myers & Perlmutter, 1978). That is, both recognition and recall are facilitated when the to-be-remembered stimuli consist of objects or properties of objects that are familiar to the child, when they fit into categories that are well known to the child, or when they relate to familiar events or experiences in the child's life.

As in other areas of cognitive development, the nature of the task appears to influence the picture one gets of young children's memory capacities. The meaningfulness and importance of the information appear crucial. Diary reports indicate that 1-year-olds remember routines and games; 2-year-olds can remember sequences of events over several months when they are salient, such as a birthday party or a trip to the zoo. Nelson (1996) labels children's constructions of familiar events "scripts" that organize experiences and help them to remember events over time. However, young children often may not distinguish between what they expect to happen on a trip to the zoo, and the specifics of a particular trip to the zoo making it difficult to assess specific recall as opposed to script knowledge, that is, the awareness of the typical sequence of events in familiar situations (Bjorklund, 2000; Daehler & Greco, 1985). Thus researchers distinguish between script knowledge and actual memory for events (event memory or episodic memory). Over the course of the preschool period, and partly based on conversations with parents about past events, children develop autobiographical memory, which reflects a coherent picture of past experiences. Autobiographical memory, however, is a combination of actual memories for past events and elaborations based on conversations with parents (Bjorklund, 2000).

There also is interest in the strategies that children use to help them remember, as well as their awareness of memory strategies or metamemory (Brown, Bransford, Ferrara, & Campione, 1983). Research suggests that even very young children use simple and concrete memory aids to help them in familiar tasks with clear goals. For example, Wellman, Ritter, and Flavell (1975) observed 3- and 4-year-olds on a memory-for-location task, in which a toy dog was hidden under one of three containers. Half the children were told to wait to find the toy, and the other half were told to remember where it was. Children given the instructions to remember used a variety of strategies, such as pointing at, looking at, or touching the appropriate container. Children who utilized some form of strategy remembered better than those who did not. Similarly, DeLoache, Cassidy, and Brown (1985) observed 18- to 24-month-olds on a memory-for-location task in which a toy cat was hidden and reached a similar conclusion. Although the strategies used by this age group are clearly concrete and external, rather than internal ones that might be used by older children, these studies provide beginning evidence for the spontaneous use of memory aids in young children.

Taken together, it is generally agreed that memory improves with development, probably as a function of cognitive and language development and the use of strategies to facilitate the organization and recall of information. Furthermore, children have an easier time remembering things that fit into their knowledge base; that is, if they can incorporate new information into a context, it is more readily assimilated and integrated into useful long-term memory. Preschoolers are just beginning to utilize strategies to facilitate memory, but these tend to be very concrete and tied to familiar situations. Moreover, there is growing evidence that parents facilitate the development of certain kinds of memory, especially script knowledge and autobiographical memory. Although it is difficult to link memory development to specific clinical problems, it seems obvious that memory abilities are a necessary and fundamental component of all other aspects of cognitive and social development. Mastery of the environment, the development of a sense of self, language development, and self-regulation all depend to some extent on children's ability to learn from past experience. Similarly, peer relations and relationships within the family will be shaped to some extent by children's abilities to remember past events and to develop expectations about the behaviors and personality characteristics of others.

EXPLORATION AND ENVIRONMENTAL MASTERY

In addition to the reciprocal vocalizations that precede language development and some signs of recognition of the familiar, young infants show interest in and engagement with the environment in the first few months of life. As infants' motor skills improve to permit visually directed reaching and the purposeful grasping of objects, interest in the physical world becomes a central focus of their waking hours. Infants reach for, examine, mouth, drop, and bang objects—all part of the early repertoire of exploratory behavior. With somewhat more advanced motor and cognitive abilities, two objects are banged together, objects are placed one inside the other, and containers are filled and emptied as infants practice emerging skills; they experiment with gravity and also explore the size, shape, texture, and taste of various inanimate objects. The increasing complexity of early play and its importance for early cognitive development has been described in detail by Piaget and others (see Rubin, Fein, & Vandenberg, 1983). In this context, infants learn about cause–effect relations and their ability to control some aspects of their environment.

As infants become mobile, they are in a position to explore ever-widening areas and to exert more control over things that capture their interest. At this point in development, some parents begin to have difficulties balancing their own needs for order and control, as well as their concerns for their infant's safety, with the infant's need to explore. Parents sometimes find that their cuddly infant is now determined to open every cupboard and drawer and that they are unable to keep up with the flurry of activity. Whereas some parents appropriately view this as an important developmental phase, others may begin to engage in battles with their child, and it is at this point that some parents, rightly or wrongly, become concerned about overactivity. At the other extreme are temperamentally withdrawn, passive, or timid babies who rarely venture out to explore (Kagan, 1997) . These infants may have more limited experiences as a result of their lack of interest in mastery, and this may influence their later cognitive and social development.

There is general agreement that, despite biologically based individual differences in exploration and consistent with Piaget's emphasis on intrinsic motivation, young children are biologically primed to explore and master the environment, that curiosity about the world is a normal and healthy facet of children's behavior. Mastery is most clearly illustrated by the tendency of infants and toddlers to repeat and practice newly acquired skills, such as climbing stairs or stacking objects. Interest has focused on individual differences in engagement with the environment, or mastery motivation, which encompasses both persistence in exploration and exploratory competence (Yarrow et al., 1983). In addition to temperamental differences, early caretaking experiences are thought to be one determinant of variations in mastery motivation. For example, attachment theorists consider maternal responsiveness to affect infants' exploratory competence. They argue that infants and toddlers who feel secure and nurtured will have more energy available to invest in exploration and more curiosity about the world. Sure of their mothers' availability, they will use her as a secure base for exploration, returning from time to time to check in with her, but showing interest in independent play and curiosity about new and interesting objects (Ainsworth et al., 1978).

Other aspects of maternal behavior also appear to be related to mastery motivation and exploratory competence. For example, mothers who provide the infant or toddler with opportunities to explore by the way they structure the environment and by providing age-appropriate and interesting toys, who support autonomy by permitting independent play and rewarding success experiences, and who encourage exploration without being intrusive or controlling appear to raise toddlers who are more invested in environmental mastery and more adept at negotiating the environment (Cassidy, 1986; Frodi, Bridges, & Grolnick, 1985). On the other hand, parents who are unable to tolerate their young child's tendency to explore or who are overly directive and controlling, thereby thwarting the child's independent attempts to learn about the world, may be setting the stage for a variety of subtle problems, both social and cognitive. It appears that toddlers' ability to master the physical environment has implications for their more general feelings of self-worth and autonomy, another major developmental issue of toddlerhood. In addition, with development, exploration gives way to pretend play, which is also seen as central to both cognitive and social development.

PRETEND PLAY

The development of pretend play is intertwined with the development of language and representational abilities, and observations of the play of toddlers and preschoolers provide a window into their spontaneous language, thought, and role taking. Numerous theorists emphasize the importance of play in young children's development (Garvey, 1990; Rubin, Fein, & Vandenberg, 1983; Howes, 1988). Erikson (1963) saw play as one means by which the young child begins to master the environment, whereas Piaget saw pretend play as enhancing cognitive and social development by allowing the child to experiment with deferred imitation, role taking, and other more advanced cognitive skills, thereby consolidating newly assimilated cognitive schemas. Others have emphasized pretend play as a social activity that facilitates symbolic development and contributes to the development of the self-concept (Howes, 1988; Garvey, 1990) and to more general social competence in the peer group (Rubin et al., 1983). Pretend play is also used as a therapeutic tool to understand the concerns and conflicts of young children. Further, more advanced and elaborated pretend play is associated with greater competence in other areas, including language, creativity, and social skills.

Pretend play first emerges, in rudimentary form, at about 13 months of age, when children can be observed to make believe that they are engaged in a familiar activity, such as eating, drinking, or sleeping. Such acts are usually short-lived, and they rely on concrete props, for example, a cup or a toy cup, if the act is drinking. By 18 months, the child is able to act on another object in pretend play. Instead of feeding herself, she will feed her doll. Rubin et al. (1983) refer to this as the shift from self-referenced to other-referenced play. At the next level, that of active other, the child pretends that the doll is the active agent, that is, that the doll is feeding itself. Studies reviewed by Rubin et al. (1983) indicate that children's play follows this developmental sequence from 12 to 30 months of age. Furthermore, as a more advanced play form emerges in the child's repertoire, earlier forms disappear. In addition, early symbolic play consists of single events, but as play becomes more complex in terms of who is the active agent, it also incorporates more complex sequences of actions and activities. The doll is not only fed, but burped, bathed, and put to bed. Thus the child is also practicing familiar sequences of events or scripts that figure prominently in his or her understanding of the world (Nelson, 1996; Rubin et al., 1983). Children also are better able to use substitute objects as props in play, an advance that illustrates another facet of representational ability. A block can stand for a cup, and the child can make believe that the doll is drinking from a cup. Most 24-month-olds are able to incorporate both sequential actions and substitutions in their play.

Pretend play, especially early on, often occurs in the context of parent–child or child–older sibling interactions (e.g., Youngblade & Dunn, 1995). The complexity of early pretend play relies considerably on the skills of a more sophisticated play partner who can maintain the theme of the play; very young children, who might not engage much in symbolic play alone or with age-mates, may follow the lead of an adult or older child, and in this context they are learning to represent their world in more varied ways. Pretend play often also involves shared positive affect, thereby enhancing social and emotional understanding, as well as social relationships.

After the third birthday, pretend play takes up an ever-increasing portion of children's spontaneous play time with peers. According to Rubin et al. (1983), in group situations, such as preschools, children rarely engage in solitary pretend play, but cooperative dramatic play sequences are common. Furthermore, children who are familiar with one another are more likely to engage in pretend play than newly acquainted preschoolers (Gottman & Parkhurst, 1980), presumably because a certain level of comfort is necessary before children are willing to move beyond their own identities and let their imaginations take over. Garvey (1977) observed pairs of acquainted 3- to 5-year-olds in a laboratory playroom well equipped with toys likely to elicit pretend play. She reported that fairly complex dramatic sequences were evident even in the 3-year-olds but that older children participated in longer and more elaborate pretend interactions. Most of the imaginary play of preschoolers revolves around a relatively limited number of common themes that are well known to children, reflecting their social milieu and shared social knowledge. According to Garvey (1977), children tended to take on particular types of roles: relational or family roles predominated (mommy, daddy, baby), followed by functional roles, that is those defined by an activity or occupation, such as teacher, bus driver, or doctor. Children across the 3- to 5-year age range took on these roles. Four- and 5-year-olds were also more likely to play imaginary characters such as a dragon or Bat man. All of these forms of dramatic play require a transformation of identity. Garvey also observed play sequences in which the child played him- or herself, but incorporated absent characters; for example, she describes a delightful sequence in which a 4½-year-old engages in a long telephone conversation with an imaginary friend about a sick teddy bear. In this instance, the prop (toy phone) appeared necessary to scaffold the pretend sequence in the absence of role adoption and a willing play partner.

Pretend play usually involves the assignment of complementary roles, a plan of action, and the use of props (Garvey, 1977). The adoption of complementary roles implies perspective-taking ability, as does the give and take necessary for truly interactive sociodramatic play. Further, children often switch back and forth between the pretend characters and their real selves, with the real self narrating or directing the play (e.g., "Now the mommy is going shopping," or "You say, 'Don't do that!' Okay?"). These shifts are usually indicated by voice changes (the child's real voice for the directions and a high-pitched baby voice or a grown-up voice for the role, depending on whether the character is a baby or a mommy). In addition, dramatic play sequences involve not only complex sets of role-appropriate interactions but also exaggerated affect expression, such as mock anger or concern, and other modifications in speech. For example, a child playing "mommy" will often talk in shorter sentences to the "baby," consistent with the way adults talk to infants. These shifts also indicate that the play is pretend; older preschoolers may also make this explicit by specifically asking a peer to pretend something. Here, too, there is evidence not only of perspective taking but also of a clear distinction between fantasy and reality, although it has been erroneously assumed that preschoolers have difficulty distinguishing between the real and the make-believe. Although this may be the case when they are observing the fantasy of others, for example, on television or in a movie, they certainly are aware of the differences when they themselves are engaged in the pretend activities.

The pretend play described by Garvey (1977, 1990) and others (Rubin et al., 1983) reflects a large store of knowledge about people, relationships, and activities, as well as an ability to step outside the self and practice various roles. When younger children engage in these forms of sociodramatic play, they are likely to follow social conventions quite literally, and any variation from traditional expectations is likely to provoke a discussion about what is appropriate ("Daddies don't cook!"; "My daddy does!") or to result in a switch in roles or a change in the activity. Older preschoolers are better able to adapt to a wider range of variations in a particular role. Moreover, role enactments in older children are more reciprocal; younger children may act out their roles, but they tend to do so with less attention to the other's behavior and verbalizations (Rubin et al., 1983). Finally, older preschoolers are more likely to negotiate role assignments and to reassure each other that it's "just pretend," something that 2-year-olds and young 3-year-olds do not appear to do.

These advances appear to be important hallmarks of normal cognitive and social development. Children integrate experiences, express feelings, practice roles, resolve disputes, and differentiate between reality and fantasy in the context of sociodramatic play. In clinical practice, play therapy is based on the premise that the themes expressed in children's play mirror their feelings, conflicts, preoccupations, and interpretations of reality, much of which they are not capable of expressing directly (e.g., Axline, 1969). Despite the emphasis on play therapy and the reliance on fantasy play in both the assessment and treatment of psychological distress in preschoolers, surprisingly little systematic research has been conducted on the fantasy play of clinically identified preschool children (Rubin et al., 1983). Thus it is unclear whether some disturbed preschoolers show delays in the development of pretend play, are reluctant to engage in fantasy, or use fantasy as a way of escaping from an unsupportive or threatening environment. Despite the reliance on fantasy in clinical practice, it is not known, except at an anecdotal level, whether some children really do express their concerns through play or what the implications of individual differences in this are for understanding and treating problems. However, because the development of pretend play is associated with major advances in language abilities and other symbolic processes, as well as with other changes in the quality of peer interactions, it seems logical to hypothesize that extremely bizarre fantasy play or the inability to engage in pretend play might be a signal of "development gone awry." For example, preschoolers who engage in extremely aggressive or disorganized fantasy play may be indicating that they are having difficulties coping with new expectations, environmental changes, the control of negative emotions, or other stresses or developmental transitions; or the disorganized play may be a marker of serious problems. At the other extreme, children who are unable to engage in pretend play may lack certain symbolic or language abilities, raising concerns about cognitive-developmental delays; or they may be showing signs of social withdrawal and emotional constriction.

In summary, the appearance of pretend play marks another major advance in cognitive and social-cognitive development. By early in the second year, children are beginning to use their representational and emerging language abilities in their play. By age 2, they are engaging in more complex representational and sequential activities. By late in the third year, role playing allows children to engage in a variety of sociodramatic play sequences that are thought to enhance social-cognitive abilities such as role taking and perspective taking, as well as awareness of self–other differentiation and feelings of self-esteem. The failure of children to engage in pretend play by age 4, or their tendency to engage in highly aggressive or bizarre fantasy play, may be an indicator of problems in development or adaptation.

THE DEVELOPMENT OF SELF-AWARENESS AND A SENSE OF SELF

At the same time that toddlers are engaged in intense exploration of the environment and beginning to engage in symbolic play, they are grappling with another major developmental accomplishment, the establishment of a sense of self. Harter (1998) emphasizes the importance of considering cognitive, social, and affective development together in trying to understand the emergence of a sense of self. One phase of the sense of self is the establishment of autonomy, the realization that one can act independently and have effects on other people and on objects. It is the combination of the need to explore and the need to test the limits of one's independence that is often termed the "terrible 2's." Exploratory competence and mastery of the environment have roots in early infancy and are associated with the quality of the early mother–infant relationship. Similarly, theorists interested in the development of self-awareness emphasize the role of the early caretaking environment in facilitating the emergence of a sense of self and in determining the nature of individual differences in self-concept. A thorough discussion of the major theories is beyond the scope of this chapter; interested readers are referred to Harter (1998).

Theorists since the turn of the century have emphasized the role of social interaction in the development of self-identity and self-esteem (Harter, 1998). Most theorists, whether they espouse a cognitive-developmental perspective (Lewis & Brooks-Gunn, 1979), favor attachment theory (Bowlby, 1969), or work from more psychodynamic orientations (Erikson, 1963; Mahler, 1968), also emphasize the importance of the caretaking environment and the role that responsive caretakers play in the child's development of self-esteem, an independent identity, and an awareness of the self as an active agent who can have an impact on the environment, both physical and social. Erikson (1963) proposed that basic trust derives from responsive early care, which in turn permits secure toddlers to assert their independence without fear of rejection and to feel competent about their ability to exert some control over their environment. From the perspective of cognitive-developmental (Lewis & Brooks-Gunn, 1979) and attachment theories (see Bretherton, 1985), infants' experiences with consistent, responsive, and contingent care set the stage for the development of expectancies about the predictability of others and their availability, which in turn influence feelings of self-efficacy. The infant whose signals are responded to promptly and consistently learns that he or she has control over the social environment. On the other hand, infants whose signals are often ignored or who are responded to inconsistently learn that their needs and behaviors do not have an effect on the behavior of others, and they do not learn to expect that their needs will be met. Their internal working models (Bretherton, 1985) or schemas of the self and relationships, which develop from their past experiences with unresponsive or rejecting care, lead them to perceive themselves as incompetent and unworthy and to view others as untrustworthy, leaving them with few resources and limited motivation to assert their independence. In Erikson's terminology, a child's lack of basic trust in early caregivers is translated into fearfulness, incompetence, and feelings of limited control in toddlerhood. Instead of feeling autonomous and able to cope with a range of new challenges, such toddlers may be expected to doubt their abilities and to feel shame, both as a result of their own perceived ineptness and of the anticipated rejection by significant others who have failed to support their developmental needs.

Before toddlers can assert their independence and autonomy, they must develop a sense of self that is independent from primary caregivers. Harter (1998) integrates current thinking in developmental psychology to propose several stages in the development of a sense of self. In early infancy, predictable features of the caregiving environment and the establishment of routines of feeding, sleeping, and awake time are coordinated with the infant's basic perceptual and feeling states to reflect what Sroufe (1990) calls *physiological regulation*. This process forms the basis of a rudimentary sense of regularity and organization for the infant. In the period from 4 to 10 months, the infant becomes more differentiated from primary caretakers, and this is reflected in behaviors such as visual following and distress at separation. Further, emerging attachment behaviors, such as proximity seeking and calming on reunion, appear to signal some primitive awareness of the infant's sense of self as distinct from mother. At this time, infants also develop a sense of agency, reflected in their reactions to their own motor movements, for example, gleeful reactions to kicking a mobile on their own or acting physically on other objects by throwing, banging, and mouthing; then repeating the action over again. Thus they are beginning to recognize that their behavior has independent effects on other people and objects. This awareness emerges at the same time that infants also begin to engage in more complex reciprocal play and turn taking with adults and to show awareness of the permanence of objects and people who are not in their immediate view. These newly emerging skills also signal the infant's awareness of the self as an active agent. As in the earlier stage, however, self-efficacy requires the cooperation of caregivers and familiar, predictable routines; social play and shared positive affect are important as well. This is partly due to the salience of emotional experiences and the regular patterning of reciprocal exchanges with caregivers, what Sroufe (1990) calls *psychological regulation*. These experiences form the child's early representations of the self and relationships, which later become the internal working model discussed by Bowlby (1969).

By the end of the first year, as the attachment relationship is consolidating, the self as an active and independent agent is also consolidating. Infants use the mother as a base for exploration, moving away to act on the environment, again illustrating something about the emergence of the self. Shared interactions with the caregiver, including mutual positive affect, joint attention, and social referencing, can be seen as signs of the infant's sense of the self in relation to the caregiver; these mutually regulated behaviors are also seen as precursors of the awareness of the inner states of others, what has come to be called *theory of mind* (Bjorklund, 2000; Harter, 1998; Thompson, 1998).

Harter (1998) distinguishes between the self as an active, independent, causal agent (the "I self") and the self as an object of self-knowledge (the "me self"). This parallels other aspects of social and cognitive development in which active, overt, or concrete advances precede more symbolic and internal representational ones. By about 12 months of age, infants begin to recognize that they can have effects on the environment that are different from the effects that others can have, an awareness that is also probably enhanced by their increased mobility and their beginning ability to communicate their wants with rudimentary language. As representational skills become more sophisticated, during the first half of the second year, toddlers begin to have some awareness of specific features of the self (the me self). For example, toddlers can recognize themselves in mirrors or in pictures and begin to identify body parts on the self and others. By the later half of the second year, toddlers can also appreciate unique features of the self and can label pictures of themselves by name, gender, and other simple attributes. This also implies an ability to conceptualize "me" from "not me" and, therefore, to recognize that others possess attributes that are different from one's own. However, at this stage, toddlers would be likely to have only a relatively rudimentary appreciation of this concept and to recognize only concrete and obvious attributes such as gender, size, and age (baby, child, adult).

In a longitudinal study of development in toddlers over the second year, Kagan (1981) defined several converging signs of growing self-awareness, as well as awareness of others as distinct individuals. He emphasized increases in "mastery smiles" that indicate satisfaction with one's own accomplishments, as well as distress at the inability to carry out an adult's request, thereby eliciting feelings of incompetence. Kagan also noted, by the latter half of the second year, an increase in children's interest in directing adult activity in game-like interactions, another indication of toddlers' growing sense of autonomy and self-efficacy. Further, Kagan documents the increased use of self-descriptive speech from 22 to 27 months, including descriptions of ongoing activities, statements specifically referring to the self using "I," "me," and "mine," and references to internal states (e.g., *want, hurt, like*). During the 18- to 30-month period, toddlers are also are beginning to internalize adult standards, to have a sense of what constitutes appropriate behavior in certain situations, and to show rudimentary self-evaluative emotions such as pride and shame (Lewis, Alessandri, & Sullivan, 1992). In addition, these emerging aspects of self-awareness develop in conjunction with advances in language development and the verbal representation of events, enhanced self-control and the ability to meet standards, and memory (including episodic memory for past events and scripts for expected behaviors in familiar situations; Harter, 1998). Thus individual differences in self-awareness are partly a function not only of the child–caretaker relationship but also of variations in language competence, memory development, and self-regulatory skills.

As a sense of self develops and children become more autonomous and aware of the effects their behavior can have on others, they also can become more difficult to control. Parents often are uncertain about how to cope with this developmental transition, because once cooperative and positive youngsters may go through a period of irritability and anger reflected in frequent tantrums, crying spells, and oppositional behavior. At this point, children may be oppositional just for the sake of saying "no!" and parents may waffle between flexibility and rigid limit setting. It is likely to be helpful for parents to recognize that this is a normal developmental phenomenon; that their children are experimenting with limits, their own and others', as well as asserting their independence, sometimes by failing to go along even with things they want to do. Parents who feel comfortable setting limits may have an easier time with this developmental phase, because testing often indicates a young child's need for some guidelines about acceptable behavior from significant others, although they need limits that are flexible and not confrontational. When parents let their toddlers gain control, either by engaging in a battle of wills, by failing to set clear and consistent limits, or by not setting any limits at all, they may be encouraging increasingly defiant behavior. Other parents may overreact to defiance from their toddler. When parents have difficulty tolerating challenges to their authority, they may set limits that are too harsh, leading to escalating confrontations that may have a negative effect on the quality and tone of the parent–child relationship. The difficulties of this developmental period are often exacerbated by the birth of a sibling, which may further fuel a toddler's tendencies to be noncompliant, negative, and attention seeking. The way that parents handle this difficult period of development may set the stage for continuing conflict, at least over the short term, as the child may become increasingly demanding in the face of either lax, inconsistent, or very strict limits.

As children mature, however, this phase of negativism and noncompliance is usually replaced by a more reasonable period of increased interest in the world and in peer relationships. The terrible 2's have been successfully negotiated, and the child's self-awareness continues to become both more complex and more differentiated as social comparisons are made and children become increasingly aware of the thoughts and feelings of others. The development of peer relationships and social-cognitive awareness become primary.

SELF-REGULATION

Closely related to self-awareness and the development of autonomy and independence is the development of self-regulatory ability. Indeed, self-control or self-regulation obviously depends on self-awareness and one's sense of self, because self-awareness and self-reflection would appear to be necessary for the internal regulation of behavior. Self-regulation, like self-awareness, is seen as developing through qualitatively distinct phases, with children moving from concrete and externally mediated control attempts to more internally mediated self-regulation (Eisenberg & Fabes, 1998; Kopp, 1982, 1989). There is general agreement that self-regulation, whether it is defined in terms of compliance, modulation of behavior, control of emotion, inhibition of situationally inappropriate behavior, control of attention, or the ability to wait for desired events, is partly a function of individual differences in temperament (Rothbart & Bates, 1998). It also depends, however, on the awareness of what constitutes acceptable behavior, and it derives from socialization experiences (Eisenberg & Fabes, 1998; Kopp, 1982, 1989).

It is important to point out that most conceptualizations of behavior problems in childhood focus on deficits in self-control. For example, Achenbach and Edelbrock (1978), in their description of childhood disorders, discuss patterns of overcontrol (e.g., social withdrawal) and undercontrol (e.g., overactivity, aggression, noncompliance). It is well known that in early childhood the bulk of problems about which adults complain are characterized by undercontrol, and these problems can be construed as failures to develop internalized standards of socially appropriate behavior and/or to use these standards to guide behavior. Block and Block's (1980) theory of personality development likewise focuses on ego control as one major dimension of personality functioning. Overcontrolled individuals are tight and lack spontaneity, whereas undercontrolled individuals tend to be explosive, active, and aggressive. Both individual child characteristics and patterns of childrearing are implicated in the development of ego control.

There has been a recent upsurge of interest in self-regulation and its development, with a particular emphasis on emotion regulation (Thompson, 1994), as well as a growing interest in children's compliance and noncompliance. Kopp (1982, 1989) has outlined a theoretical model of the cognitive and social antecedents of self-control in infancy, as well as of its emergence during toddlerhood and the preschool period. Consistent with a transactional model of development, Kopp (1982, 1989) suggests that early modulation of behavior, as well as later self-regulatory abilities, derive both from individual differences in infant characteristics that have biological/constitutional roots and from the quality of caretaking. With development, as self-regulation becomes more internalized, socialization processes within the family and cognitive processes within the child become especially salient determinants of individual differences in self-control.

Kopp proposes that modulation of physiological arousal in the early months and infants' organized responses to environmental stimuli during the first year depend largely on constitutional factors and parents' abilities to provide predictable routines, to respond appropriately to infants' communications, and to prevent overwhelming frustration.

Through most of the first year, infants are able to modulate their reactions when supported appropriately by parents, but their behavior does not have an intentional quality, and it is dependent on ongoing events. By the end of the first year, however, infants begin to comply with parental requests and can even anticipate the need to perform or inhibit particular motor acts, such as not touching something dangerous or fragile. Kopp argues that certain cognitive developmental advances, in object permanence and recognition memory, must necessarily precede the emergence of this early form of control, which involves compliance with social demands and the expectations of caregivers, goal-directed behavior, intentionality, and rudimentary awareness of the self. It is assumed that this form of self-control occurs in only a limited number of situations that are quite predictable and that they are associated with relatively clear external controls. Further, although children know that they should not do certain things, they are not likely to understand the reasons for the prohibitions.

Anyone who has ever been around toddlers can think of examples of this form of control, for instance, the child who knows that the stove or a valuable china teapot is off-limits. The self-initiated and coordinated behaviors that characterize certain games, particularly when turn taking and complementary roles are involved, also require control over one's behavior, as well as some degree of self-awareness and anticipation of the reactions of the partner (Brownell, 1986; Kopp, 1982, 1989). Furthermore, there is accumulating evidence that the strategies parents use to gain compliance and direct behavior are important determinants of children's willingness to comply (Kochanska, 1997; Maccoby & Martin, 1983). Thus firm, clear, consistent, and appropriate limits appear more effective than inconsistent, ambiguous, or harsh attempts at control. For some children, gentle guidance is effective, whereas for others more clear-cut limits are needed (Bates et al., 1998; Belsky, Woodworth, & Crnic, 1996; Crockenberg & Litman, 1990; Kochanska, 1995)

Kopp (1982) notes that true self-control emerges by the end of the second year, as children are able to comply with expectations and can inhibit impulses in the absence of external constraints. This advance in behavioral control appears to depend on more advanced representational thinking and more complex memory development, including evocative or recall memory. Both are seen as cognitive prerequisites if children are to begin to monitor their own behavior in accordance with social rules in the absence of constant adult reminders. Language development also plays a role. In the second year, children use language to describe their ongoing behavior, and this may sometimes aid them in initiating or inhibiting a specific behavior (Kagan, 1981). Kopp (1982) distinguishes between the early, self-generated self-control of which toddlers are capable and which tends to be relatively inflexible and tied to specific situations and the more advanced self-regulation of the preschooler.

By about age 3, children are able to engage in more complex, adaptive, and long-term self-regulatory behaviors. Kopp suggests that this form of self-regulation may involve self-reflection and planning strategies. Language may also be used to verbalize plans or prohibitions, and, therefore, advances in language development may aid in self-regulation. Certainly, the complex routines that preschoolers follow and their ability to function cooperatively with peers and teachers in nursery school and day care suggest fairly marked gains in socially appropriate regulation of self-help skills and social interaction. At this stage, too, children are able to apologize for transgressions and to recognize when others are behaving in unacceptable ways, suggesting both some degree of self-reflection and the internalization of standards of behavior. Throughout the preschool years, children acquire ever greater control over impulses and more awareness of the limits of socially acceptable behavior. Related to these advances are the development of conscience and morality (Kochanska, 1993), the idea that behavioral control and definitions of right and wrong often involve more than social convention; that is, they stem from higher precepts, such as not harming others or violating their trust.

Individual differences in child personality and childrearing strategies appear to be associated with differences in self-regulation (Eisenberg & Fabes, 1998; Kochanska, 1993, 1995, 1997; Maccoby & Martin, 1983). For example, children who are more irritable and easily aroused may have a more difficult time controlling impulses and tolerating frustration, and these difficulties may be exacerbated if their parents are themselves impatient and explosive. Studies suggest that children show developmental changes in compliance and noncompliance strategies; for example, younger children may ignore parental requests or simply say "no." These behaviors have been considered indices of emerging self-assertion (Crockenberg & Litman, 1990; Kuczynski, Kochanska, Radke-Yarrow, & Girnius-Brown, 1987); preschool children may be more likely to engage in negotiation. Moreover, Crockenberg and

Litman distinguish between age-appropriate attempts to establish autonomy and outright defiance that reflects clearly negative and problematic behavior. A growing body of research also indicates that parental behavior that is harsh and power assertive is more likely to elicit angry defiance (Crockenberg & Litman, 1990; Kuczynski et al., 1987), especially among toddlers who are themselves more irritable and difficult to manage (Belsky, Woodworth, & Crnic, 1996).

As already noted, behavior problems in early childhood and beyond often reflect difficulties with internalized standards of behavior as indexed by noncompliance, overactivity, aggression toward peers, defiance of authority, inattention, and a limited ability to tolerate frustration or delayed gratification. Findings from longitudinal studies also suggest that early deficits in self-control may persist (e.g., Block & Block, 1980; Richman et al., 1982), although clinically significant difficulties tend to reflect a constellation of problems that may indicate a generalized lack of internalized standards and concern for the rights and/or feelings of others. Although relatively little is understood about the processes that influence the development of self-regulatory abilities in clinical populations of young children, it appears that, over and above children's temperamental characteristics, parental approaches to discipline, parental strategies of conflict resolution and self-control abilities, and the quality of relationships within the family are all relevant to understanding children's problems in the early development of self-control.

SOCIAL UNDERSTANDING
AND PERSPECTIVE TAKING

The development of a sense of the autonomous self and the ability to regulate behavior and emotional reactions are closely related to the development of social understanding and the ability to recognize that others have thoughts, feelings, desires, and knowledge that are different from one's own. The awareness of internal states in the self and in others has come to be called *theory of mind* (Bjorklund, 2000), suggesting that young children develop a coherent set of expectations about other people based on awareness of themselves and their experiences in regular interactions with familiar adults and peers. Bjorklund (2000) defines theory of mind as "developing concepts of mental activity" (p. 214). This broad area encompasses a range of social-cognitive advances that include awareness of one's own feelings and their causes (Saarni, Mumme, & Campos, 1998), as well as metacognition, or awareness of cognitive processes such as attention, memory, and thinking (Bjorklund, 2000). Research on the development of social understanding, both in the laboratory (e.g., Denham & Auerbach, 1995) and in the natural environment (e.g., Dunn, Bretherton, & Munn, 1987; Dunn, Brown, & Beardsall, 1991), indicates that adult conversation and scaffolding play a role in children's developing ability to recognize their own emotions and understand not only their causes but also their effects on others. For example, Dunn et al. (1987) studied mothers and children's naturally occurring conversations during toddlerhood and the preschool period. Mothers often elaborated on ongoing events and labeled emotions during emotionally arousing interactions, especially mother–child or sibling conflicts (see also Chapter 5). Children whose mothers provided more interpretation of events and their impact on the self and others were more advanced several years later on laboratory tasks assessing emotional understanding (Dunn et al., 1991). Awareness of one's own emotional experiences and their causes appears to be a prerequisite for the ability to recognize emotions in others and to feel empathy or sympathy for others in distress (Eisenberg & Fabes, 1998; Saarni et al., 1998).

Of particular importance to cooperative interactions with others, both adults and peers, is the ability to read social cues, interpret facial expressions of emotion, and infer what others are thinking and feeling. Young infants mirror the emotional reactions of others, but it is not until the end of the first year that children have a rudimentary awareness of others' feelings. By the second year, with the emergence of language and a sense of self, children's ability to read some basic facial expressions and infer basic emotions in others are evident (Saarni et al., 1998). Given the functional importance of emotion for social communication, children seem to learn to read emotion cues in face and voice earlier than they can infer other sorts of less emotion-laden information, such as thoughts and intentions. For example, children have a harder time taking the perspective of another when the task involves memory and reconciling what they know with discrepant information given to another child. Much recent research on theory of mind has relied on false-belief tasks. For example, a child may be shown candy that is removed from its likely place (e.g., a candy jar) and placed in an unlikely place (a crayon box). When asked where another child will go to look for the candy, 3-years-olds will identify the unlikely place because they know that the candy is there and because they are unable to take the perspective of the child who does not have the privileged information (i.e., the real location of the candy). However, 4-year-olds will correctly respond that the other child will go to the wrong place (candy jar) to look for the candy. Studies using a variety of false-belief tasks administered to children in different cultures have found that a transition takes place between ages 3 and 4 in the ability to understand that the other child has information that is different from one's own (Bjorklund, 2000). Convergent findings across different types of tasks suggest that there is a common underlying cognitive skill that explains children's ability to succeed on perspective-taking tasks that require appreciation of differences in knowledge. In particular, it has been suggested that the ability to deal simultaneously with contradictory information may play a role in success on these tasks ("What I know is different from what he knows").

The ability to consider the thoughts, feelings, and wishes of others, even when they differ from one's own, is a prerequisite for harmonious social interaction. In adult–child encounters, adults often take the lead in explaining or elaborating why one course of action is preferred over another, as well as noting the consequences of different behaviors (e.g., Dunn et al., 1987; Kuczynski et al., 1987; Zahn-Waxler, Radke-Yarrow, & King, 1979). In peer interactions, the more skilled children who can manage these challenges on their own are more likely to have an easier time cooperating during play, especially sociodramatic peer play that involves role taking, role assignments, turn taking, and other skills that depend on the ability to coordinate activities with another and anticipate the other's behavior. The complex set of cognitive and social-cognitive skills that are called perspective taking or theory of mind, then, are important for social relations and appear to depend to some degree on earlier socialization experiences. They also emerge in conjunction with rapid advances in language and memory development during early childhood.

SUMMARY

In this chapter, some of the major advances in cognitive and social development that occur during toddlerhood and the preschool years have been described. It should be evident from this discussion that exploration and pretend play, self-regulation and self-awareness, and memory and language development are all intricately intertwined, with advances in one domain partly tied to advances in another. Thus, for example, the ability to engage in pretend play implies some degree of stable self-image that permits the child to switch roles; the ability to engage in a mutually regulated interaction with another also rests on self-regulatory ability, memory, and language, as well as a common core of organized knowledge about the social world. Moreover, it appears that participation in pretend-play sequences with other children also serves to enhance self-awareness, social knowledge, perspective taking, and self-control. It also seems clear that the preschooler, although limited to some degree by experience and cognitive structures, is much more sophisticated about the world than earlier theorists believed (e.g., see Bjorklund, 2000, and Flavell's, 1963, discussion of Piaget) . In particular, observations of children's spontaneous behavior in a range of social and problem-solving situations indicates that preschoolers are much less egocentric than was suggested even 20 years ago. Finally, individual differences in these various developmental achievements appear to depend, in part, on biological predispositions but also on environmental factors, particularly parental tolerance, sensitivity, and the provision of appropriate stimulation, scaffolding, and opportunities to learn about the world.

When children's development in one or more of these domains does not proceed smoothly, this may reflect a transient problem or reaction to a difficult developmental hurdle. However, a potentially benign or transient problem may have wider ramifications for a child's functioning. For example, a child who is having difficulty grappling with issues of separation and autonomy may also develop problems in self-regulation and in the peer group, but such problems may be more likely if parents deal with early conflicts over separation in an angry and authoritarian manner (Calkins, 1994). When parents are sensitive to developmental stresses, they can often help young children overcome potential difficulties and move on to the next developmental task. Unfortunately, not all parents are equally skilled at anticipating their children's developmental needs or appropriately interpreting irritable, explosive, or withdrawn behavior. Conversely, not all children respond equally well to parental attempts at protecting them from frustration. Although many children progress despite less than optimal support from parents, others have a difficult time coping with the frustrations of development in the absence of, or in spite of, help and guidance from significant adults. In some children, then, potential problems with autonomy, self-control, or mastery may be exacerbated by parental insensitivity, ignorance, or rejection, leading to increasingly more severe problems or problems that surface each time the child confronts a new developmental challenge. Other children may have difficulty at some developmental transition points, even with adequate to excellent parenting. However, the way that families manage the developmental tasks of toddlerhood and the preschool years may have longer term implications for their children's development in middle childhood and beyond.

CHAPTER 3

Clinical Issues

ANNOYING BEHAVIOR OR A PROBLEM?

Jenny is riding a tricycle around the preschool classroom when Jerry arrives. Jerry wants it! He watches Jenny for a few seconds as she rides around the room, then dashes over to her and tries to push her off the bike. The teacher intervenes.

Alan's mother just had a new baby, and Alan has been particularly moody and unpredictable. One minute he is clingy and tearful, the next he is wild and defiant, throwing toys and disobeying.

Sarah is a leader in the classroom and is always the one to be the "mother" in the playhouse at nursery school. When Sandra wants to take turns, Sarah protests and refuses to play with Sandra, roughly pushing her out of the way. Sandra goes off tearfully to tell the teacher.

Jeffrey has been in preschool for a week and has refused to talk to or play with the other children. In fact, the teacher has never heard him say a word to anyone but his mother. He has consistently ignored the overtures of other children and spends his time either hovering at the edge of a group of children, watching their play, or off by himself in a corner playing with trucks. When the teacher attempts to engage Jeffrey in group activities, he withdraws even more.

Jill and her mother are in the supermarket, and Jill is reluctant to stay in the shopping cart. It's no fun going shopping if you can't run around and touch things! When her mother insists that she sit in the shopping cart, Jill begins to throw groceries from the basket all over the floor of the meat department while crying and screaming. Her mother is mortified as people walk by and stare disapprovingly.

These are all familiar scenes to anyone who has had contact with young children. Most people would not consider these toy struggles, temper tantrums, or signs of sibling jealousy to be anything but typical behaviors. Indeed, studies suggest that these and a range of other behaviors that are troubling or annoying to adults are very common in the general population of preschoolers. But when do temper tantrums or fights between peers become problems worthy of concern? Is Jeffrey's social isolation just an indication of excessive shyness in a new and overwhelming situation, something he will soon overcome if left to adapt slowly? Or is it a sign of a potentially more serious difficulty in relating to others? If Jill was having frequent tantrums and was finally referred to a psychologist, would the behavior then become a symptom of a psychological disturbance? When an annoying behavior becomes something a parent cannot handle, does that make it a symptom of a child's behavior disorder or of a parent's problems setting limits? How does one distinguish among *annoying behavior, age-specific problems*, and *symptoms of disorder*? In an attempt to provide some conceptual clarity, the terms *worrisome* and *annoying behavior* are used throughout this chapter to refer to typical and age-appropriate behavior that may concern some parents; *age-specific problem* and *problem behavior* are used to indicate an exaggeration in the frequency and/or intensity of typical behavior to an upsetting degree, something which may or may not be a sign of a more serious difficulty to come; and *symptom* or *symptomatic behavior* are utilized to designate a problem of probable clinical significance.

These three degrees of troublesome behavior overlap considerably, and it is difficult, if not impossible, to clearly differentiate them. Furthermore, different observers may interpret a particular behavior differently, giving the same behavior a different meaning or developmental significance. For example, toy struggles in preschool are seen by some psychologists as an important developmental step in learning the rules of social exchange and sharing. Parents, on the other hand, may become upset by frequent squabbles over toys between peers or siblings and worry that their child is not learning to share. Toy struggles, in and of themselves, therefore, might be considered either annoying but healthy behaviors or age-specific problems, depending on the point of view of the observer. However, when they occur in the context of frequent aggressive encounters with other children, disobedience, and temper tantrums, toy struggles might be seen as a symptom of a more serious problem warranting treatment. Similarly, tantrums may be the hallmark of a two-year-old's struggle to assert herself and establish some degree of independence and autonomy. Or, in the context of a variety of other problem behaviors indicative of more widespread aggression, noncompliance, and anxiety, the tantrums may be seen as symptomatic behavior. As a first step in attempting to differentiate between age-related behaviors and behavior problems in young children, a number of studies have assessed the frequency of behaviors considered annoying or problematic by adults; some of these studies have also looked at age changes and sex differences in target behaviors in an effort to clarify systematic variations in irritating or upsetting behaviors.

HOW COMMON ARE PROBLEM BEHAVIORS?

Epidemiological studies and large-scale surveys have been conducted to examine frequencies of occurrence of specific potentially problematic behaviors in representative samples of children. Thus researchers have asked parents and preschool teachers to rate large numbers of annoying and/or worrisome behaviors typically shown by children. These studies have found that most of the behaviors of interest, that is those that might be considered symptomatic of disorder in some contexts (e.g., not listening, being overactive, fighting with other children, worrying, or being shy), are very common. Thus many if not most children will exhibit these behaviors some of the time, in specific situations or at a particular period of development, although only a few children will show these behaviors at high intensities and/or frequencies. Other symptomatic behaviors are quite rare, exhibited by very few children, even at low frequencies (e.g., stealing, bizarre mannerisms), and, when they are observed, they are more obviously indicative of a problem.

Most studies of this type have been conducted on children of preschool age or older, although a few have included younger children. It is not surprising that the nature of parental concerns about young children parallels expected developmental changes. Jenkins, Bax, and Hart (1980) examined parental concerns in a representative sample of parents of children ranging in age from 6 weeks to 4½ years. In infancy, concerns were relatively rare, with worries about sleeping, feeding, and crying predominant. Between ages 1 and 2, the total number of parental concerns began to increase somewhat, with feeding and sleeping difficulties still the major focus. Difficulties with bowel and bladder control emerged as parental worries at age 2. The number and intensity of parental concerns peaked at age 3, when the major complaints revolved around difficulties with management and discipline.

Other studies have likewise found that parents of young children frequently report concerns about toileting, eating habits, and sleeping problems. Relatively high proportions of parents of 3-year-olds also complain of more general problems with noncompliance, limited self-control, and poor relations with siblings and peers (Earls, 1980; Koot, 1993; Richman, Stevenson, & Graham, 1982). For example, in an epidemiological study of 705 3-year-old children in London, Richman et al. (1982) reported that 12.9% were described by their mothers as overactive and restless, 10.7% were seen as difficult to control, and 9.2% were seen as attention seeking. In a large-scale screening study of daycare attendees in rural Vermont, Crowther, Bond, and Rolf (1981) reported even higher rates of overactivity, low frustration tolerance, frequent fights with peers, and inattention in 3-year-old boys. Koot (1993) studied a representative community sample of 469 2- and 3-year-olds in Holland. Roughly 25% of parents rated their toddlers as often defiant, demanding, unable to wait, and unable to sit still. It seems unlikely that such a large proportion of young children is showing clinically significant symptoms. Rather, these studies suggest that many of the behaviors that may indicate problems are also extremely common in the general population.

Both cross-sectional and longitudinal studies also reveal that the nature of children's problem behaviors changes with age. Thus, as noted previously, management difficulties appear to peak at age 3 and to become less troublesome thereafter. According to both maternal and teacher reports, other specific behaviors, including fears and worries, tantrums, overactivity, attentional problems, and fighting with peers, seem to decrease in both frequency and severity over the preschool years in non-clinical samples (Coleman, Wolkind, & Ashley, 1977; Crowther et al., 1981; MacFarlane, Allen, & Honzik, 1954). Thus these findings from large-scale studies indicate that some problem behaviors show age-related decreases; these findings have been interpreted to suggest that problems in preschoolers generally are likely to be outgrown and often reflect age-appropriate manifestations of difficult behavior.

Sex differences in the frequency and intensity of problem behaviors have also been examined. In general, boys are more likely than girls to be described as aggressive, overactive, inattentive, and disobedient, although findings are inconsistent about the age at which sex differences first appear. Several studies of preschoolers have found only trivial sex differences in parent reports of specific problem behaviors (Campbell & Breaux, 1983; Earls, 1980; Koot, 1993; Richman et al., 1982; Shaw et al., 1998). Crowther et al. (1981), on the other hand, reported that sex differences were apparent by age 3 on a large number of potentially symptomatic behaviors. Teachers rated boys in day care as showing more destructive behavior, disruptive behavior, noncompliance, and peer problems, and lower frustration tolerance than girls. Although sex differences in young children's behavior require further research, Crowther et al.'s (1981) findings are consistent with a large number of studies of school-age children that indicate higher rates of aggressive and overactive behaviors in boys (Achenbach, 1991; Offord, Boyle, Fleming, Munroe-Blum, & Rae-Grant, 1989).

Taken together, these studies indicate that specific behaviors that are considered indicative of psychological disturbance in some contexts are very common in the general population, that certain behaviors show age-related increases or decreases, and that sex differences are sometimes found in the frequency and severity of annoying or worrisome behavior.

DIMENSIONS OF BEHAVIOR
PROBLEMS IN YOUNG CHILDREN

The foregoing discussion should make it obvious that isolated behaviors rarely reflect significant disturbance. Thus researchers have looked for clusters of behaviors that may occur together and may define a typology of disorder. Across the age span from toddlerhood to adolescence, two major classes of problem behavior have been identified in children (Achenbach, 1991, 1992): those characterized by undercontrol and those characterized by overcontrol. Behaviors characterized by *undercontrol* are typically high in annoyance value and/or the potential to hurt others. These behaviors have been termed *externalizing* because they are expressed outward against others or have an impact on the child's environment. Examples include overactivity, tantrums, fighting, destructive behavior, and disobedience. Behaviors reflecting *overcontrol* also tend to cluster together. They have been termed *internalizing* because they are reflected in social withdrawal, fearfulness, unhappiness, and anxiety and represent self-focused expressions of distress. Unfortunately, internalizing behaviors are often ignored or not recognized by adults in the child's environment because they are usually less dramatic and less irritating to others than externalizing symptoms are.

Hundreds of studies have confirmed these general clusters of behavioral symptoms, although specific behavioral manifestations may vary as a function of age and developmental level. It is not clear whether these rather global typologies of internalizing and externalizing symptomatology are sufficiently precise in their characterization of young children's problems to facilitate decisions about treatment or predictions about prognosis or whether specific subtypes of internalizing and externalizing disorders must be the focus of clinical decision making. It is likely that problems appear more global in early childhood and become more specific and differentiated with development.

A RELATIVE DEFINITION OF PROBLEM BEHAVIOR

The studies that examine the prevalence of specific behaviors do not allow us to define normality or abnormality objectively, but they do place problem behaviors in an appropriate developmental context. Knowing that 3-year-old Jamie is very aggressive in preschool and that aggression in preschool is common among 3-year-old boys may lead us to conclude that Jamie's behavior is merely typical and need not be a cause for parental concern beyond attempts to handle it in the present situation. However, such an evaluation will depend on factors in Jamie's family and peer group, on Jamie's overall pattern of behavior and its intensity in a variety of situations, and on changes in his behavior over time. Isolated behaviors are usually less of a cause for concern than those that occur together with other maladaptive behaviors or within a troubled family milieu. Similarly, even if we know that separation distress is quite rare by age 4, its presence does not permit us to conclude that a serious problem exists with long-term consequences for the child's development until other associated factors have also been examined. The presence of a disorder or an incipient disorder cannot be determined on the basis of one or two annoying or upsetting behaviors. The emphasis must be on the pattern of behavioral disturbance rather than on specific symptoms. That is, the frequency, intensity, and constellation of symptomatic behavior is relevant to a determination of whether a clinically significant problem exists, as is the wider family and social context of the behavior.

Assessment of problem behavior is further complicated by differences in perceptions and interpretations of children's behavior, as well as the variability in the behaviors children display in different settings and with different people. Thus a child's toy struggles with peers, temper tantrums, or separation distress may worry one parent and be dismissed as typical behavior by another. In many families, fathers and mothers appear to perceive their children's behavior differently, as evidenced by the only modest agreement between parents on rating scales describing children's behavior (e.g., Achenbach, McConaughy, & Howell, 1987; Koot, Van Den Oord, Verhulst, & Boomsma, 1997). In addition, children behave differently with different adults and in various settings. Thus, for example, data on a community sample participating in the NICHD Study of Early Child Care (NICHD Early Child Care Research Network, 1998) indicated very low agreement between mothers and caregivers asked to rate children on the Child Behavior Checklist/2–3 at 24 and 36 months. This may reflect both different perceptions of what constitutes problem behavior and the fact that children behave differently in different settings. For instance, one child may be cooperative with new people or in preschool but noncompliant at home, whereas another is sociable at home but shy and withdrawn in preschool. Thus it is necessary to assess a child's behavior from multiple perspectives, that is, within a developmental framework and from the vantage point of several significant adults in the child's environment. A relatively comprehensive assessment is needed if an accurate picture of the child's functioning is to emerge.

As already noted, the developmental supports available to the child from within the family must also be considered in an evaluation of problem behavior. Are parental expectations unrealistic, thereby exacerbating conflict during a difficult developmental transition? For example, are parents too rigid and demanding in setting limits at a time when the toddler is attempting to establish independence and autonomy, thereby creating a "battle of wills" that leads to frequent temper tantrums and bouts of noncompliance? Conversely, are parents reluctant to set limits for fear of thwarting their child's sense of self at a time when firm, consistent, but flexible guidelines are more congruent with the child's developmental needs? Are parents who are overwhelmed with their own problems unable to provide a stable, nurturing, and structured environment that fosters exploration and the development of self-awareness and self-control? Or is the child's behavior being misinterpreted as a problem by parents who lack an understanding of normal development? This is not to imply that parental management practices are always inappropriate. It is obvious that some extremely skilled and patient parents have children who at one time or another are extremely difficult to control. However, parental attitudes and management practices are a central aspect of the assessment process.

In summary, particular behaviors may be typical or may be indicators of a potential problem. Assessment must focus on the child in a developmental and family context. It ultimately involves a decision as to whether the behaviors in question are age appropriate, typical, and likely to be outgrown or the sign of a "clinically significant" problem. If the clinician judges the problem to be clinically significant, does it correspond to the usual patterns of aggressive or withdrawn behavior observed in young children? What meaningful clinical decisions can be made about treatment? Of course, before an assessment can be conducted, someone in the child's immediate environment, usually a parent or preschool teacher, must be sufficiently concerned about the behaviors in question to make a referral to a mental health professional.

FACTORS INFLUENCING REFERRAL

Many children with problems, especially young children who are not attending day care or preschool, probably do not reach mental health practitioners. Conversely, anyone who has worked with young children and their families has seen children with age-appropriate difficulties who were brought in for help because of parental concern. Factors influencing referral patterns are complex and have not been investigated extensively. Thus most of what follows is a distillation of clinical experience and is not based on empirical findings. However, it seems obvious that some combination of family, child, social, and cultural factors must converge to lead to referral in some cases and to work against referral in others.

At the first level, child behavior is obviously relevant. Children whose behavior is annoying to others are more likely to be referred than children whose behavior, even though equally disturbed, is quieter and less overt. Thus children who are aggressive, disobedient, and overactive are more likely to be seen as a problem by parents or child-care workers than are quiet, withdrawn, and fearful children. Furthermore, it is likely that parents will seek help more readily if their child's exasperating behavior is apparent outside the home as well. Thus the child who throws temper tantrums at home but is well behaved and cooperative around other adults will be less likely to be referred for help. But once a parent's concern is corroborated by the preschool teacher or the pediatrician—that is, when the behavior is both sufficiently annoying to others and evident across situations (e.g., home and preschool/child care)—help seeking is more likely. Further, when the behavior problems are accompanied by cognitive and/or language delays, parents may be more motivated to seek help in order to understand the severity of the cognitive problem and to obtain remedial intervention. Clinically, it appears that cognitive and learning problems may be less threatening than behavioral ones or may be viewed by parents as more likely to require treatment.

Parents' previous experience with children, their implicit theories about the nature of development, their levels of tolerance for children's behavior, their developmental expectations, and their own definitions of "normality" will also influence their assessment of the need to seek help. Thus, for example, the parent who believes that early signs of disturbance are possible indicators of more serious, long-term problems (a continuity view) may be more likely to seek help than a parent who sees problematic behavior in preschoolers as merely a difficult phase of development (a discontinuity view). Similarly, parents with more limited tolerance for rambunctious and exuberant behavior may be more likely to seek a referral than parents who are more child centered and tolerant of high levels of noise and activity.

In my own work, I have been struck particularly with the wide variation in parents' knowledge of normal development and expectations for their children's behavior. Tolerance levels, developmental expectations, and experience with children appear to interact in complex ways. Parents with unrealistic expectations and low tolerance may make excessive maturity demands on their preschooler that may tax their child's competence or self-control, and they may seek help to "make their child behave." For example, parents with limited exposure to young children may be more likely to interpret sibling or peer squabbles as "meanness" and may have unrealistic expectations for sharing and harmony between young children. We have found sibling and peer diffi-culties to be a major concern of parents of young children. On the other hand, parents who are both tolerant and aware of developmental issues concerning sibling or peer conflicts may be overly lax about setting lim-its and allow toy struggles or other typical child conflicts to escalate to more serious fights, thereby providing inadequate guidelines for more appropriate conflict resolution. Parents with limited knowledge of de-velopment also may become unduly upset by the finicky and faddish eating habits that often characterize preschoolers, or they may worry that problems with toilet training will develop into rebellion and other more serious problems. Forcing these issues in an insensitive and heavy-handed manner can turn eating or toileting into a battleground and lead to serious parent–child conflict that may ultimately lead par-ents to seek help. Whereas a discontinuity view and moderate levels of tolerance are probably adaptive for most children and parents, it is also important that parents not overlook or rationalize away a potentially serious problem.

Parental perceptions of child behavior as either typical or poten-tially problematic will likewise be influenced by a range of other factors, including their own history of childrearing, their family history of psy-chopathology, and their own experience with the mental health system and their attitudes toward it. For example, families with a severely dis-turbed adult member, such as an aunt or grandparent, may be more likely to seek help early on, even for relatively minor problems, as a pre-ventive effort. Other families in which a close relative has a history of hyperactivity or learning problems may be more likely to dismiss the need for help with the comment that "Joey is just like Uncle George was." As Uncle George is now a successful businessman, they assume that Joey too will outgrow his early childhood problems. On the other hand, if Uncle George's early problems developed into more serious aca-demic and interpersonal ones in adolescence, they may want to prevent the occurrence of problems like those they observed in their own family of origin while growing up. Similarly, parents' willingness to seek help will be influenced by their own experiences with problems and the helpfulness or lack thereof of their contacts with the mental health sys-tem.

Additional family factors that would be expected to influence refer-ral patterns include marital status and the quality of the marital relationship, educational and occupational status, and emotional and material resources. In a large-scale study of service utilization in the Netherlands, Verhulst and van der Ende (1997) found that most families who identified problems in their children did not seek treatment. The factors that influenced help seeking included stressful family events and the severity of child problems. Although families with a history of mental health problems were more likely than other families to see problems in their children, they were not more likely to utilize mental health services. This study, however, focused on children from age 4 to adolescence, so it is difficult to draw conclusions specifically about service utilization by families of young children. Pavuluri, Luk, and McGee (1996) studied service utilization patterns specifically in preschool children screened in New Zealand. Consistent with expectation, most parents who saw their children as having problems did not seek help, primarily because they believed that the problems would be outgrown or that they should be able to handle the problems themselves. In general, low-income, single-parent families experiencing high levels of psychosocial adversity were the least likely to seek treatment.

Similar results were reported by Lavigne and colleagues (1998a), who studied service utilization in families seeking pediatric services for their 2- to 5-year-old children. Children identified as problematic through screening assessments were more likely to have been seen by a mental health professional if their problems were more serious, if they were not members of minority groups, if problems were accompanied by family conflict, or if they were referred by their pediatricians. It is also worth noting that about one-fourth of the families seeking mental health services had not screened positive for a problem; conversely, consistent with other studies, about three-fourths of the families with a child who screened positive did not seek mental health services. These data underscore the complexities in predicting service utilization in families with young children.

From a clinical perspective, family systems issues may influence help seeking, as suggested by the Lavigne et al. (1998a) data on family conflict. For example, it is not uncommon for parents to seek help with childrearing concerns as a ticket into marital or family therapy, although neither partner is willing or able to acknowledge marital problems. On the other hand, some disturbed parents with disturbed children may postpone referral because they need to feel supported before they are able to confront and deal with their child's difficulties. Still other families may avoid seeking help because they are afraid that their child's difficulties will reveal their own problems or because there is marked disagreement between the parents on the need for help. Thus a complex range of factors influences help seeking in parents of preschool children, and these are further compounded by issues of access to services in the United States.

Access to mental health services varies widely across countries and socioeconomic groups. It is noteworthy that both New Zealand (in the Pavuluri et al. study) and the Netherlands (in the Verhulst & van der Ende study) provide universal health care that includes mental health services; access and cost should not be major barriers to treatment and, therefore, cannot explain the low rate of service utilization reported. In contrast, in the United States, there are serious problems of access to mental health services for young children that have been exacerbated by the advent of managed care (American Academy of Pediatrics, 2000; Jellinek, 1999). Therefore, some families who may wish to seek help for their young children may be overwhelmed by the difficulties they face finding appropriate services or negotiating the bureaucracy, or they may be concerned about whether they will be able to afford services once they find them. Many health insurance policies do not provide adequate coverage for mental health services, and this is especially so for child mental health.

Once a referral is made, it is the task of the mental health professional to determine the severity of the problem—whether it is indeed serious enough to warrant intervention, or whether it reflects an age-appropriate struggle with a developmental transition that requires primarily parental understanding and support. If treatment does appear indicated, it will be necessary to decide whether the parents, the child, or the family should be the focus of intervention and what type of intervention appears most relevant (e.g., parent education, family therapy, etc.). These issues are addressed more fully in Chapter 7.

ATTEMPTS TO DEFINE
CLINICALLY SIGNIFICANT PROBLEMS

Clinicians agree that a definition of disorder in young children must include a pattern of symptoms that has been troublesome for some time, that is evident in more than one situation, that is relatively severe, and that is likely to impede the child's ability to negotiate the important developmental tasks necessary for adaptive functioning in the family and the peer group. Thus it is not the presence of specific problem behaviors that differentiates "normal" from "abnormal," but their *frequency, intensity, chronicity, constellation*, and *social context*. In one of the examples discussed earlier, toy struggles would not be interpreted as problematic if they occurred once in a while, were of short duration, or were apparent in a preschool-age child who had few other problems. On the other hand, toy struggles might be considered more worrisome if they occurred frequently, were intense, escalated into more serious fights, and were initiated by a child who was in other ways very difficult to control and seemed to be showing a general pattern of aggression, noncompliance, and poor regulation of negative affect. Richman et al. (1982) used a combined statistical and clinical approach in an attempt to identify children with clinically significant problems. They noted that roughly 15% of their sample was assessed as showing mild problems and another 7% as showing moderate to severe problems. Children identified as evidencing moderate to severe problems were described as exhibiting a range of symptoms of relatively marked intensity that appeared to be interfering with their developmental progress and were having a negative influence on family functioning.

These data are quite consistent with more recent epidemiological studies of diagnosed disorder in preschool children (e.g., Lavigne et al., 1996), which are discussed in more detail later in this chapter, as well as with studies examining elevated scores on checklist measures such as the Child Behavior Checklist (CBCL). For example, Koot (1993) reported that about 11% of the Dutch toddlers in his community sample were rated above the clinical cutoff on the Externalizing Problems scale of the CBCL/2–3. Lavigne et al. (1996) reported that 8.3% of a sample of preschoolers attending primary pediatric care facilities received scores above the clinical cutoff (90th percentile) on the Total Problems scale of the CBCL. Gender differences were apparent, and problems were lowest at age 2 (4.7%) and highest at age 4 (13.2%). These rates, however, are higher than those obtained in the NICHD Study of Early Child Care (NICHD Early Child Care Research Network, 1998). Moreover, in the NICHD study, when agreement between both mothers and caregivers was considered, very few children actually were seen as showing serious problems at either 24 or 36 months; only between 0.5% and 1% of children were rated above the clinical cutoffs by *both* informants on the Externalizing, Internalizing, or Total Problems scales.

Stable problems were evident in only about 3% of children, according to maternal reports obtained at ages 24 and 36 months. These data indicate that sample composition, measurement instrument, age of child, and a range of other factors influence prevalence figures. Indeed, it is likely that problems become more easily identifiable and more stable after age 3 or 4.

Even if there is moderate to good agreement among clinicians about the presence or absence of a recognizable disorder in young children (Lavigne et al., 1996), accurate prognostic predictions are quite difficult to make. The teacher, the parent, and the psychologist may all agree that Jamie's behavior is disrupting the family and impairing his ability to venture into the peer group. But does that mean that in 6 months or a year he will still be having problems? There are few guidelines to assist the professional in making such judgments in the individual case. However, contrary to the popular belief that most early problems will be outgrown, there is growing evidence that although many children do overcome early problems, a significant proportion of problem preschoolers will continue to have serious adjustment difficulties at school entry and beyond (Campbell et al., 1996; Lavigne et al., 1998a, 1998b; Pierce, Ewing, & Campbell, 1999). As noted earlier, studies that examine the persistence of troublesome or annoying behavior in nonclinical samples of young children suggest that the behaviors most often disappear with development. On the other hand, longitudinal studies of young children identified as having a constellation of problems that are impairing functioning suggest that some problems do persist (e.g., Campbell et al., 1996; Lavigne et al., 1998a, 1998b; Shaw, Owens, Vondra, Keenan, & Winslow, 1996). These studies are discussed in more detail in Chapter 8. In general, however, the evidence indicates that externalizing problems are more likely than internalizing ones to persist, particularly in boys, and that family factors appear to mediate outcome (Campbell, 1995; Campbell et al., 2000). Moreover, age at first diagnosis appears related to persistence, with children who show more clearly identifiable problems at ages 4 and 5 being more likely to show persistent problems than younger children, who might well be going through a developmental phase (Lavigne et al., 1998a). In addition, sleep disturbances, especially when they are prolonged, are often associated with behavior problems in young children (Lavigne et al., 1999; Richman et al., 1982), even with indicators of family stress controlled (Bates, Viken, Alexander, Beyers, & Stockton, 2002).

DIAGNOSTIC ISSUES

The categorization of problems in young children is particularly problematic. Although behaviors rated on checklists may cluster in relatively similar ways across the age range, the usefulness of this dimensional approach to the identification of problems in young children requires more research before we can be sure of its accuracy and predictive validity. Similarly, alternative categorical approaches to diagnosis, such as DSM-IV (American Psychiatric Association [APA], 1994), are only beginning to be examined systematically with young children (e.g., Keenan, Shaw, Walsh, Delliquadri, & Giovannelli, 1997; Lavigne et al., 1996). Moreover, if both descriptive approaches are identifying children with serious problems, they should show moderate to high convergence. It is not yet clear, however, that this is the case. Keenan et al. (1997), for example, observed similar rates of disorder when both dimensional and categorical approaches were used to classify young children, but the approaches identified different children. This raises questions about the relative predictive validity of these two diagnostic systems. Moreover, if one is to utilize the DSM approach, are the categories designed for use with school-age children and adolescents applicable to preschoolers? And finally, which approach to the description and classification of young children's problems is more clinically useful and less stigmatizing? The issue of stigmatization is often overlooked; the interested reader is referred to Hinshaw and Cicchetti (2000) for an important and poignant discussion of this complex topic.

DIAGNOSTIC CLASSIFICATION USING THE DSM AND RELATED SYSTEMS

Because the mental health professions have adopted the DSM-IV diagnostic system (APA, 1994) and are required to utilize this system for reimbursement by insurance companies, this approach to diagnosis is discussed with a focus on the disorders that appear most relevant to this age group (e.g., oppositional defiant disorder, separation anxiety disorder) but that do not reflect extreme impairment and/or developmental delay (e.g., autism, pervasive developmental disorder) or grossly inadequate care (e.g., reactive attachment disorder). These more serious disorders are beyond the scope of this book, either because they reflect a more obvious biological etiology, as in autism (e.g., Rutter, 2000), or because they appear to result from gross and prolonged deprivation and serious deficits in parenting that are outside the normal range of experience, as in reactive attachment disorder (APA, 1994).

The changing diagnostic system over the past 20 years, from DSM-III (APA, 1980) to DSM-III-R (APA, 1987) to DSM-IV (APA, 1994), means that research has necessarily lagged behind the appearance of modified criteria. When the first edition of this book was published, however, few published studies existed that used categorical diagnoses with young children. Today, there is a small body of work utilizing these structured diagnostic systems (especially DSM-III-R) with preschool children and, to some degree, supporting their reliability and concurrent and predictive validity (e.g., Keenan et al., 1997; Lavigne et al., 1996, 1998a).

At the same time, however, both DSM-III-R and the revised DSM-IV continue to have limitations when applied to preschool children. Although the authors of DSM-IV wisely suggest that diagnoses of certain childhood disorders, such as conduct disorder, will generally not apply meaningfully to very young children, other disorders are described more ambiguously. However, the use of diagnostic criteria is based on largely unvalidated inclusion and exclusion criteria, especially when used with very young children. Further, the use of a diagnostic label implies "a dysfunction in the individual" (APA, 1994, page xxii), meaning that the disorder resides "in the child." This appears to "overmedicalize" and overpathologize less severe (i.e., nonpsychotic or nonautistic) problem behaviors in toddlers and preschoolers. There is particular concern about the overdiagnosis of disorders such as oppositional defiant disorder and attention-deficit/hyperactivity disorder. This is partly because DSM-III-R and its successor, DSM-IV, do not provide adequate guidelines for determining the developmental and clinical significance of the specific symptomatic behaviors that define these disorders, raising questions about their appropriateness for use with preschoolers.

In an effort to deal with this problem, the American Academy of Pediatrics (AAP, 1996) has published a companion to DSM-IV, called the DSM-PC, for pediatricians and others working in primary care that is meant to provide clearer developmental guidelines and to delineate distinctions among developmental variations in behaviors, problems that may be clearly evident but do not reach the level of a disorder, and more serious problems that warrant a diagnosis (AAP, 1996). In addition, this manual provides a discussion of children in family and neighborhood context, making it clear that children's disorders do not emerge de novo, isolated from the childrearing environment and community supports. These distinctions and clarifications, along with the detailed descriptions of clinical presentation as a function of age, are an important addition to the guidelines available to clinicians working with young children. In addition, the National Center for Clinical Infant Programs (NCCIP, 1994) has published Zero to Three, a diagnostic system for infants and toddlers. This diagnostic system includes downward extensions of some DSM-IV diagnoses, as well as a new set of diagnoses. It also includes a discussion of family issues in all their complexity, especially the realization that most problems in young children reflect disturbances in relationships with primary caregivers. Thus all diagnoses are accompanied by a characterization of relationship disturbance (e.g., overinvolved, underinvolved, angry, abusive). This is an important addition to the classification of emotional and behavioral problems in young children. Despite this strength, however, this system has its own set of problems, primarily a failure to integrate these issues into the diagnoses themselves and a lack of adequate empirical support for many of the categories. The following discussion, as already noted, attends only to the DSM-IV categories that may apply to preschool children. These are discussed from the DSM-IV perspective, with additions from the DSM-PC and the Zero to Three systems where applicable.

DSM-IV Externalizing (Disruptive Behavior) Disorders

Oppositional Defiant Disorder

Only two externalizing disorders, called disruptive behavior disorders in DSM-IV, are generally considered appropriate diagnoses for children of preschool age: oppositional defiant disorder (ODD) and attention-deficit/hyperactivity disorder (ADHD). The criteria for ODD include the presence of four out of eight symptoms of uncooperative behavior and negative affect (loses temper, argues, defies or refuses to comply, deliberately annoys others, often blames others, touchy, angry, spiteful) that continue for at least 6 months and interfere with social and cognitive functioning. Moreover, to be a symptom a behavior must "occur more frequently than is typically observed" in children of "comparable age and developmental level." Although the developmental guidelines for this diagnosis are vague, the requirements of four instead of two symptoms (as in DSM-III) and the duration and impairment criteria make the diagnosis more exclusive and mean that it is less likely to be applied to children who are going through a short-lived developmental transition. As noted in the DSM-IV manual (APA, 1994), "Because transient oppositional behavior is very common in preschool children . . . caution should be exercised" (p. 92) in making this diagnosis in young children. Still, it is easy to imagine that parents might construe some of the typical behaviors of toddlerhood, especially in families with more than one child, as meeting symptomatic criteria (annoying others, spiteful). Thus it seems necessary for the clinician to rule out, for example, typical sibling squabbles in evaluating the clinical significance of particular symptoms in young children. Given the overlap between the typical behaviors of toddlerhood and the symptoms of oppositional defiant disorder, it may be easy to overdiagnose age-appropriate, but difficult, behavior as a disorder, with all that this concept implies. The DSM-PC (AAP, 1996) provides some perspective on this issue by including discussion of a number of issues such as the birth of a sibling, family conflict, and other stressful life events, that may lead to adjustment reactions in young children, expressed as problematic behaviors that overlap considerably with the symptoms of ODD. At the same time, parents who are dealing with a very difficult developmental transition may well benefit from structured interventions geared to handling difficult children, regardless of whether they actually meet the DSM-IV criteria for a diagnosis of ODD.

Research is beginning to address questions about the applicability of this diagnosis to young children, although, unfortunately, published studies have used the DSM-III-R criteria. Most notably, Lavigne and colleagues (1996), in one of the few studies to have examined the prevalence of the DSM-III-R diagnoses in a nonclinical sample of preschool children, found that ODD was by far the most common diagnosis. In this sample of children attending primary care pediatric practices, 16.8% met criteria for at least a probable diagnosis of oppositional defiant disorder; of these, 8.1% were considered to be showing severe symptoms. More than twice as many boys as girls were considered to have ODD, with the rate peaking at age 3 and leveling off by age 5. The only other diagnosis that occurred with any frequency was ADHD, which was observed in only 2% of children and was also more common in boys. Almost all children who received an ADHD diagnosis also received another diagnosis, usually ODD. This is consistent with the view that ADHD and ODD may not be distinct clinical entities in very young children. In another study examining the frequency of DSM-III-R diagnoses in a relatively small sample of low-income children at age 5, Keenan et al. (1997) reported that 8% were diagnosed with ODD and 5.7% with ADHD. These two studies indicate that it is possible to diagnose these two disruptive disorders in preschool children reliably.

Moreover, follow-up data provided by Lavigne and colleagues (Lavigne et al., 1998a, 1998b) indicate that about 50% of the children with disruptive diagnoses at intake, initially seen between ages 2 and 5, were likely to continue to receive a diagnosis at subsequent follow-up assessments 1 to 3 years later. Children who were younger at the time of initial assessment were more likely to outgrow their problems, suggesting that this diagnosis becomes more valid by age 4 or 5, when real problems can be more easily differentiated from transient age-related difficulties with defiance, tantrums, and the regulation of negative affect. Recall that Lavigne et al. (1996) found the highest rates of ODD at age 3, a time at which children are often struggling with issues of autonomy and self-regulation and parents may feel frustrated as their child becomes less cooperative. This suggests that the elevated rate of ODD reported in this study at age 3 includes a large proportion of false positive cases, children who were indeed experiencing a difficult developmental transition.

Attention-Deficit/Hyperactivity Disorder

When people think about the likely problems of preschool children, they think most readily of ADHD. DSM-IV included major changes in the diagnostic criteria for this disorder, making it both more difficult and easier to receive a diagnosis. The criteria were made more stringent by the addition of the requirement that the symptoms interfere with functioning across settings (home and school or day care), thereby ruling out children who might be showing situation-specific anxiety or upset that may be misconstrued as ADHD. The 6-month duration criterion also serves to rule out children who seem impulsive and overactive because they are going through a brief adjustment reaction to stressful life events, such as entering day care or coping with the birth of a sibling. At the same time, the inclusion of subtypes means that children must meet criteria for only six symptoms (as opposed to eight in prior versions of the DSM). Thus children showing six symptoms of hyperactivity–impulsivity (HI) or six symptoms of inattention (IA) meet criteria for ADHD-HI or ADHD-IA subtype. Children with six symptoms in each domain meet criteria for ADHD–combined type. Although younger children tend not to meet criteria for the inattentive subtype (Lahey et al., 1998), presumably because this set of symptoms is not that apparent until children must meet the demands of school, young children may easily meet criteria for the HI subtype, which include fidgeting, difficulty staying seated, difficulty taking turns, difficulty playing quietly, and talking excessively. This has raised concerns about the overdiagnosis of this disorder in younger children (e.g, Carey, as cited in Marshall, 2000, p. 1281). However, it is noteworthy that in the Lavigne et al. (1996) study, ADHD was not diagnosed excessively (using DSM-III-R criteria, requiring eight symptoms, but not necessarily across settings), and it rarely occurred in the absence of ODD. It should also be noted that in the DSM-IV manual a caveat is provided: "It is especially difficult to establish this diagnosis in children younger than 4 or 5 years" (APA, 1994, p. 81). However, the potential to overdiagnose this disorder in young children is a cause for concern, as the criteria that would differentiate between age-appropriate levels of activity, shifts in attention, and impatience are nowhere defined. It is indeed difficult to make a clear diagnostic decision when confronted with a rambunctious, curious 3- or 4-year-old whose parents cannot cope with his behavior.

Preschoolers, who are learning about the world and how to master its complexities, are expected to exhibit boundless energy, to attend readily to the new and novel, and to exhibit unrestrained enthusiasm and exuberance. When, therefore, does a shift in activity and interest signify curiosity and exploration, and when does it reflect a too-rapid change in focus and an inadequate investment of attention? When does excitable and impatient behavior indicate an age-appropriate need for external support and limit setting, and when does it suggest a failure to internalize standards necessary for the development of self-control? When do frequent toy struggles reflect a child's age-appropriate need for experiences in the peer group that facilitate sharing and turn taking, and when do they indicate excessive impulsivity and an inability to wait? Although the DSM-IV specifies that "developmentally inappropriate" inattention, impulsivity, and overactivity are required for a diagnosis of ADHD, this is a difficult decision to make in the absence of normative data defining age-appropriate behavior. However, as noted in the DSM-PC (AAP, 1996), a diagnosis is most likely to occur when there are also signs of either cognitive deficits or oppositional behavior. The rambunctious toddler or preschooler with a sunny disposition is less likely to meet criteria for a diagnosis of ADHD than is the child who is noncompliant and angry, consistent with Lavigne et al.'s (1996) observation that few children in their preschool sample received a diagnosis of ADHD in the absence of a co-occurring ODD diagnosis.

In the Zero to Three diagnostic system (NCCIP, 1994), both oppositional and hyperactive-impulsive symptoms are captured under the overall rubric of "regulatory disorders," which emphasizes the difficulties some young children have controlling negative mood, activity level, and attention. Recall that these characteristics are seen as important components of infant temperament (Rothbart & Bates, 1998) as described in Chapter 1. The Zero to Three system attempts to consider problematic behaviors from a developmental perspective, and despite the focus on the importance of relationships, there is still a sense that the problem is within the child; although early problems may be ameliorated by sensitive parenting, the problems are still described primarily as emerging from biological and maturational processes. Undoubtedly, this is accurate to some degree, and especially so for some young children who would qualify for such a diagnosis. However, substantial evidence also exists that parenting plays a role in the emergence and persistence of oppositional behavior (e.g., Campbell et al., 2000; Shaw et al., 1996; Shaw, Bell, & Gilliom, 2000), as do replicated findings indicating the importance of child-by-parenting interactions (Bates & McFadyen-Ketchum, 2000; see also Chapter 1 on temperament-by-parenting interactions).

These data raise questions about how much we gain from the addition of a diagnosis of self-regulatory deficits to the characterization of the disruptive behavior disorders. Moreover, in the absence of research on the reliability and validity of these categories and their developmental significance, it is not clear what they add to attempts to describe and explain problems in young children. Are these transient problems that might just as appropriately be considered in terms of parent–child problems or adjustment reactions? Does the proliferation of categories add to the tendency to overpathologize normative or transitional behavior? How do these categories relate developmentally to the DSM-IV categories of ODD and ADHD? That is how many toddlers with a diagnosis of regulatory disorder, negative–defiant subtype or motorically disorganized–impulsive subtype would ultimately receive a diagnosis of ODD or ADHD at school age? These questions obviously await further research.

Conduct Disorders in Young Children?

Although there is an alarming increase in the discussion of conduct disorder in young children, both DSM-IV and the DSM-PC indicate that this diagnosis rarely applies to children under 5 or 6. Although the rare 5- or 6-year-old may actually merit such a diagnosis, it is difficult to conceptualize the majority of symptoms of conduct disorder as applying to children younger than this. However, some attempts have been made to use this diagnosis with very aggressive and defiant preschoolers who seem more impaired than a diagnosis of ODD would suggest (Keenan & Wachschlag, 2000). The question becomes whether aggression, bullying, lying, and stealing are equivalent across developmental levels. Is hitting a child with a block the same as threatening with a knife or other weapon? As the focus of research shifts to early emerging aggressive behavior, given concerns about long-term consequences, these become serious questions with implications for prevention and treatment (Campbell et al., 2000). However, it is my view that except in very rare instances, this disorder, which entails intentional violation of the rights of others, cannot be diagnosed meaningfully in children younger than 5 or 6, and even then one can question the circumstances in which such a diagnosis is appropriate.

DSM-IV Internalizing (Emotional) Disorders

Much less is known about the internalizing disorders, reflecting anxiety, social withdrawal, fearfulness, and sad mood, in young children than about ODD and ADHD. The reason is partly that these behaviors must be more extreme than externalizing behaviors are for them to be noticed, and partly that they are often short-lived and transient. Thus, for example, many children show specific fears, such as fear of animals, the dark, or monsters (Campbell, 1986), and these are often age-related fears that do not impair functioning. Thus it is unlikely that most children with specific fears would meet diagnostic criteria for a specific phobia. Indeed, in the Lavigne et al. (1996) study, out of 510 children, only 2 met criteria for a simple phobia. In fact, Lavigne et al. (1996) comment on the very low rate of internalizing or emotional disorders in their sample. This finding is consistent with the caveats and developmental guidelines discussed in the DSM-PC, which notes that many of the symptoms of depression (e.g., sad mood, eating or sleeping problems) and anxiety disorders (worry, avoidance of social activities, shyness) are quite common and that they may also be relatively brief reactions to specific life events or changes.

Moreover, in DSM-IV, with the exception of separation anxiety disorder, the other internalizing disorders (social phobia, generalized anxiety disorder, depression) use criteria meant to cut across the age range from childhood to adulthood; there is almost no discussion of developmental differences in clinical presentation. Discussion is provided in the DSM-PC, but it is of interest that the behaviors that may indicate fear, anxiety, or depression in young children, such as crying, tantrums, clinging to an adult, or avoiding interactions with unfamiliar people, are behaviors that may be triggered by a range of situations. Therefore, in the absence of a prolonged period of symptomatic behavior that interferes with the child's ability to progress developmentally and to interact in the peer group, it is difficult to arrive at a specific diagnosis, except possibly the diagnosis of adjustment reaction or separation anxiety disorder (see the next section). The category of adjustment disorder (NCCIP, 1994) is really meant for subsyndromal reactions that are described as short-lived responses to clearly identifiable stressful events. The absence of an obvious diagnosis need not imply that parents will not benefit from some guidance about how to handle their child's distressed behavior; but the question of whether the behavior is serious enough to warrant a diagnosis merits some thought.

Separation Anxiety

Separation anxiety is the only anxiety disorder that is specific to childhood. It is described in DSM-IV (APA, 1994) as "developmentally inappropriate and excessive anxiety concerning separation from home" (p. 113) or from "major attachment figures." Among the eight symptoms defining this disorder are "recurrent excessive distress" in anticipation of separation, worry about losing the attachment figure, school refusal, and fear of being alone or of sleeping alone. Nightmares and physical symptoms may also be present. Only three symptoms of 4 weeks' duration are required for a diagnosis, although the disturbance needs to cause significant distress and/or impairment in functioning. Developmental guidelines are not provided. However, it is suggested that separation anxiety is most likely to develop after some life stress, such as the loss of a relative or pet, a major illness, or the move to a new neighborhood. In young children, then, who do not have the cognitive capacities to understand sudden and/or dramatic life change, it is not clear when we can reasonably talk about a "disorder," as opposed to an appropriate reaction to a stressful, confusing, and/or frightening event. Because young children may not be expected to cope easily with certain kinds of stressful events or to readjust quickly to major life change but instead may need the close support of an attachment figure to help them make the necessary transitions, the expression of anxiety through nightmares, physical symptoms, or separation protest may be adaptive rather than pathological. Thus, a 3-year-old who shows a major reaction to a loss or other major life change or upsetting event, expressed as clinginess, crying, and other signs of separation distress, may be behaving in very predictable ways that clearly do not warrant a diagnosis of a psychiatric disorder. On the other hand, in the absence of any identifiable event in the life of a young child who becomes virtually panic stricken at the prospect of separation, such a diagnosis may be warranted; at the least, this fearful and incapacitating behavior may be evidence that something serious is going on in the family. It also seems reasonable that this diagnosis is less apt in 2- and 3-year-olds than in older preschool children, although in the face of a catastrophic event, such as the loss of a parent or family separation, such a reaction may not be unsurprising even in somewhat older children, who may be concerned for example, with being abandoned by the remaining parent.

It is interesting and appropriate that the Zero to Three system does not even mention separation anxiety as a disorder in its own right, because in infants and toddlers this would be an inappropriate diagnosis. Instead, the symptoms of clinginess and upset are more likely to reflect serious problems in the family and the child–caregiver relationship, if not outright deprivation or neglect. Similar comments can be made about the inclusion of mood and anxiety diagnoses in Zero to Three. Prolonged sad mood, excessive fear of strangers, excessive separation distress, and other intense fears are unlikely to occur on their own in very young children in the absence of a major loss, traumatic event, or neglectful or abusive care or in the context of a more serious disorder such as autism or reactive attachment disorder.

Parent–Child Problem

In recognition of the fact that many problems in young children reflect problems in the parent–child relationship or in parents' approaches to childrearing, the DSM also includes "parent–child relational problem" as another "condition" that may warrant clinical attention and be the focus of treatment. Surprisingly, this condition merits only a brief paragraph in the DSM, and it is not discussed explicitly in the DSM-PC despite the fact that this is a very common presenting complaint in pediatric primary care. Indeed, in the Lavigne et al. (1996) study, parent–child problem was the second most common classification (4.6%) after oppositional disorder, and it was more than twice as common as ADHD. In addition, dramatic differences appeared as a function of age. In the sample of 2-year-olds, 9.2% presented with a parent–child problem as the terrible 2's emerged, but by age 4 only 2.8% were considered parent–child problems, and by age 5, only one parent–child dyad was so classified. Because many problems of early childhood revolve around the quality of the parent–child relationship and issues of limit setting and control, and because this is by far the most widely researched area of early childhood social development, this topic clearly deserves more attention in diagnostic manuals for clinicians working with young children.

Summary

Although several diagnostic and dimensional assessment systems are now in widespread use with toddlers and preschoolers, it is difficult to make a blanket statement about which system is preferable. The dimensional approach of Achenbach (1991) that relies on the assessment of particular symptom clusters via parent and teacher rating scales has the benefit of a large empirical and cross-cultural database. On the other hand, structured interviews and the use of DSM-IV categories, especially when guided by the DSM-PC, may provide a more integrated picture of problems. At this stage of our knowledge, both are useful, although neither has adequately grappled with the developmental appropriateness versus clinical significance of behavioral clusters in very young children. Moreover, although there is accumulating data on the reliability of these measures with young children, validity issues require further work, especially in view of the large numbers of false positives that are often identified in screening and diagnostic assessments (Bennett,

Lipman, Racine, & Offord, 1998). With this in mind, I now turn to my own research on hard-to-manage preschool children to illustrate some of the issues described in prior chapters.

OVERVIEW OF LONGITUDINAL RESEARCH ON PROBLEM PRESCHOOLERS

When the first edition of this book was written more than 10 years ago, there was almost no research on problem preschoolers. The pioneering work of Naomi Richman and colleagues (1982) was my primary source of information. Over the past decade, interest in the emergence and manifestations of behavior problems in young children has grown, and I hope that my work has contributed to the concern about identifying problems early. Indeed, the work of Lavigne et al. (1996, 1998a, 1998b), Shaw et al. (1996, 1998, 2000), and Speltz et al. (1999), to name but a few, attests to the burgeoning interest in "early starters," as well as in those with more transient adjustment reactions and difficulties with transitions.

In an effort to identify early behavioral markers for attention-deficit disorder and related externalizing behavior problems in young children and to understand more about the early developmental course of problem behavior, my students and I began a study focused on the early identification and follow-up of hard-to-manage preschool children in 1979. Two cohorts of children were followed longitudinally into middle childhood. We were initially quite concerned about the ethical implications of this work, because we worried about overpathologizing the difficult behavior of young children. For example, we were uncomfortable acknowledging that a particular child was a problem for fear of fueling a self-fulfilling cycle of negative parental perceptions, discipline problems, harsh childrearing practices, and escalating conflict. On the other hand, after years of clinical work with school-age children and their parents, we were convinced that some problems could be identified early and that parents could be given some support and guidance in dealing with hard-to-manage preschoolers who are capable of creating chaos in a family. We were also convinced that some hard-to-reach school-age youngsters developed problems partly as a result of insensitive and inappropriate childrearing, excessive stress in the family, and a generally unhealthy psychological environment that failed to support them through difficult periods of development. Clearly, child character-istics were also important. As we got to know the families in our stud-ies, the complexity and multiple determinants of these early-emerging problems became increasingly clear; their developmental course and outcomes also reflect complex transactions among a constellation of factors that are probably different for each child and family. This view now seems self-evident to students of developmental psychopathology and is generally accepted in the research (e.g., Cicchetti & Cohen, 1995; Cummings et al., 2000) and clinical (AAP, 1996) communities. However, when we began this work, this view was not widely accepted.

But, even today, the biological revolution in psychiatry threatens to reduce much of child psychopathology to neurotransmitter imbalances (e.g., Pliszka, McCracken, & Maas, 1996) and genetic determinism (Harris, 1998). It is certainly important to understand the underlying pathophysiology of disorder, as well as genetic contributions to child-rearing and to maladaptive patterns of behavior. Nevertheless, an over-emphasis on biological determinism runs the risk of encouraging an overreliance on medication as the treatment of choice for young chil-dren (Coyle, 2000) in the absence of adequate appreciation of other fac-tors in the child's life that require intervention if healthy development is to proceed. Therefore, although the developmental psychopathology perspective is widely accepted, the medical model perspective on chil-dren's problems is also widespread. In a sense, this perspective is reflected in the DSM approach to the diagnosis of disorders, which are conceptualized as within the individual child rather than as the out-come of a developmental and transactional process (Sroufe, 1997; Cummings et al., 2000).

Over the course of about 15 years, we have collected a huge amount of empirical data on the children and families who have partici-pated in our studies, much of which has been reported in journal articles and book chapters (Campbell, 1991, 1994, 1997; Campbell, Breaux, Ewing, & Szumowski, 1986; Campbell & Cluss, 1982; Camp-bell, Breaux, Ewing, & Szumowski, 1984; Campbell, Ewing, Breaux, & Szumowski, 1986; Campbell, March, Pierce, & Ewing, 1991; Campbell et al.,1994; Campbell et al., 1996; Campbell, Szumowski, Ewing, Gluck, & Breaux, 1982; Pierce et al., 1999). This work has been conceptualized within a transactional model meant to examine changes in children and families over time in an attempt to understand the different develop-mental pathways followed by children who look hard to manage in the early preschool years. I first describe the research in general terms and then present descriptions based on prototypic children that are meant to illustrate the types of problems that are apparent in early childhood. They illustrate different patterns of childhood symptoms, styles of family functioning, and strategies of childrearing that presumably set the child on a particular developmental pathway as a preschooler and ultimately also affect academic and social competence at elementary school age. They also suggest different initial causal mechanisms and different maintaining factors. Although etiological formulations remain speculative, it is generally agreed that similar clinical pictures may develop from diverse causes (Cicchetti & Rogosch, 1996).

Identification and Initial Assessment

The children in our first study did not consist of a representative sample of preschoolers who were difficult to handle. Because we were concerned about the ethics of labeling young children, we initially decided to recruit children through pediatric offices and preschools but to insist that parents initiate contact with the project. Thus our sample was composed of a self-selected group of parents who were seeking help because of problems managing their toddlers or young preschoolers. Parents with concerns about their child's activity level, defiance, poor impulse control, and difficulty playing alone were invited to participate in a study of development; parent training groups were offered as an incentive. Children with grossly delayed language development, psychotic-like symptoms, clear indications of brain damage, sensory impairments, or a Stanford–Binet IQ below 75 were excluded from the sample. Children between 25 and 47 months of age who were in good physical health made up the sample of 46 parent-referred problem youngsters and 22 controls. Details of sample recruitment may be found in Campbell et al. (1982).

Initial assessment data on each child were collected during a home visit, two visits to our laboratory playroom, and a visit to the child's preschool classroom. Assessments included a structured interview administered to the child's mother, a series of questionnaires describing child behavior that were completed by both parents and by preschool teachers, observations of the child in the laboratory during free play, structured tasks, interactive play with the mother, and a naturalistic observation of the child's interaction with peers and teachers in nursery school.

In addition, intelligence was assessed with the Stanford–Binet, and a delay task was administered as one index of impulse control. Measures of activity level, attention, compliance, and aggression were derived from the observations and questionnaires. A developmental and family history was obtained from a structured interview. Children were assessed again at ages 4 and 6 on parallel but age-appropriate measures. They were followed up again at age 9, with an emphasis on the children's behavior at home and school, as assessed by a structured interview with their mothers and questionnaires completed by mothers and teachers. At age 13, further follow-up data were obtained from interviews and questionnaires administered to mothers and to the adolescents themselves.

Initial parent reports indicated group differences on rating scales assessing hyperactive–distractible behavior and aggressive–noncompliant behavior; groups did not differ on scales assessing anxiety. Independent laboratory observations revealed that the free-play behavior of problem youngsters was less focused and directed to toys than the play of comparison children. The play of the problem children also was characterized by more shifts in activity from object to object and by more involvement with objects in the room other than toys. Parent-referred problem children also moved around more and were less attentive during structured tasks than comparison children. They were more impulsive on a laboratory task assessing delay capacity in which they were required to wait for a signal before finding and eating a cookie hidden under one of three cups (Campbell et al., 1982).

Those parent-identified hard-to-manage children who attended preschool were rated by their teachers as more hyperactive and aggressive than comparison children but, consistent with parental reports, not as more anxious. Observations in their preschool classrooms indicated that they were also more aggressive with peers; problem boys were less compliant with teacher requests than were other children in the sample. Problem and control groups did not differ in their tendency to approach peers or to play cooperatively (Campbell & Cluss, 1982). It should be noted that teachers were informed only that children were in a study of the development of preschoolers and that no mention was made of problem behavior.

Although the families of the problem children were, on average, from lower social classes and were experiencing higher levels of psychosocial stress—including parental illness, marital dysfunction or disruption, financial difficulties, or problems with extended family—there were wide individual differences on these background measures. Finally, on measures of mother–child interaction obtained during a relatively unstructured free-play period, problem children showed only a nonsignificant tendency to be more noncompliant or aggressive in their play. Mothers of hard-to-manage children were more likely than mothers of control children to be negative and controlling during this play observation (Campbell, Breaux, Ewing, Szumowski, & Pierce, 1986).

Age 4 Follow-Up

Parent report and laboratory measures were repeated 1 year later, when children were 4. As is often the case in longitudinal studies, differential attrition occurred. Families lost to follow-up were primarily from the problem group; even within this group, they tended to be the most distressed and dysfunctional families in the sample (Campbell et al., 1984; Campbell, Ewing, et al., 1986). This means that many of the more difficult children in the sample or those who would be expected, on theoretical and clinical grounds, to have the worst outcomes were among the children most likely to drop out of the study. Indeed, those families lost to follow-up differed significantly from those who remained in the study in both social class and level of psychosocial stress (Campbell, Ewing, et al., 1986). Despite this differential attrition, groups continued to differ at the age 4 follow-up assessment.

Children who were identified as problems at age 3 continued to be rated as significantly more hyperactive and aggressive at age 4, but not as more anxious. They also were less focused in their play, and they moved around more during structured tasks. On a laboratory task that required them to delay searching for a cookie hidden under one of three cups until they received a signal from the experimenter, problem youngsters were still more impulsive. It is also important to note that, despite these continued group differences, most children improved relative to their own initial performance, as evidenced by parallel developmental progressions in the two groups. Thus, as a group, the problem children became somewhat less active and impulsive, relative to their performance 1 year earlier, on several laboratory measures. These data indicate that children identified as hard-to-manage at age 3 continued to have more difficulties than comparison children when followed up 1 year later; thus, problems in the group as a whole did not appear to reflect only age-related activity or a transient developmental phenomenon. Further, within the problem group, children tended to maintain their rank order, with more active and impulsive 3-year-olds remaining more active and impulsive than their peers at age 4. For example, within the problem group, maternal ratings of aggression–hostility at age 3 and age 4 were significantly correlated, as were ratings of activity level; activity shifts during free play, observed at ages 3 and 4, were likewise related, as were impulsive responses on the cookie task.

Early predictors of maternal ratings of problem behavior at age 4 were also examined. Lower social class and more negative and controlling maternal behavior observed in the laboratory at age 3 predicted higher ratings of hyperactivity and aggression at age 4. In addition, boys who had been more noncompliant and aggressive during play with their mothers at age 3 and who had been rated by their mothers as more symptomatic at initial assessment continued to be rated as more active at age 4; negative child behavior and early aggression ratings, but not gender, also were associated with aggression ratings at age 4. These findings underline the relatively high degree of continuity in problem behavior, particularly in the context of a more negative mother–child relationship (Campbell, Breaux, Ewing, Szumowski, & Pierce, 1986).

Cohort 2

In a second longitudinal study, we focused only on boys, most recruited from local preschools and child-care centers and rated by their teachers or caregivers as overactive, impulsive, and inattentive. Boys rated high by their teachers were matched with classmates who were below our cutoffs for elevated symptom levels. A second group of parent-referred children was also included. As before, boys rated high on symptoms of ADHD (inattention, impulsivity, overactivity) were also rated high on measures of aggression and noncompliance. Moreover, most of the children rated high by teachers also received elevated ratings from parents, regardless of referral source (Campbell et al., 1991). Careful observational measures across home, school, and laboratory settings (by observers blind to group assignment or behavior in other contexts) were consistent with our data on our first cohort: problem boys (n = 69) were more impulsive, active, and disruptive when observed at home during a structured task, in the laboratory during free play and structured tasks, and in their preschool classrooms or child-care settings than were comparison boys ($n = 42$; Campbell et al., 1994). However, problem severity and its persistence over time were clearly related to indicators of family adversity (e.g., single-parent status, lower educational level, maternal depression, stressful life events) and to observations of negative maternal control in the laboratory during a toy-cleanup procedure (Campbell, 1994, 1997). To illustrate these issues more fully, four prototypic children are described next.

CHILD 1: JAMIE L.

Jamie was briefly introduced earlier. His mother called the project after seeing our descriptive poster in her pediatrician's office. Jamie was then 3½ years old. During the telephone screening, Mrs. L. stated that she was calling the project because of Jamie's problems in preschool, primarily aggression with peers and wild and uncontrollable behavior. His preschool teacher had recently asked her to consider removing him from school. Jamie's mother also complained about his frequent temper tantrums and defiance ("He doesn't take 'no' for an answer"), his overactivity ("always on the go; constantly moving"), and his tendency to get overexcited and out of control, especially when around other children.

During the home visit, Mrs. L. was interviewed about Jamie's early development and current behavior. He was born full term, weighing over 7 pounds, but with some mild delivery complications. Jamie was described as an active infant who cried a lot and was difficult to calm. He was irregular in his sleeping patterns and tended to require less sleep than his mother expected, taking short naps but not sleeping for long periods. Feeding, however, was not a problem. Jamie could be calmed somewhat in early infancy if he was held and walked, but by 6 months of age he resisted physical contact. His parents first became worried about a problem when he was just over 1 year old. Their concerns focused on his high activity level and his difficulty settling down. By age 3, their concerns also included his aggression with peers, short attention span, excitability, and discipline problems.

These middle-class, well-educated, professional parents were extremely patient with Jamie and set clear and relatively consistent limits. They avoided the use of physical punishment, which they saw as upsetting to Jamie and which could lead to even poorer control than a firm but calm approach would. Thus they gave him a clear warning before sending him to his room to calm down. They also used a good deal of verbal reasoning with explicit rules. Mrs. L. noted that Jamie became easily upset by changes in routine and that he did best when he was well prepared ahead of time for something new.

Jamie and his 1-year-old brother lived with both parents in a quiet, residential neighborhood. Their mother had taken a break from her career to stay at home with her children. Her husband was likewise very involved with the family and spent evening and weekend time with the children; this also served to give Mrs. L. some needed time away from them. The marriage seemed stable, and the climate of the home was warm and relatively relaxed, under the circumstances. Jamie was clearly the main source of stress in the family because he needed frequent monitoring, direction, and supervision. Mr. and Mrs. L. agreed that Jamie was difficult, and they used similar methods of discipline with him. They both were feeling frustrated and defeated by the time they contacted the project.

Jamie was an appealing youngster with red hair and freckles. He greeted the home visitors enthusiastically and quickly struck up a conversation with the examiner. On the Stanford–Binet, he scored in the superior range of intelligence, and his good language and reasoning ability were especially noteworthy. Despite his cognitive strengths, the examiner noted his short attention span, fidgetiness, need for structure, and tendency to leave his seat frequently. These observations were consistent with his behavior during the laboratory assessment of free play, during which he shifted activities frequently and spent much of his time engaged with objects other than toys, such as locked cabinets. He was also more impulsive than average on the cookie task. During unstructured play with his mother, Jamie was moderately noncompliant, but Mrs. L.'s calm, warm, positive but firm approach was very effective in keeping him involved in elaborate and creative fantasy play. She was especially skilled at redirecting him to a new activity or at elaborating on his ongoing fantasy play as ways of keeping him focused. Despite Jamie's difficult behavior, Mrs. L. did not become confrontational. Jamie was eventually enrolled in a more structured preschool program, and his parents participated in a parent training group.

When Jamie was followed up at age 4, he showed some improvement in his ability to focus attention and to control himself, although he was still difficult to discipline, restless, easily bored, and aggressive with peers. In the interim the family had moved to a new house, but otherwise the family situation was unchanged. His parents felt more comfortable about their methods of handling Jamie and were continuing to set firm and consistent limits and to support each other. Jamie was still active during free play in the lab, although he was able to control himself better on structured tasks, such as the cookie delay task.

In terms of the issues delineated earlier in this chapter, Jamie's behavior seems to be more than just annoying; he is not merely showing age-appropriate behavior that is misconstrued by intolerant parents. Indeed, his parents appear especially sensitive and supportive of him. Noteworthy are the severity and patterning of Jamie's problem behaviors, a mixture of high levels of hyperactivity, aggression with peers, and noncompliance. Further, his difficulties are apparent across situations—home, school, and lab—and persistent from ages 3 to 4.

It is difficult to arrive at a satisfactory etiological formulation of Jamie's problems, except by exclusion. Family disruption, poor child-rearing, or other environmental explanations appear inaccurate and inappropriate. Although Jamie appears to have been active, irregular, and difficult to console from early infancy, the notion of a poor match between child temperament and family environment (Thomas et al., 1968) does not seem to apply. Indeed, we were struck by the incredible patience of Jamie's parents and their ability to be firm but loving. It is hard to imagine what Jamie's behavior would have been like if, indeed, he had been born into a less stable, adaptive, and concerned family. It is hard to come up with predisposing factors except those reflected in Jamie's early problems with sleeping and consolability and the continuity noted over time in his excitability and problems with self-regulation, which may be indicative of a constitutional basis for his problems, consistent with the NCCIP diagnosis of self-regulatory difficulty. Jamie continued to have difficulties at home, at school, and with peers, despite his parents' concerted efforts to deal constructively and sensitively with his problems.

CHILD 2: ANNIE J.

Annie was also introduced at the beginning of this book. Her mother called the project when Annie was 2½ after seeing our poster in her pediatrician's office. Mrs. J. expressed concerns about Annie's high energy level, tantrums, sleep problems, and fearfulness. She found Annie particularly difficult to discipline and seemed at a loss about how to handle her daughter's behavior. At the initial interview, Mrs. J. complained about Annie's impatience, low frustration tolerance, difficulty playing alone, lack of concentration, and fussiness. However, she also reported that Annie could amuse herself for up to 20 minutes at a stretch and enjoyed watching *Sesame Street*, suggesting that her attention span and ability to play alone were well within the typical range for a child her age. Mrs. J. was a highly anxious woman with doubts about her own competence. She questioned her own ability to manage Annie and noted that she and her husband disagreed on the best approach to childrearing. Mrs. J. had tried a number of different disciplinary approaches by the time she called the project, including reasoning, smacking, and time-out. When interviewed, her current approach was threatening to spank Annie with a wooden spoon and screaming at her when she misbehaved. Annie, in turn, was fighting back by screaming and smacking her mother and by throwing things. Despite this negative approach, Mrs. J. seemed unable to enforce limits, so that when a battle ensued between Annie and Mrs. J., Annie often won. Her tantrum behavior was clearly paying off. Annie's father appeared to be calmer, firmer, and less negative with her, as well as less easily manipulated, and, consequently, he did not elicit this explosive behavior from her. Mrs. J. also reported that she perceived Annie's difficult behavior as purposely provocative. When first seen, Annie was not yet toilet trained and was still in diapers; she was still drinking from a bottle, and she was sitting in a high chair for meals in order to keep her under control. Because she was not yet in preschool and had had only limited peer experiences, it was not possible to assess Annie's social behavior in another setting.

According to maternal report, Annie was born full term after a long and difficult delivery. Mrs. J. also reported pregnancy complications. She noted that she had been concerned about behavior problems from early infancy because Annie never slept much as an infant (although she also reported that Annie slept through the night for 6 or 7 hours from about 6 weeks on). Mrs. J. also reported feeding problems, a high activity level, and difficulty soothing Annie, who did not like to be held or cuddled. However, further inquiry did not clearly substantiate these patterns.

Annie was then the only child of college-educated parents in their late 20s. Her father worked in a managerial position; her mother had stopped working just prior to Annie's birth and was home with her full time. The marriage was stable on the surface, with the exception of parental disagreements over Annie. No marital problems were acknowledged. However, Mrs. J.'s high anxiety level, anger and frustration with her daughter, intense concern, quite negative perceptions, and low self-esteem caused us to wonder about maternal depression and about the marital relationship as well.

Annie was an attractive little girl with blond hair and blue eyes. She was quite fussy and clingy during the home visit, demonstrating separation distress prior to the administration of the Stanford–Binet and insisting that her mother remain with her. The examiner noted that Annie was frequently out of her seat, was quite distractible, and refused to attempt several items. The test, though incomplete, revealed that she was functioning at least at the upper end of the bright normal level and probably higher. During the visit to the laboratory, Annie was frequently out of her seat and off task during structured activities; she was impulsive on a delay task; and she shifted activities frequently during free play, showing relatively limited involvement with toys and somewhat disorganized play. When asked to play with her mother, Annie was active, demanding, irritable, and noncompliant; her mother was seen as controlling and directive, as intruding inappropriately into Annie's play, as tending to nag, and as lacking in warmth. Overall, the quality of the interaction was fraught with tension and conflict over who was in control.

Mrs. J. described Annie as a difficult infant, and we did observe the overactivity and noncompliance she reported. However, the inconsistencies in Mrs. J.'s reports of Annie's behavior and her inability to set firm limits or provide opportunities to facilitate Annie's development were all indications of problems with childrearing and in the mother–child relationship. Annie probably was somewhat difficult and irritable as an infant, although it is also possible that she was a relatively easy baby with an overanxious, unsure mother who was insensitive to her signals and unable to meet her needs early on. It was quite clear from the interview material that Mrs. J. was not well informed about what to expect from a young infant; her expectations were at times unrealistically high (sleeping, attention span), at others unrealistically low (toilet training, weaning, experiences with peers). It was also apparent that

Mrs. J. was ineffective, inconsistent, and quite harsh in setting limits. Although she was intensely concerned about her daughter, she was not warm or affectionate. Indeed, project staff had the impression that Mrs. J. was extremely critical of and negative about Annie, an impression that has persisted over the years. The early history, paired with Annie's separation problems and her mother's high level of anxiety and tendency to infantilize her daughter, clearly suggest relationship difficulties, including an insecure (resistant) attachment. This impression derives from a consideration of Mrs. J.'s intense but insensitive and unresponsive behavior and Annie's apparent difficulties gaining comfort from her mother (Ainsworth et al., 1978; Carlson & Sroufe, 1995). By age 2½, Annie was locked in an ambivalent struggle with her mother over her needs for autonomy and independence, which were in conflict with her unmet needs for nurturance and support.

This troubled mother–daughter relationship probably was not helped by the fact that Mr. J. had a much easier time with Annie. He was warmer with her and less negative and controlling, and she responded by being more affectionate and agreeable. At the completion of the assessment, we recommended that Mr. and Mrs. J. attend a parent training group that focused on normal developmental expectations for toddlers and preschoolers and on setting firm, positive, and consistent limits. We also suggested that Annie be given the opportunity to play with other children. We also worked with Mr. and Mrs. J. on toilet training, as this area had become the focus of considerable parent–child conflict. Annie's parents eagerly followed our suggestions, but they had a difficult time thinking in developmental or psychological terms. They were not willing to accept a referral for additional help outside the project.

When Annie was followed up 1 year later, she had improved somewhat, according to maternal report. Similarly, observational measures suggested some improvement, although Annie was still less focused in her play than many other children in the sample. Mrs. J. also reported that Annie was toilet trained and not drinking from a bottle any longer. She also had been enrolled in a preschool program several mornings a week. There she reportedly was doing well with her peers, and she loved going. The teacher saw no problems with her. However, the interview revealed that Mrs. J. still saw Annie as requiring a good deal of structure, as defiant, and as difficult to control. Mrs. J. complained of having particular difficulty when she took Annie shopping, expecting her to wait patiently and not to touch things, another example of inappropriate expectations. In addition, sleep problems were reported, with Annie going into her parents' bed several times a week; eating had also become an area of conflict, with Annie refusing certain foods and her mother trying to coax her to eat and at times feeding her. In addition, Mrs. J. had been briefly hospitalized during the interim for a medical problem, and Annie had begun to wet her bed in response to her mother's departure.

Thus problems with developmental tasks continued to be in evidence, fueled by the parents' difficulties conceptualizing their daughter's psychological needs or helping her to negotiate issues of separation–individuation and the establishment of autonomy and independence. It is particularly significant that Annie was able to separate successfully enough to attend a preschool program and that her teacher found her eager to play with other children and to participate in structured activities. With the appropriate emotional support provided by the preschool teacher, Annie was able to begin to reach out to others and to develop appropriately in certain areas.

Significantly, although Annie appeared to have relatively severe difficulties at age 3, and although according to maternal report, her earlier behavior had been quite problematic, she had made notable gains by age 4. Despite these gains, Mrs. J. still complained about a range of difficulties with Annie, although these difficulties appeared to be specific to her relationship with her mother and did not spill over to affect her school adjustment. Thus her problems were not cross-situational. Further, the pattern of her symptoms suggests a mixture of anxiety and high activity level rather than aggressive behavior. Her activity level may well reflect her high level of anxiety, whereas maternal reports of defiance and oppositional behavior may reflect inappropriate expectations or Annie's attempts to separate and gain control, as well as a coercive pattern of interaction between mother and daughter (Patterson, 1980). Annie's problems generally suggest a poor fit between her own developmental and emotional needs, possibly a somewhat fearful, inhibited, and irritable temperamental style (Rothbart & Bates, 1998), accompanied by poor regulatory skills, and her mother's harsh disciplinary style, unrealistic expectations, and lack of warmth and acceptance. This pattern of mother–daughter conflict and negative maternal perceptions has persisted, although Annie also continues to function well at school and with peers.

CHILD 3: ROBBIE S.

Mrs. S. called the project when Robbie was just 3, reporting that she was "at her wits' end" and no longer knew how to deal with her son's high activity level. She reported that he could not sit still, was up at 6 A.M. "running the halls," that he was moving all the time, and that he had an attention span of "less than 20 seconds." She also noted that he was unable to entertain himself, except in the bathtub.

During the intake interview, Mrs. S. reported that she had first become concerned about Robbie's high activity level and sleep difficulties when he was 9 months old but was reassured by her pediatrician that his behavior was not that atypical and would be outgrown. She noted that he was still a restless sleeper who moved around a lot during sleep and that he slept for relatively brief periods. By age 3, he was no longer taking afternoon naps. She described Robbie as unable to relax and unable to focus on one toy for more than a few seconds, tending instead to move rapidly from one toy to another during play. He was not at all interested in stories or other sedentary activities. Mrs. S. described relatively violent temper tantrums that included throwing things, hitting and kicking, screaming, and crying, but she noted that Robbie was not aggressive around other children. Mrs. S. was firm but patient with him; she set clear guidelines for acceptable behavior and did not give in to his tantrums. She was also quick to praise his good behavior and to provide rational reasons for limits and prohibitions. Mr. S., on the other hand, was quite inconsistent, sometimes giving in to Robbie's tantrums, sometimes becoming very angry and harsh with him.

Robbie was born full term after a long and difficult labor, but there were no indications of fetal distress. Despite sleep problems and a high activity level, he was described as a cuddly infant without feeding or other difficulties. Robbie is the younger of two children. His 6-year-old sister was reported to be developing normally. Both parents graduated from high school and were employed in managerial positions. Robbie's mother returned to work when he was 6 weeks old, placing him in family day care. He was still in the same day care setting when he was first seen in the project.

At the time of the home visit, Robbie greeted the tester with an impish grin and proceeded to show her his trucks. Robbie was an extremely outgoing and engaging child with curly, blond hair and green eyes. He readily separated from his mother but left the test session from time to time to "check in" with her and tell her what he was doing. His language was somewhat immature and difficult to understand, but Robbie was a bright youngster and caught on quickly to task demands, performing in the bright normal range. He was frequently out of his seat during testing, but he was relatively easy to redirect with the introduction of a new task.

During the observation of free play in the laboratory, Robbie shifted activities frequently, playing only briefly with any one toy. He was much more interested in manipulating forbidden objects (the video camera, microphone, locked cabinets) and climbing into the sink. He was at the extremes on measures of activity and inattention derived from these observations. In addition, on a delay task that required him to wait for a signal from the experimenter before finding and eating a piece of cookie, Robbie made several impulsive responses. He was frequently out of his seat and off task during structured tasks. Thus, during a laboratory assessment of activity level, attention, and impulse control, Robbie confirmed his mother's reports of problematic behavior. During the mother–child play interaction, Robbie was able to focus attention on toys for much longer and was even able to complete several tasks. His mother provided him with a good deal of structure, support, and positive feedback while firmly and consistently enforcing limits. The relationship between Robbie and his mother seemed warm and positive.

There was little doubt from Robbie's history and behavior at initial intake that he was showing early signs of problems that might well reflect attention-deficit/hyperactivity disorder. However, several issues complicate the formulation of his difficulties. First, Robbie had been in day care from 6 weeks of age until age 3 in a setting that appeared to provide adequate physical and emotional care but inadequate cognitive stimulation or organized activities with age-mates. Second, there was a significant family history of antisocial behavior and what appeared to be bipolar disorder in first-degree relatives of both parents. Third, Robbie's parents had an extremely poor marital relationship, with frequent arguments and much tension. Finally, Robbie's father was inconsistently and intermittently involved with him. Mr. S. showed brief periods of great interest and concern but would then withdraw and ignore Robbie, rebuffing his overtures.

Mrs. S. was very eager for help and support. She attended a parent training group faithfully and completed all homework assignments with incredible thoroughness. She was already utilizing most of the disciplinary approaches discussed in the group but seemed to derive a good deal of satisfaction and comfort from discussing Robbie with the other parents. She also felt vindicated by the support of the group leaders. Mr. S. blamed Robbie's problems on his wife's "laxness" (i.e., her use of reasoning and time-out, rather than physical punishment), and she was clearly concerned about whether or not she might be the "cause" of his difficult behavior. Mr. S. refused to accompany his wife to any of these sessions.

Robbie changed child-care arrangements several months after entering the project. He moved from the family day-care home to a well-run day-care center with age-appropriate structured activities and a good staff-to-child ratio, where he could play with other children his own age. Robbie adjusted well to this new setting, got along well with other children, and became more manageable at home. For example, he would come home exhausted from day care and began to sleep through the night. Bedtime was no longer a struggle.

At the age 4 follow-up, Mrs. S. reported that Robbie's behavior continued to improve. His mother saw him as much more manageable and as able to entertain himself for brief periods of time. She reported that he got along well with the other children in child care and loved going. Although he still had relatively regular temper tantrums, Mrs. S. felt much more in control of the situation. She was explicit and consistent in setting limits and able to ignore tantrum behavior. Laboratory observations likewise suggested some improvement in Robbie's self-control, as reflected in more focused play and less impulsivity.

Despite these apparent improvements, there had been a number of significant changes in Robbie's life. The marital situation further deteriorated, and his parents separated just prior to his fourth birthday. Robbie was, not surprisingly, confused about the situation; unfortunately, the conflict between his parents became increasingly intense, and Robbie became the focus of their anger and resentment. This situation has steadily worsened. In particular, Mr. S. threatened Mrs. S. with a custody suit. When Robbie was 5, Mrs. S. called asking for a referral for Robbie, who was wetting his bed, having nightmares, and wanting to sleep with her. He was also having angry outbursts at home and getting into fights with his sister, as well as with other children at school. He and his sister had, unfortunately, been put into the position of message carriers between their warring parents. Robbie was seen in play therapy for a number of months in an attempt to help him deal with his confused and intense feelings of anger and betrayal, as well as his concerns about being abandoned. Like many youngsters his age facing parental separation, his ambivalence about his absent father was intense (Wallerstein & Kelly, 1980); he longed for and worried about his father and fantasized about reunion but was often reluctant to visit and adamantly refused to leave his mother on several occasions.

It appeared that we were dealing with a youngster whose initial difficulties reflected a combination of temperamental difficultness and family tensions. His problems appeared to have been exacerbated by the continuing instability in his life. Initial problems appeared relatively severe and apparent across situations, although his good adjustment to day care and his lack of aggression with peers were noteworthy. The nature and severity of Robbie's problems appeared to wax and wane in tandem with environmental stress and instability, factors which are likely to predict later outcome. Continued follow-up has revealed persistent problems that appear to worsen when family stress intensifies; Robbie also has had a good deal of difficulty coping with the demands for conformity, achievement, and compliance required in school.

CHILD 4: TEDDY M.

When Teddy was just under 2½, Mrs. M. called the project to seek help. She was concerned particularly about Teddy's high activity level, short attention span, excitability with peers, and difficulty amusing himself. He was not, however, described as either aggressive with peers or difficult to discipline. During the interview, Mrs. M. also noted concerns about Teddy's low frustration tolerance and his lack of sustained involvement in play. Although she described him as able to play alone for as long as 30 minutes on some construction activities, she was concerned about his tendency to move quickly from one activity to another and to show little interest in many of his toys.

Teddy was described as a somewhat irritable infant who cried a lot when tired and required more than an average amount of sleep. He was not a cuddly baby, and, when upset, he was described as quite difficult to console, sometimes crying for 30 minutes at a time. When distressed, Teddy did not like to be held, and he generally resisted physical restraint. He was also quite active as an infant and walked early. Feeding was not a problem. Teddy was a full term infant, delivered without complications. There is nothing remarkable in his developmental or family history.

Mr. and Mrs. M. were both college educated, and Mr. M. was employed at a managerial level in a local business. Mrs. M., a former nurse, remained home full time with Teddy and his 5-year-old brother. She reported that she was able to discipline Teddy effectively, relying primarily on reasoning and sitting him on a chair in time-out. The marriage appeared to be stable, and Mr. M. was quite involved with the children. There were no problems noted with their older child, who was described as much easier to care for as an infant and much less active than Teddy as a toddler and preschooler. Teddy was only 28 months old when first seen in the project, and he was not attending any organized preschool.

Teddy was a cute youngster with brown hair and brown eyes. At first he was somewhat shy with the tester, but after a few minutes of play and conversation with his mother present, he warmed up and showed interest in the "games" she had brought. Teddy was cooperative during the administration of the Stanford–Binet, and he performed at the bright normal level. The examiner did not find him particularly fidgety or inattentive, and he remained seated for the entire 30-minute testing session. During the laboratory assessment of free play, Teddy showed interest in the toys and became particularly involved with a family of dolls and a pounding toy, spending most of his time with one or the other of these. He did explore other toys and the room in general, but he was much more focused on specific toys than the other three children described previously. Although Teddy was impulsive on the cookie-delay task, he was neither fidgety nor inattentive during structured tasks. During the mother–child play interaction, Teddy was engrossed with a toy workbench, and he played relatively independently. His mother, though warm and supportive, was quite directive. Based on the laboratory assessment and our observations of Teddy during the home visit, we did not see him as more active or distractible than the average 28-month-old. Both parents attended a parent training group, where we hoped that exposure to other parents of children with more severe problems would place Teddy's behavior in a more appropriate developmental perspective.

When seen for follow-up 1 year later, Teddy was still described by his mother as somewhat restless and inattentive on interview; she also expressed some concern about his difficulty sharing toys and his emerging verbal defiance. However, she saw these as only mild problems. The laboratory assessment did not suggest that Teddy was particularly active, inattentive, or impulsive. Although he changed activities fairly often during free play, he was not impulsive on the cookie task and he was attentive and organized on other structured tasks.

Teddy seems to be a good example of a child who was developing normally, although he may have been somewhat more difficult than average in infancy. Alternatively, he may have been merely more active and less cuddly in infancy than his brother, something for which his parents were not prepared. In either event, it appears that Mr. and Mrs. M had high expectations and they sometimes misinterpreted Teddy's age-appropriate activity level, relatively short bouts of sustained play, and limited ability to share toys as problems. Mr. and Mrs. M. were seen as somewhat demanding, although they were also warm and loving. This type of early parent–child mismatch has the potential to lead to overly harsh discipline or to parent–child conflict that escalates and leads to more serious later problems. However, Teddy's family was a stable, caring, and concerned one and his parents were firm but not overbearing in their approach to childrearing.

The pattern of Teddy's behavior is also worth considering. Not only were his symptoms relatively mild, but parental complaints of hyperactivity and inattention were not combined with concerns about aggression toward peers or high levels of oppositional or impulsive behavior. His behavior was also not problematic in many situations, and he did not become more difficult to manage with development. Rather, parental concerns at age 4 were somewhat different from their initial complaints and focused on age-appropriate manifestations of development. Thus, from the start, Teddy looked more like a comparison youngster than a child with a clinically significant problem that was likely to persist and/or escalate in severity. Continued follow-up was consistent with this interpretation.

SUMMARY

In this chapter, several clinical issues were discussed. Differences between age-specific problems and signs of more serious, potentially persistent problems were addressed. In particular, drawing on data from epidemiological studies, it was concluded that problem behaviors are very common in the general population of nonreferred children and that many troublesome behaviors also show age-related developmental change. The social and developmental context in which problem behavior occurs was seen as crucial in determining whether an annoying or worrisome behavior should be considered merely typical, an indicator of a difficult developmental transition, or a sign of a potentially significant problem. It was concluded that symptoms that clustered together and appeared to interfere with developmental progress were particularly worthy of concern. Several factors influencing referral were also noted, and patterns of behavioral disturbance in young children were described.

Diagnostic issues also were addressed. It was concluded that the developmental guidelines contained in DSM-IV are inadequate but that, when they are used in conjunction with the more elaborate descriptions of problem severity, family and social context, and developmental manifestations contained in the DSM-PC, more appropriate and more cautious diagnostic decisions can be made. Closer examination of the diagnostic criteria for attention-deficit/hyperactivity disorder, oppositional defiant disorder, and separation anxiety disorder, however, indicate that many of the behaviors that define these disorders may be age-appropriate behaviors or typical ways of reacting to stress in young children. Therefore, the need for caution in the use of these diagnostic labels was seen as important. Although some 3- and 4-year-olds may well meet criteria for these disorders, there is also the danger of overpathologizing the typical behaviors of young children; the use of a diagnostic label, with the implication that the problem is "within the child," is often misleading, unnecessarily upsetting to parents, and potentially stigmatizing. The need to consider developmental appropriateness, as well as family and social context when making a diagnosis, cannot be overemphasized.

An attempt was then made to illustrate these issues by describing our longitudinal research on hard-to-manage preschoolers. Comparisons between problem youngsters and comparison children at intake and after a 1-year interval indicated that parental concerns were likely to be confirmed by data obtained from other sources and that problems persisted in some children. Four prototypic children from the study were then described in more detail in order to provide illustrations of the nature of early symptomatology in young children whose parents found them difficult to manage in toddlerhood and the early preschool period. In each instance, problems of one sort or another appeared quite early, at least by the child's first birthday; some relatively significant problems also were found to persist at the age 4 follow-up. In particular, the constellation of hyperactivity, impulsivity, inattention, defiance, and peer aggression was associated with continued externalizing problems. Sleep problems were also often evidenced. The relative contributions of child characteristics, parental expectations and management strategies, and ongoing family stresses to problem identification and persistence appeared to vary somewhat from one child to the next, illustrating different patterns of symptoms, as well as different pathways to early difficulties.

In one instance, child problems appeared to be rather isolated symptoms in a well-functioning family. Unrealistic parental expectations, probably paired with a child's fearfulness and negative affect, appeared to be associated with problems in a youngster whose difficulties were not clearly atypical initially. A negative mother–child relationship was associated with an uncertain outcome at age 4. With another child, high parental expectations were associated with positive parenting and a good parent–child relationship. The outlook for this child appeared to be good. In yet another, the relative contributions of endogenous child characteristics and family dysfunction were more difficult to disentangle, although severe family disruption led to the appearance of new symptoms. Symptoms of anxiety and sadness were especially apparent in association either with severe mother–child conflict or marked family disruption, although in most instances both externalizing and internalizing symptoms occurred together.

These clinical vignettes also illustrate the observation that particular symptoms appear to become salient at different stages of development, sometimes as exaggerations of normal developmental tasks. Thus sleep and feeding problems and consolability appear especially noticeable in infancy; activity level becomes particularly important as children become mobile and exploratory around the first birthday. By age 2 or so, compliance with requests and ability to play alone also become important, as parental expectations change with the child's growing cognitive and self-regulatory abilities. Peer relations, the ability to play cooperatively with other children and to share toys without eruptions of excessive aggression, become noteworthy at about age 3, as children show more focused interest in peers in more formalized preschool and day-care programs. By age 4, children seem to be able to cooperate better in the peer group and to function more independently at home, although issues of noncompliance and self-regulation are still primary parental concerns.

CHAPTER 4

Family Factors
and Young
Children's Development

In this chapter, I argue that a variety of family factors have an effect on young children's early development and later functioning and adjustment. I focus on observable and measurable aspects of the family environment, recognizing that this emphasis on family factors cannot disentangle genetic from environmental influences. Rather, it is assumed that parenting behavior and childrearing strategies, and even the effects of family turmoil and dysfunction, to some extent reflect the co-occurrence of genetic and environmental influences, as well as gene–environment interactions. However, the elucidation of these complex and poorly understood processes is beyond the scope of this book. Moreover, with few exceptions, the issues and processes under discussion in this chapter have not been studied with genetically informed designs, such as twin or adoption studies, that permit one to tease apart the effects of parent–child similarity in personality, emotion regulation, and cognitive functioning that derive from shared genes from those that reflect relationship history, childrearing practices, and socialization strategies. Clearly, relationship quality and childrearing practices are themselves influenced by parental temperament and personality, and they are also reactions to children's behavior and developmental level. As such, they must reflect a mix of genetic predispositions in both the parents and the children, as well as environmental events, some of which are also partly a function of genetically mediated behaviors.

Some readers may think that I have placed undue emphasis on mother–child interaction to the exclusion of fathers throughout this chapter and the book as a whole. Unfortunately, this reflects the state of the research literature on early parenting and socialization, which is almost exclusively focused on maternal behavior (Cowan, 1997; Lamb, 19987b; Parke & Buriel, 1998; Thompson, 1998). Finally, some readers may think that I put too much emphasis on parenting behavior, especially relationship quality and limit setting, in discussing both early development and the emergence of behavior problems. In my view, this seems both inevitable and appropriate given the focus on infants and young children. Regardless of how initial patterns of behavior emerge in dyadic parent–child interactions, despite bidirectional and transactional processes, parents do have more control and power than the infant in shaping early infant and child behavior, except in the most extreme circumstances of a severely impaired or intensely irritable and unconsolable infant. It is the parent who must respond to the distressed infant or redirect the toddler about to get into trouble. Although parental success will be partly determined by child characteristics and relationship history, the parent is still the one responsible for infant caretaking and child well-being. Thus, although it is recognized that the child contributes to his or her own development and socialization experiences, in infancy and early childhood the parents are still seen as responsible for scaffolding their child's cognitive and social advances by providing appropriate support, stimulation, and opportunities for optimal development.

Given these caveats and qualifications, this chapter focuses on the following family processes and characteristics: (1) childrearing practices and parental expectations, which to some extent determine the nature and quality of the child's socialization experiences; (2) aspects of family structure and family relations, which influence the child both directly, through their impact on the climate of the home, and indirectly, via their effects on childrearing and parental availability and support; and (3) the family's social context, which also affects the child both directly and indirectly via its influence on the parents. Each of these factors is addressed in turn. Where appropriate, clinical vignettes are used to illustrate significant interactions among family, child, and parenting factors.

THE ROLE OF PARENTS IN SOCIALIZATION AND SOCIAL DEVELOPMENT

Clinical wisdom, empirical data, and common sense converge to emphasize the central role that parents play in children's socialization and social development. From the earliest days of life, parents are responsible for meeting the infant's needs for protection, nurturance, and physical caretaking. They must help the newborn infant adapt to life outside the womb, for example, by establishing smooth caretaking routines, by helping the young infant regulate sleep–wake cycles and negative arousal, and by protecting the infant from overstimulation (e.g., Kopp, 1989; Sroufe, 1979). Over the course of the first year, parents must function primarily as caretakers and nurturers, with the goals of protecting their young infants from harm, providing for their physical needs, and fulfilling their needs for social, affective, and cognitive stimulation. By the end of the first year, as children begin to develop language, symbolic thinking, a sense of self, and the ability to act on their environment in effective ways, the responsibilities of parents shift from primarily providing nurturance and protection to caregiving that is balanced by limit setting and the use of effective control strategies. At this developmental stage, parents must confront the difficult but rewarding tasks of teaching children the rules of appropriate social behavior, of helping them to master the rules of social exchange and of the physical world, and of facilitating the internalization of values and morals.

It seems obvious that some children are easier to socialize than others (Kochanska, 1997; Maccoby & Martin, 1983). For example, individual differences in infant characteristics, such as irritability and consolability, or in activity level will make some children more difficult to satisfy or to control than others. Similarly, some parents seem to have an intuitive sense of how to gain their child's cooperation, whereas others attempt to control their young children in ways that limit their success from the start. There is a growing body of evidence linking qualitative features of the early mother–infant relationship to later social and cognitive competence (e.g., Carlson & Sroufe, 1995; Thompson, 1998). This work underscores the importance of parental responsiveness and availability, as well as warmth and sensitivity. Research on childrearing practices also indicates that positive, nonconfrontational approaches that are basically educative tend to be more effective than controls that are inflexible and harsh (e.g., Belsky et al., 1998; Crockenberg &

Litman, 1990; Kochanska, 1997; Zahn-Waxler et al., 1979). In addition, children learn through observation and imitation. Thus parental actions and emotional expressions also provide models for children's behavior, including their responses to parental control, their internalization of values, goals, and moral standards, and their behavior with others in their social network.

The Quality of Parenting and Infant–Parent Attachment

As noted in Chapter 1, attachment theorists (Ainsworth et al., 1978; Bowlby, 1969; Carlson & Sroufe, 1995) see the quality of the early mother–infant relationship as the prototype for all later relationships and as forming the groundwork for later cognitive and social development. In addition, they argue that maternal warmth and sensitivity to infant signals are important determinants of early mother–infant interaction that, in turn, will influence the quality of the attachment relationship that develops over the course of the first year. Thus mothers who are able to read their infants' social and distress signals and are then available to respond promptly and appropriately will be more likely to raise infants who are securely attached. Because securely attached infants have a history of positive interactions with mothers who are accessible and responsive, they have learned that the world is predictable and supportive and that they have some control over events; they are able to reach out to explore, partly because the world does not seem to be a threatening place and partly because they have learned that they will be protected when in distress or danger. This feeling is akin to what Erikson (1963) termed a sense of basic trust. According to attachment theory, secure infants have learned that their communications lead to responses from others, fostering a sense of self-efficacy, what some theorists see as the underpinnings of basic motivation (Hunt, 1961; White, 1959) and an emerging sense of self (Thompson, 1998).

On the other hand, when parents are insensitive and unresponsive, infants learn to expect that their needs will not be met, that the world is neither predictable nor supportive. Such infants will develop insecure patterns of attachment, reflected in avoidant and socially withdrawn behavior, angry, resistant behavior, or disorganized behavior suggesting anxiety and fear. Some insecurely attached infants are less likely to venture out to explore the environment, presumably because their parents have not provided them with consistent protection from harm or with comfort when they are frightened or upset, what Ainsworth and others (Ainsworth et al., 1978; Bowlby, 1969) have termed a secure base for exploration. Other insecure infants may focus their attention on objects that seem more predictable and under their control rather than on social interactions with people, which have been frustrating, unpredictable, and/or unsatisfying for them. Because they do not expect to be comforted when distressed, insecurely attached infants may ultimately learn to avoid or resist contact with unavailable or frustrating parents, especially when under stress. Still other infants have been so traumatized by harsh parental treatment that their behavior seems bizarre, and when they are upset they do not seem to know where to turn for comfort (Carlson & Sroufe, 1995), appearing disorganized and unable to cope with stress. Although data are consistent with attachment theory, it should be noted that maternal sensitivity and responsiveness account for a reliable but small proportion of the variance in attachment security and that other aspects of maternal and paternal behavior, as well as the wider family context and aspects of child personality, undoubtedly play a role in the development of attachment quality (Cowan, 1997; De Wolff & van IJzendoorn, 1997; Thompson, 1998).

Some studies indicate that insecurely attached infants tend to be more noncompliant with maternal requests and prohibitions than securely attached infants. They also exhibit less interest and flexibility in problem-solving situations, are less adept at eliciting help and support from their mothers when confronted with difficult problems to solve, and are less socially competent with peers (Carlson & Sroufe, 1995). Sroufe (1983) and others (e.g., Bretherton, 1985) argue that the absence of a secure attachment, which derives initially, at least in part, from insensitive and unresponsive maternal behavior, has ramifications for the infant's social development and capacity to cope with developmental challenges such as environmental mastery, independence and autonomy, and the ability to function well with other children. Thus parental responsiveness, availability, and sensitivity in the first year of life are seen as influencing the quality of the early parent–infant relationship, which, it is argued, in turn is important for social adaptation and socialization in the toddler and preschool years. As children begin to develop a sense of themselves and to function more independently, their internal working model of relationships, their ability to regulate emotion, and their emerging social understanding, derived in part from the quality of their early attachment, will influence their coping strategies in other contexts (Carlson & Sroufe, 1995; Thompson, 1998). There is some empirical support for this position, but it is not without its critics (e.g., Lewis et al., 2000; Thompson, 1998). The important role of concurrent parenting and family climate cannot be overlooked (e.g., Cowan, 1997; Lamb, 1987a; Lewis et al., 2000; Thompson, 1998).

As noted in Chapter 1, there is also debate about the role of infant characteristics in the establishment of a secure attachment. It seems logical that infants who are extremely difficult to care for will be less likely to elicit sensitive and responsive caregiving. Furthermore, with some especially difficult infants, even the most sensitive caretakers may prove ineffective. Research findings linking infant irritability to the quality of later attachment have been equivocal, with some studies (e.g., Crockenberg, 1981) finding a relationship between infant difficultness and insecure attachment and others supporting Sroufe's (1985) argument that caretaking sensitivity overrides infant characteristics in determining the quality of the attachment relationship that develops (e.g., Bates et al., 1985). It is my view that quality of caregiving and child characteristics both are significant in determining outcome, although with either very neglecting or rejecting caretaking or extreme infant irritability, problems are more likely to be in evidence.

If insecurity is associated with less adaptive functioning in the mother–toddler relationship and in the peer group, it seems logical that it may also predict obvious behavior problems that reflect maladaptation above and beyond problems in specific developmental transitions. Several studies have examined the relationship between insecure attachment in infancy and later behavior problems. Sroufe (1983) studied an inner-city sample of mothers and children living in poverty and reported that insecure attachment was associated with a variety of internalizing and externalizing problems in preschool. Lewis et al. (1984) followed a sample of middle-class infants until age 6. Insecure attachment predicted behavior problems, but only in boys and only in the context of ongoing family stress and disruption. In contrast, Bates and associates (Bates et al., 1985; Bates & Bayles, 1988) found a relationship between infant difficultness and problem behaviors at ages 3 and 6, but no relationship between attachment security and behavior problems at either age. In the NICHD Study of Early Child Care (NICHD Early Child Care Research Network, 1998), maternal sensitivity, but not insecure attachment at 15 months, predicted ratings of behavior problems at 24 and 36 months. In two more recent studies of high-risk samples of young children living in poverty, disorganized attachment in toddler-hood, but not other patterns of insecurity (resistant, avoidant), pre-dicted higher rates of aggressive and disruptive behavior at age 5 (Lyons-Ruth, 1996; Shaw et al., 1996). In the Shaw et al. study, data were consistent with a transactional model. Toddlers who were seen as more problematic at age 2 *and* who also were disorganized during reunions with their mothers during the Strange Situation (Ainsworth et al., 1978) were most likely to receive elevated aggression ratings at age 5. Shaw et al. (1996) and Lyons-Ruth (1996) also provide data consistent with a multiple or cumulative risk model. Although in both studies disorga-nized attachment was a significant predictor of later problems, other family and parenting factors were also strong predictors of behavior problems, including maternal hostility, maternal psychosocial prob-lems, and parental disagreements over childrearing. Thus most studies linking insecure attachment to later behavior problems suggest that in-secure attachment is a risk factor for later problems only in concert with other adverse circumstances in the family. By itself, insecurity cannot be considered a harbinger of later risk.

One recent study examined attachment security and parenting in young boys showing clinically significant levels of aggressive and non-compliant behavior (DeKlyen, Speltz, & Greenberg, 1998; Speltz et al., 1999). Youngsters with behavior problems were more likely to be inse-curely attached to one or both parents than comparison boys. Indeed, only 28% of the problem boys were securely attached to both parents, in contrast to 75% of the comparison boys. However, attachment security in this study did not predict severity of behavior problems, either con-currently or 2 years later. Because attachment is measured differently in preschoolers than it is in infants, the very behaviors that index insecu-rity in the preschool period (e.g., manipulative and coercive behavior) may also be reflections of the behavior problems themselves. This study, then, provides some interesting and provocative data, but it does not clarify the role of attachment as a presumed risk factor for later behav-ior problems in clinically referred samples.

In line with the transactional and ecological perspective, early rela-tionship problems in some mother–infant dyads appear to persist and continue to be associated with difficulties as the child grows older, espe-cially if mothers are inflexible, inconsistent, rejecting, or disengaged and their children are angry and uncooperative. Other mother–child dyads probably overcome early difficulties as the child's needs change and the parents become more able to respond appropriately, either because they are better able to cope with an older child or because of decreases in external stresses that had taxed their limited resources. In still other instances, the possible negative impact of a poor mother–child relationship may be ameliorated in part by a warm affective bond and positive experiences with other adults: father, grandparents, or a caring babysitter. Thus an insecure attachment may be one ingredient in the mix of factors predicting behavior problems in young children. However, as noted by Lewis et al. (1984), behavior problems do not inevitably signal an insecure attachment; conversely, an insecure attachment need not produce behavior problems. Moreover, it is especially important to consider other aspects of the parent–child relationship, as well as the necessary changes that must occur in that relationship as the child's needs change with development (Cummings et al., 2000; Thompson, 1998).

Childrearing Practices and Socialization

Positive Limit Setting and Young Children's Compliance

Much of the work on parent–child relations has focused on associations between childrearing practices and on children's development of cooperation and self-control. The focus in infancy is almost exclusively on the quality of caregiving, but by toddlerhood, the focus shifts to include parents' ability to set limits and to provide guidelines for acceptable behavior. Studies generally find that children tend to be compliant most of the time, although the relationship between child compliance and parental behavior is clearly a transactional one, with children's past behavior influencing the nature of future parental prohibitions and with parenting behavior contributing to children's willingness to cooperate. Thus the quality of the ongoing mother–child relationship appears to play a role in the development of children's compliance. As noted earlier, several studies have found that toddlers who are securely attached to their mothers are also more compliant with maternal requests and less likely to refuse to cooperate with prohibitions. However, their mothers, in turn, are less restrictive and less likely to set arbitrary or punitive limits. That does not mean that these mothers never get angry and that their children are always well behaved. Rather, studies suggest that mothers who have harmonious relationships with relatively cooperative toddlers and preschoolers have not only a history of positive interaction but also a hierarchy of behavioral control strategies that they apply based on the situation. For most situations, they can obtain compliance with a request and an explanation (Crockenberg & Litman, 1990; Kochanska, 1997; Maccoby & Martin, 1983).

Mothers use a range of positive control strategies with good effect, including anticipating trouble, diverting or redirecting attention, providing choices and explanations, enlisting cooperation, and suggesting rather than demanding. Numerous studies indicate that these approaches are associated with child compliance and that physical restraints, threats, and negative prohibitions are more likely to elicit both immediate noncompliance and ongoing power struggles (Belsky, Woodworth, & Crnic, 1996; Crockenberg & Litman, 1990; Kochanska, 1997). Furthermore, mothers who are able to set priorities appear to have an easier time. Thus it seems important to childproof the house and to ignore minor infractions of household rules in favor of more serious violations that involve safety hazards or that impinge on the rights of others. In one study (Zahn-Waxler et al., 1979), mothers who had clear priorities about what was and was not a serious transgression and who responded selectively to misbehavior with strong prohibitions paired with explanations had toddlers who exhibited more prosocial behavior and were more likely to make reparations for harm caused to others. Mothers who used more frequent prohibitions and failed to pair them with explanations and reasons had toddlers who were more likely to ignore maternal commands and less likely to behave prosocially. Kochanska (1997) has found that children who have a warm and positive relationship with their mothers are more likely to want to comply, and she has termed this "committed compliance," as distinct from children who comply out of fear of negative consequences. Committed compliance and a positive relationship are also seen as underlying self-control more generally and the development of conscience (Kochanska, 1997; Patterson, DeBaryshe, & Ramsey, 1989).

In general, then, studies indicate that limit setting is more effective when it occurs in the context of a positive mother–child relationship and provides educative guidance and clear expectations than when it is punitive and apparently arbitrary. This approach has been termed *authoritative* (as opposed to *authoritarian*) childrearing by Baumrind (1967), and it is characterized by respect for the child's rights and feelings, along with clear guidelines and expectations for mature and socially appropriate behavior. The ability to set appropriate limits and to engage in authoritative parenting undoubtedly depends on parental personality style, the understanding of young children's developmental needs, and age-appropriate expectations. In this context, it is worth noting that studies reveal that the terrible 2's are rarer than popular writings suggest (e.g., Belsky, Woodworth, & Crnic, 1996; Minton, Kagan, & Levine, 1971) and that extreme child noncompliance in the late toddler and early preschool periods often occurs when parents use inappropriate childrearing practices or fail to establish firm, consistent, child-centered controls (Belsky, Woodworth, & Crnic, 1996; Crockenberg & Litman, 1990).

Limit Setting with Hard-to-Manage Children

Although positive approaches to obtaining compliance and setting limits on child behavior may work with most children, mothers of children with behavior problems routinely complain that "nothing works!" Of course, by the time such children reach the clinician, the escalating, negative, and coercive cycle described by Patterson (1980) is well established, and it is difficult, if not impossible, to tease apart the direction of effects. These mothers may be utilizing harsh and negative disciplinary practices because their initial attempts at more low-key and subtle approaches proved frustrating and ineffective with angry, defiant, or inattentive children; or parents' initially harsh and demanding limit setting may have either inaugurated or escalated the cycle of child noncompliance. In either case, it is clear that patterns of child noncompliance and negative maternal control are highly correlated and built up over time, reflecting a history of ongoing negative and coercive transactions.

Several studies have examined disciplinary encounters with children identified as difficult or highly active. For example, it has been reported that toddlers who had been rated as difficult to handle in infancy were more likely to initiate behaviors that were forbidden or troublesome and, in general, to test limits at age 2 (Lee & Bates, 1985). Their mothers were more likely to employ power-assertive disciplinary techniques in response to these provocations, leading to a cycle of coercive and conflicted interactions. Gardner (1987, 1989) conducted naturalistic observations at home and found that mothers of highly aggressive preschoolers were more negative, less likely to engage their children in positive and proactive exchanges, and less likely to follow through when they did issue a prohibition than mothers of matched control children. In a second study of 3-year-olds with elevated behavior problem ratings who were observed in the laboratory during a toy cleanup procedure, Gardner, Sonuga-Barke, and Sayal (1999) did not find that mothers of problem children were less positive or child-centered in comparison with mothers of control children, but they did find that mothers of problem preschoolers were less likely to use proactive strategies such as anticipating trouble and redirecting activities. Rather, they were more likely to intervene in a reactive fashion after their children became noncompliant. Moreover, this interactive style predicted continuing problems at age 5, suggesting that it reflects a mutually antagonistic style of interaction that may resemble the coercive processes described by Patterson (1980). Speltz, DeKlyen, Greenberg, and Dryden (1995) also found that mothers of clinically referred preschool children with behavior problems were more negative and critical during an observation in the laboratory than mothers of comparison children.

In our own work (Campbell, Breaux, Ewing, Szumowski, & Pierce, 1986), we observed mother–child interaction during an unstructured play situation. Mothers of hard-to-manage toddlers and preschoolers redirected play activities more often than control mothers and provided more negative control statements; problem youngsters were more active and engaged in more aggressive play than controls. In our second cohort, mothers of hard-to-manage preschoolers were more negative and controlling when observed during a compliance task (toy cleanup), despite the fact that their children were not markedly more noncompliant than controls (Campbell, 1994). Finally, studies comparing clinically diagnosed hyperactive preschoolers and their mothers with control dyads indicate that hyperactive children are more negative and noncompliant during both free play and more demanding structured situations and that their mothers are more directive and less rewarding of independent play and compliance (Mash & Johnston, 1982). Patterson (1980) has conducted observations in the homes of families who sought help with management of aggressive preschoolers. His findings highlight the reciprocity inherent in these aversive interactions, as well as the child's typical role as initiator.

The Role of Fathers in Families with Hard-to-Manage Children

Parents often report that hard-to-manage children comply more readily with fathers than with mothers and that they are more likely to listen to their mothers when fathers are present. Both of these parental perceptions of child compliance patterns have been confirmed by observational studies conducted in the homes of young children (Lytton, 1980; Patterson, 1980). Patterson suggests that in two-parent families without behavior problem children mothers are the principal caretakers, although fathers contribute to childrearing both directly and indirectly, by supporting mothers in their childrearing and socialization efforts. However, in families with children who are difficult to control, mothers are more likely to function as "crisis managers" who must cope on a daily basis with a range of childrearing dilemmas and conflicts. Often fathers in such families withdraw to avoid dealing with unpleasant situations. This exaggerated role differentiation vis-à-vis childrearing is consonant with the complaints of many mothers of children with behavior problems who report feeling isolated and demoralized by their lonely battles for compliance and control (Mash & Johnston, 1983). On the other hand, in some families with preschoolers who have behavior problems, fathers are involved in childrearing, and there is evidence that negative and harsh control by fathers also is predictive of more severe problems as assessed not only by parents but also by teachers (DeKlyen et al., 1998).

When fathers severely curtail or ignore their childrearing responsibilities, there are obviously numerous ramifications throughout the family system. Their wives are likely to feel unsupported and abandoned by their husbands, fueling feelings of anger, resentment, and frustration. Such feelings may well be expressed in inconsistent, lax, or overly harsh discipline that further exacerbates the child's problems, as well as the ongoing hostilities between mother and child. Lack of paternal involvement in childrearing not only leaves the mother as the sole and unsupported agent of socialization but also deprives the young child of important experiences with an alternative role model and source of nurturance. Thus the psychological unavailability of some fathers of problem preschoolers, even in two-parent families, may contribute to the intensity and duration of mother–child conflict and to more general and persistent problems in socialization.

Lamb (1987b) emphasizes the important role played by fathers in helping children, especially young boys, establish sexual identity, internalize standards for behavior, and develop the capacity to regulate their own behavior. In addition, as noted earlier, the nature of father involvement in childrearing can have an indirect effect on the mother–child relationship, as well as on the quality of marital interaction (e.g., Belsky,

1984). Fathers who spend time with their preschoolers are cementing the father–child relationship and contributing to their children's sex role identity, cognitive and social development, and sense of self-worth. They also are indirectly supporting their wives in their childrearing efforts, something that may also strengthen the quality of both the marital relationship and the mother–child relationship. This aspect of parenting and marital interaction has been studied recently under the rubric of "coparenting," with obvious relevance for understanding children's adjustment (e.g., McHale & Rasmussen, 1998).

It should be emphasized that these comments apply whether the family functions as a "traditional" one (in which the mother has the major responsibility for childrearing and sex-role differentiation within the family is quite clear-cut) or a more "contemporary" arrangement (in which both parents share the childrearing, household chores, and career roles *relatively* equally). From the perspective of the child, the important factor is the degree to which both parents are involved in childrearing and how much they support each other in their childrearing efforts. Children can adapt to a variety of family organizations and structures provided they have a strong relationship with one, or preferably both, parents.

Mechanisms

The work reviewed so far makes it clear that parental behavior, in the context of other aspects of family functioning, is an important piece of the puzzle, accounting for variations in young children's cooperation and overall adjustment. What mechanisms may account for some of these associations? Several have been proposed. Attachment theorists suggest that the internal working model of the relationship and a child's sense of well-being derived from a secure attachment account for the association between childrearing and children's outcomes (e.g. Carlson & Sroufe, 1995). Others agree that the quality of the early parent–child relationship sets the stage for either harmonious interaction or frequent conflict (Kochanska, 1997; Maccoby & Martin, 1983; Patterson et al., 1989). It may be that the positive qualities of parental behavior that are associated with a secure attachment in infancy are modified and expanded as sensitive, responsive parents adjust to the differing requirements of toddlers and preschoolers and rely on proactive limit setting and gentle guidance to socialize their children (e.g., Crockenberg &

Litman, 1990; Kochanska, 1997). Conversely, some insensitive, irritated, or rejecting parents may have an especially difficult time coping with the transition from infancy to toddlerhood, when more active engagement and monitoring are required, and they may set harsh and inflexible limits on their toddlers, with few attempts to explain the reasons for their prohibitions and punishments. However, something about the quality of the parent–child relationship remains an important correlate of the child's adjustment. Such parent–child interactions are also likely to reflect aspects of the temperament or personality of both parents and child. Thus genetic predispositions in both the child and parents are undoubtedly accounting for some of the covariation in child behavior and parental control (Collins et al., 2000; Rutter et al., 1997). Modeling of parental problem solving and styles of emotion regulation are also important to consider, although again both gene–environment correlations and gene–environment interactions are relevant here as well.

Clinical Implications

Several of the children discussed in Chapter 3 illustrate the complex interactions between child characteristics and childrearing practices in contributing to the possible onset and persistence of problems or to the amelioration of early difficulties. In all four examples, infant difficultness of varying severity was reported, as indexed by behaviors such as excessive crying and unconsolability, irregular sleep patterns, and feeding problems. These reported behavior patterns probably reflect some endogenous infant characteristics, as well as parental expectations and interpretations of infant behavior (Bates, 1987). Parental approaches to dealing with these early difficulties appeared to set the stage for the development either of harmonious parent–child relations despite the problems or of an extremely tense and troubled relationship. Parents' philosophy of childrearing, flexibility, and the general affective tone of the relationship also were associated with the nature of mother–child disciplinary encounters later on during the preschool period. The nature and extent of paternal involvement in childrearing also seemed to contribute to the quality of the mother–child relationship, as well as to general family climate.

For example, Jamie L. was described as an irritable and fussy infant who was difficult to calm and who required little sleep. However, his parents appear to have handled his early demandingness with sensitivity and patience. Although at age 3, when he was seen in our project, he was quite noncompliant, aggressive, inattentive, and impulsive, the quality of the mother–child relationship did not appear to be seriously impaired. We were impressed with his mother's patience and supportiveness and with the warmth that characterized their interaction during play. Unlike some mother–child pairs in our study, Jamie and Mrs. L. did not become involved in negative, conflicted, and escalating coercive cycles of behavior. Mrs. L. realistically perceived Jamie as difficult to handle, but she also recognized his intelligence and creativity, and the positive affective bond between them was unmistakable. Mrs. L. remained patient and calm in her disciplinary encounters with Jamie. She was able to set clear and firm limits while also permitting him some degree of autonomy, for example, by providing alternatives and reasons. Mr. L. was also very involved in childrearing and provided his wife with needed time away from this difficult and demanding youngster. It appears that these parents were coping extremely well with Jamie's difficulties and that they provided an optimal environment for his growth and development, despite his problems with self-control and social interaction.

In contrast, Annie J.'s difficulties appeared to be related to a troubled mother–child interaction that began in early infancy. In speculating about the early development of Annie's problems, it is tempting to hypothesize that, based on maternal report and observed behavior in toddlerhood, Annie developed an insecure, resistant attachment to her mother. This troubled relationship was reflected in her excessive anxiety, clinginess, and separation distress and in the absence of warmth and reciprocity observed in their interaction. Furthermore, Mrs. J.'s relative insensitivity to Annie's needs as a 2½-year-old and her ineffective management strategies make it likely that she was not particularly sensitive or accurate in interpreting Annie's social communciations when she was an infant. This hypothesis gains support from Mrs. J.'s inconsistent reports and somewhat distorted expectations. Annie's role in this situation is less clear. She may indeed have been a difficult infant, as Mrs. J. described, or she may have developed into a demanding and whiny youngster as her needs were constantly frustrated by a mother who was intrusive but not warm and affectionate and who was also highly anxious and insecure in her new role, as well as ignorant of the needs of young infants. This interpretation is consistent with the views of Greenberg, Speltz, and DeKlyen (1993), who suggested that behaviors labeled by mothers as discipline problems in early childhood may, instead, reflect the frustrated attempts of toddlers to gain attention and nurturance from unresponsive or rejecting caregivers.

By the time Annie was a toddler, she and her mother were locked in a daily struggle for control. Mrs. J., unable to set firm, consistent, and reasonable limits, tended to be inconsistent, unpredictable, and overbearing, resorting to power-assertive disciplinary methods such as threatening and shouting. However, these methods proved ineffective, serving only to fuel Annie's noncompliant behavior. Furthermore, in the absence of a close, positive mother–daughter relationship, Annie had little incentive to respond cooperatively to Mrs. J.'s requests and tended to vent her frustration and confusion by challenging her mother's authority. Mrs. J., in turn, anticipating a struggle, approached Annie in ways guaranteed to elicit anger and defiance. Interparental disagreement over childrearing and interparental inconsistency probably contributed to this troubled mother–child relationship. Finally, inappropriate developmental expectations appeared to exacerbate interactive problems, as well. Mrs. J.'s beliefs about appropriate behavior and her negative perceptions of Annie seemed quite resistant to change. Although Mr. J. was involved in some caretaking and although he tended to see Annie in a more positive light than did his wife, it does not appear that his involvement was sufficient in either quantity or positivity to counteract the problems in the mother–daughter relationship. Furthermore, there is some suggestion that marital tension contributed to maternal insensitivity, impatience, and anger that was directed primarily at Annie.

Although high standards for behavior and somewhat inappropriate developmental expectations also characterized Teddy M.'s parents, they were able to modify their perceptions and to gain greater understanding of his developmental needs. Their ability to change their expectations may well have averted the development of more serious problems. Further, changes in both Teddy and his parents occurred in the context of a positive parent–child relationship and parental unity concerning childrearing expectations and goals.

These clinical examples support suggestions from both our own work (Campbell, 1995, 1997; Campbell et al., 1996) and that of others (DeKlyen et al., 1998) that high levels of ongoing parent–child conflict and negative maternal attitudes are associated with the onset and persistence of problems in young children. Alternatively, changes in parental attitudes and expectations can ease parent–child conflicts. Yet some problems do persist despite optimal childrearing efforts.

FAMILY CLIMATE

Not surprisingly, parent–child conflict rarely occurs in isolation from other factors. Numerous studies indicate a relationship between a disturbed family environment and children's problems (see reviews by Campbell, 1995; Cummings et al., 2000; Davies & Cummings, 1994; Emery, 1999; Fincham & Osborn, 1993; Parke & Buriel, 1998). In general, childhood problems, especially externalizing problems in boys, are associated not only with parent–child discord but also with marital distress, separation and divorce, parental psychopathology, maternal depression and general malaise, and more general family stresses, including unemployment and poor housing (Greenberg et al., 1999; McLoyd, 1990, 1998; Sameroff et al., 1993). The nature of these relationships is complex, with both high levels of marital conflict and critical parenting occurring together, as well as with other indicators of family adversity. Many of these indicators of family climate are highly intercorrelated with each other, as well as with methods of childrearing; and they may have direct effects on the child, as well as indirect effects mediated through less involved or more negative parenting (e.g., Webster-Stratton & Hammond, 1999). Thus the association between children's problems and any one risk factor can rarely be examined in isolation from other associated factors. In addition, as noted earlier, each of these factors will have complex ramifications throughout the family system, impinging on the child both directly and indirectly through its effect on parents and siblings.

Marital Distress and Conflict

A relationship between marital distress and childhood problems has been established in numerous empirical investigations (e.g., see Cummings et al., 2000; Emery, 1999; Fincham & Osborn, 1993; Hetherington, Bridges, & Insabella, 1998; Parke & Buriel, 1998, for reviews). In general, studies suggest that boys are more vulnerable to the effects of marital discord than girls are and that the result is more likely to be acting-out, undercontrolled behavior characterized by noncompliance and aggression than overcontrolled behavior characterized by social withdrawal and anxiety. This conclusion may be premature, as overcontrolled behaviors are more likely to be overlooked and less likely to lead to clinic referral. In addition, as Emery (1999) has suggested, boys may be more readily upset by family conflict and may express this in a range of symptoms, with externalizing ones most easily identified. Longitudinal, prospective studies do indicate that both interparental disagreement over childrearing and marital discord are precursors of childhood problems (Block, Block, & Morrison, 1981; Richman et al., 1982; Shaw et al., 1996), and it has been suggested that overt marital hostility and anger are more closely associated with children's externalizing problems than marital distress per se (Davies & Cummings, 1998; Fincham & Osborn, 1993). Thus it is well established that marital turmoil can lead to problems in children, and it is likely that a tension-ridden and conflicted home environment will have both direct and indirect effects on children, especially preschool children.

For example, Cummings, Zahn-Waxler, and Radke-Yarrow (1981, 1984) studied young children's reactions to expressions of anger and affection in the home and noted that even very young children responded with anxiety, overt distress, and anger to expressions of anger by others, whether they themselves were involved in the conflict or were merely bystanders. Some toddlers attempted to comfort a distressed adult or to reconcile angry individuals. When older children (6–7) were witnesses to confrontations between adults or between adults and children, they were even more likely to attempt to protect one member of the couple or to mediate the dispute. There is little doubt that young children are highly responsive to the intensity and quality of the affective exchanges that occur in their immediate environment, especially among close family members.

When children witness frequent arguments and interparental strife, feelings of anxiety and insecurity are likely to result, children's perceptions of themselves and of their parents are likely to be affected, and the nature of family interaction patterns is likely to be changed. For example, children who attempt to intervene in parental disputes and are unsuccessful may feel both guilty and incompetent. If, in fact, the child is the focus of the parental discord, as is often the case, the child may feel even worse. Even very young children may be enlisted as the ally of one parent against another, possibly also contributing to feelings of anger and guilt. Such feelings may be expressed in a variety of ways, including social withdrawal and tearfulness, aggression toward others, or anger and noncompliance. These responses may be mediated through the emotional contagion observed in very young children, as well as through imitation and modeling. Because parents serve as the most important agents of socialization, parents' styles of solving interpersonal problems and regulating negative emotions may become models for their children. In this manner, children may imitate hostility and anger, having learned that this is a usual and acceptable way to deal with interpersonal disputes. The preceding constitute some of the direct effects of marital discord on children's behavior.

Davies and Cummings (1994, 1998) have proposed the "emotional security hypothesis" to account for some of the findings linking marital discord to children's problem behavior. Briefly, it is suggested that high levels of conflict between parents undermine children's feelings of safety and security and that they develop internal working models of family relationships as anxiety producing, possibly because they worry about family stability or about being the brunt of parental anger. Moreover, the experience of interparental anger forces young children to regulate their own negative emotions, which they may do by withdrawing, intervening, or expressing anger and hostility themselves. In any case, the high levels of negative emotion aroused in a tense and conflict-ridden family, especially one in which the children often witness parental arguments and/or physical abuse, tax the ability of young children to cope with their high levels of negative emotion and also undermine feelings of safety and support in the family context. Such feelings then may lead to symptomatic behavior, either anxiety, sadness, and withdrawal; acting-out, explosive behavior; or a combination of both. Like attachment theory, this perspective is based on the idea that the family should serve as a safe haven and source of support for young children, and it recognizes that anger, conflict, and physical aggression will undermine feelings of safety, comfort, and trust. Family conflict may also interfere with young children's attempts to regulate their own negative emotions. Thus the link between marital discord and children's problems is partially mediated by children's emotional reactions to conflict and their immature attempts to cope with their own feelings, as well as to make sense of the feelings of those around them.

In addition, there are pervasive effects that are indirect, mediated by the impact of marital distress on the parents and their ability to fulfill parental roles. Parents, when they are engaged in constant bickering, may have little tolerance left for the typical behaviors of young children. They also may have less energy available to provide emotional and instrumental support to children, leaving the children feeling frustrated, unloved, or neglected. These feelings may trigger defiance, demandingness, and anger in some children; sadness, fearfulness, and withdrawal in others; or a combination of angry outbursts and social withdrawal in still others. Further, some distressed parents may unrealistically expect young children to meet some of their own emotional needs, those that would be more appropriately met by their spouses or other adults. Finally, parents, preoccupied with their own problems, may become ineffective and inconsistent disciplinarians, further contributing to the development of behavior problems in their children. Thus, by draining parental resources, marital dysfunction may take its toll on the children by leaving them bereft of adequate parenting. Younger children are likely to be especially vulnerable because they are in need of more sustained involvement and cognitive and social stimulation from parents and because they are less able to separate themselves from parental squabbles by spending prolonged periods of time away from home with peers.

More recent research on marital conflict has moved from a general focus on distress to interest in more specific aspects of the marital relationship that may be especially relevant to understanding the effect of marital conflict on young children. Belsky (Belsky, Woodworth, & Crnic, 1996) and others (e.g., McHale & Rasmussen, 1998) have discussed "coparenting," or the degree to which parents work together, support each other, and share childrearing goals or, conversely, the degree to which either one parent must shoulder most childrearing tasks or to which there is conflict over discrepant childrearing styles and goals. Not surprisingly, studies indicate that low levels of coparenting are associated with problems in young children (Belsky, Woodworth, & Crnic, 1996; McHale & Rasmussen, 1998). In a related vein, Jouriles and colleagues (1991) have studied parental disagreements over childrearing that appear to predict children's externalizing problems over and above general levels of marital distress. This finding was recently confirmed by Shaw et al. (1996) in a sample of low-income families with young children.

The relationship between marital discord and children's problems is frequently a bidirectional one. The association between parental reports of marital conflict and child behavior problems may reflect the fact that having a difficult child can increase tensions within a family. The child's problem behaviors may elicit latent marital conflicts, become the focus of marital disagreements, or exacerbate already existing marital dysfunction. For example, parents may engage in intense disagreements over how to handle a difficult child (e.g., Jouriles et al., 1991), with one parent advocating sterner discipline than the other. Conflict over childrearing may become the overt focus of anger and discord, masking other ongoing problems in communication that are more subtle or more threatening to confront. The child's difficulties also may bring other problems to the fore. For instance, conflicts over finances, in-laws, or the distribution of responsibilities may become more salient as children's needs change and they become more demanding or as their problems worsen. Parents may also use a child's problems to dramatize other marital issues or to retaliate against the spouse. In clinical interviews, it is not uncommon to witness one parent assigning blame to the other for the child's difficulties or for parents to engage in mutual recriminations. A mother may attribute a child's problem behavior to lack of paternal involvement, or a father may blame his wife's laxness or incompetence for his child's lack of control or problems with peers. Negative rather than supportive interactions between parents regarding a child's problems are a clear signal that marital stresses are relevant to an understanding of the child's difficulties, whether they appear to figure as an etiological factor or a factor contributing to environmental stresses that exacerbate and/or maintain ongoing problems within the family system.

Marital Separation and Divorce

Although some children may fare better in a harmonious one-parent family than in a discordant two-parent family (Emery, 1999), especially when one parent is seriously disturbed or abusive (Wallerstein & Kelly, 1980), accumulating evidence also links marital disruption to both short-term stress reactions and longer term adjustment difficulties in children (Emery, 1999; Hetherington et al., 1998; Parke & Buriel, 1998). For example, studies confirm that separation and divorce are more common in the lives of young children with problems than in those of controls or nonreferred age-mates. Both clinical descriptions (Wallerstein & Kelly, 1980) and more controlled studies (Hetherington,

1989; Hetherington et al., 1998) suggest that preschool children, especially boys, have a particularly difficult time adjusting to parental divorce, reacting with nightmares, regression, guilt, fear of abandonment, and intense longing for the absent parent. Boys may have an especially difficult time partly because they are most often losing the same-sex parent and partly because they are more vulnerable to problems (Hetherington, 1989).

The negative effect of marital separation on children, in addition to the separation itself, also is likely to be a reaction to other life changes and losses that occur in tandem with the loss of the departed parent. Marital separation usually occurs in the context of a number of pervasive life changes (Hetherington et al., 1998), such as a decline in living standards, changes in living arrangements, a move to a new neighborhood, and changes in relationships with both parents. Thus the young child may have to adapt to altered routines, a new babysitter or childcare setting, a new school, and the establishment of new friendships while coping with the loss or partial loss of both parents. Both Hetherington (1989) and Wallerstein and Kelly (1980) describe the diminished ability of angry, depressed custodial mothers to provide adequate parenting in the immediate aftermath of the separation, the time at which the preschooler is especially vulnerable to feelings of loss, rejection, guilt, and self-blame.

These changes in family structure and functioning are also associated with increased mother–child conflict (Hetherington, 1989; Wallerstein & Kelly, 1980), especially between custodial mothers and their preschool sons. The combined effects of a distressed youngster, mourning for the absent father, and a depressed, angry, and overwhelmed mother result in heightened conflicts over discipline, and these negative interactions spill over to the preschool classroom, in which young children from divorced or separated families also are more likely to get into conflicts with peers and to demonstrate a diminished capacity for independent and creative play. Although preschoolers of both sexes show profound reactions to the initial separation, girls and their mothers are more likely to reestablish harmonious relationships by 18 to 24 months postdivorce, whereas mother–son conflict is more likely to persist.

It is clear from the extensive literature on the impact of divorce that young children show particularly dramatic reactions to family breakup, that reunion fantasies persist for many years, and that the capacity of young children from divorced families to adapt to change ultimately depends on the ability of both parents to maintain strong, positive, and supportive relationships with their children, while also shielding them from interparental conflict. When children are cut off from contact with the noncustodial parent, when they are enlisted as allies of one parent against the other, or when they are used as message carriers, the likelihood is high that problems will be both prolonged and severe.

Clinical Implications

The case of Robbie S., who was introduced in the previous chapter, illustrates a number of these themes. Despite a good relationship with a competent and devoted mother, Robbie and his sister became the focus of early marital conflict, with their unpredictable and often unavailable father blaming Mrs. S. for Robbie's difficulties. Once his parents separated, Robbie became embroiled in their battles as a message carrier, and he contributed to the heightened tension by provoking both parents with stories of the other. Clinically, Robbie exhibited all the symptoms described by Wallerstein and Kelly (1980), including regression, self-blame, fear of abandonment, intense concern about the absent father, and elaborate reunion fantasies. These themes were apparent in his play and conversations. Furthermore, reunion fantasies appeared to spur him on to provoke his parents, as their only communication consisted of mutual recriminations about who was to blame for Robbie's ongoing difficulties. As conflict between his parents intensified, Robbie's problems became more serious, spilling over to his once good relationship with peers and resulting in poor school achievement. Robbie's problems appear to have stabilized at a fairly severe level, clearly fueled by his troubled family situation and by his difficulty adapting to parental divorce.

Parental Psychopathology

Numerous studies have demonstrated a link between psychological problems in parents and difficulties in their preschool children. These range from studies in which maternal self-reports of depressive symptomatology and somatic complaints have been correlated with other indicators of child functioning (e.g, NICHD Early Child Care Research Network, 1999) to more detailed clinical studies employing careful diagnostic appraisal of parents (e.g., DeMulder & Radke-Yarrow, 1991;

Sameroff, Seifer, & Zax, 1982; Teti, Gelfand, Messinger, & Isabella, 1995). In general, the focus has been on maternal depression, although a few studies also have examined mothers with schizophrenia and other diagnoses (Goodman & Brumley, 1990; Sameroff et al., 1982). Longitudinal studies of mentally ill parents document a relationship between parental psychopathology and young children's early development and psychosocial adjustment (DeMulder & Radke-Yarrow, 1991; Sameroff et al., 1982; Teti et al., 1995). In general, these studies indicate that infants, toddlers, and preschoolers with seriously disturbed parents show less adaptive behavior with parents and peers when observed at home, in settings with other children, and in the laboratory. In addition, the severity and chronicity of the parental disturbance may be more important than specific diagnosis (NICHD Early Child Care Research Network, 1999; Sameroff et al., 1982).

The mechanisms and processes linking maternal psychiatric disturbance to children's difficult behavior are, of course, multifaceted. Underlying genetic vulnerabilities are likely to be important, but research on young children has focused on more proximal mechanisms, most notably the parenting behavior of depressed women (e.g., Campbell & Cohn, 1997; Field, 1992; DeMulder & Radke-Yarrow, 1991; Teti et al., 1995). For example, women who are depressed are less involved, responsive, or sensitive with their infants and toddlers (e.g., Campbell, Cohn, & Meyers, 1995; DeMulder & Radke-Yarrow, 1991; NICHD Early Child Care Research Network, 1999). Moreover, by toddlerhood, mothers must put effort into setting limits and modeling appropriate social behavior, something that may be especially difficult for seriously depressed women with few psychosocial resources. On the other hand, many women who are depressed function adequately as parents (e.g., Campbell & Cohn, 1997; Frankel & Harmon, 1996). Attempts to reconcile these conflicting findings have emphasized the severity and chronicity of the maternal disorder (e.g., Campbell et al., 1995; Frankel & Harmon, 1996; NICHD Early Child Care Research Network, 1999) and the fact that maternal depression often co-occurs with other risk factors, such as marital distress, low social support, and financial difficulties (Cicchetti, Rogosch, & Toth, 1998; NICHD Early Child Care Research Network, 1999). More chronically depressed women coping with more psychosocial stress are less likely to respond sensitively to their infants or to use proactive and consistent controls with their toddlers (Zahn-Waxler, Iannotti, Cummings, & Denham, 1990); their children are more likely to show disorganized patterns of attachment (Campbell et al., 2001; Cicchetti et al., 1998; Teti et al., 1995), less co-operation across settings with parents, caregivers, and peers, and poorer cognitive development (NICHD Early Child Care Research Network, 1999).

Even in the absence of serious psychopathology, mothers who report more depression and anxiety also are more likely to seek pediatric (Wolkind, 1985) and mental health services (Shepherd et al., 1971) for their children. It appears that maternal mood influences both the quality of caretaking and a woman's interpretation of and tolerance for her preschooler's behavior. Women who feel fatigued, dispirited, and unsupported have less tolerance for the typical behavior of preschool-age children, which may lead them to label even age-appropriate behavior as problematic and to seek help for problems that other parents would just ignore.

Taken together, these studies indicate a link between parental psychological distress, especially depressed mood and other psychiatric disturbances, and young children's social-emotional development. As already documented, it is generally accepted that the development of children's problems derives from a transactional process by which children with genetic vulnerabilities to disorder are raised in disturbed environments in which a number of developmental needs are inadequately met. In considering the phenomenology of maternal depression, it is possible to speculate about the ways in which symptoms of ongoing and severe depression may interfere with parenting. Lack of energy, negative and irritable mood, feelings of despondency, and flat affect may be reflected in less engagement and warmth; less responsiveness; less proactive limit setting, teaching, and conversation; poorer modeling of positive and effective conflict resolution strategies; and more anger directed at the child or other family members. In this way the link between maternal depressive symptoms and children's problem behavior is partially mediated by harsh, insensitive, or uninvolved parenting (Harnish, Dodge, Valente, and the Conduct Problems Prevention Research Group, 1995; NICHD Early Child Care Research Network, 1999), as well as other problems in the family systems of depressed women (Cummings & Davies, 1999).

The work of Cummings and Davies (1999) also suggests that disturbed parents would be expected to elicit a range of negative emotions in their children, because young children tend to mirror the affective exchanges of those in their immediate environment. Their children may be less empathic and prosocial with peers, and they are likely to develop lower self-esteem and feelings of self-efficacy. These direct effects of living with a disturbed parent are thought to interact with biological factors to produce disturbances in offspring.

In addition, however, maternal depression is associated with more general risk factors, such as psychological disturbance in the spouse, more marital discord and divorce (Cicchetti et al., 1998), and less social support (NICHD Early Child Care Research Network, 1999), further compounding the effect of parental illness on the child. Thus the young child with a severely disturbed parent is also more likely to be deprived of support from a second, intact and emotionally competent parent who might compensate for the inadequacies of the ill parent. There is some evidence that other adults can buffer young children from the negative impact of poor parenting. In addition, other adults can serve as role models and can provide sufficient support to poorly functioning parents to help them overcome some of their deficits. However, the increased social isolation and lack of support from other significant adults often experienced by children living in disturbed families also may compound the effects of poor parenting and inconsistent discipline. In this manner these more general factors also may be contributing to the association between parental psychiatric disturbance and poor child outcomes, in line with multiple-risk models (Cicchetti et al., 1998; Sameroff et al., 1993).

Clinical Implications

Both Robbie's and Annie's problems may have resulted in part from the effect of psychological disorder on parental behavior (both childrearing and family conflict) in interaction with biological vulnerabilities. Annie's mother did not acknowledge problems in herself or her marriage, although she appeared highly anxious and somewhat depressed. It is not inconceivable that her relatively negative perceptions of Annie and her poor tolerance for her daughter's behavior partly reflected her own feelings of anger, despair, and helplessness in the face of marital problems and/or her own depression. Robbie's family had a positive history of depression and antisocial behavior. In addition, his father appeared quite impaired, although he did not have a history of psychiatric contacts. In our formulation of Robbie's problems, it was logical to consider the possibility that a biological vulnerability to disorder was interacting with the severe psychosocial stress Robbie was under, thereby exacerbating and maintaining his symptoms.

SOCIAL CONTEXT

As noted in Chapter 1, a variety of other environmental factors also have both a direct effect on the child and an indirect influence mediated through the parents. These have been discussed in detail by Bronfenbrenner (1986) in the context of an ecological model of development. Relevant factors that influence the quality of a preschooler's life, such as the availability of social support for the family and material and community resources, must be considered here. These include financial resources, quality of housing, nutrition, the quality and availability of health care, parental educational levels, the nature and stability of parental employment, the quality of child care or preschool programs, and the presence in the community of extended family members or close friends.

Social Support

The availability of social support from family members or friends appears to be especially important for the mental health of adults and for optimal child development (Brown & Harris, 1980; Cochran & Brassard, 1979). Women who feel supported by others are better able to cope with difficult and irritable infants (Crockenberg, 1981). Women who consider their support adequate also are more responsive to their infants' communications (Crnic, Greenberg, Ragozin, Robinson, & Basham, 1983). Conversely, socially isolated women with limited social support and few friends are more likely to perceive their children negatively and to engage in coercive interactions that have the potential to become abusive (Wahler, 1980). Social support in the form of assistance with child care, advice, modeling of caretaking, and limit setting, as well as more general emotional support, should all have an effect on parental behavior.

In addition, Cochran and Brassard (1979) emphasize the role of extended family and adult family friends in facilitating cognitive and social development in young children by direct social interaction with them and by indirectly modeling skills for parents. Other familiar and caring adults in the child's environment may take over important care-taking functions when a parent is ill or otherwise incapacitated. Studies suggest that other adults in the child's social milieu may serve a buffering role, protecting children from the negative effects of parental unavailability occasioned by mental illness, divorce, or other mental stresses.

The Quality and Availability of Child Care

As more and more mothers of infants and preschoolers juggle careers and family responsibilities, the importance of adequate, accessible, and affordable child care also becomes crucial to child and family well-being. The substitute caregiver becomes an integral member of the child's social network, with an important role to play in providing nurturance and socialization experiences. The effect of child care on the development of infants and toddlers has become a highly volatile and contentious issue. For example, Belsky (1988) has argued that infants placed in more than 20 hours per week of nonparental care during the first year are at risk to develop insecure attachments to parents, as well as a range of later difficulties, including poor self-regulation, noncompliance, and aggression toward peers, that are possibly mediated by the insecure attachment to parents. Others have countered that a more contextual view is necessary and that the effects of child care cannot be determined without also examining family factors and quality of care, as well as child characteristics (Clarke-Stewart, 1989; Hungerford, Brownell, & Campbell, 2000; Lamb, 1998). The debate has focused on the relative importance of such factors as age of entry into care, quality of care, type of care, and hours in care, in tandem with an examination of parental behavior and other family factors that may mediate or moderate the effect of child-care experiences on young children (NICHD Early Child Care Research Network, 1997b, 1998, 2001).

Thus any report of purported negative effects of child care must take into account structural and process aspects of child-care quality (e.g., child-to-caregiver ratio and group size, caregiver training, staff turnover, caregiver responsiveness, sensitivity, and age-appropriate stimulation), as well as other child-care parameters, as these factors have been shown to influence children's development (Hungerford et al., 2000; Lamb, 1998; NICHD Early Child Care Research Network, 2002b).

In addition, family factors such as social class and educational level, parental involvement, and marital status influence the nature of the care parents seek for their children and interact with child-care quality to determine outcome (e.g., Howes & Olenick, 1986; NICHD Early Child Care Research Network, 1997a, 1997b). Although Belsky has emphasized the potential negative effects of day care (Belsky, 1988, 2001), others have noted that there are positive benefits when children are in high-quality programs (Lamb, 1998; Ramey & Ramey, 1998). These include greater competence with peers, improved sociability and prosocial behavior, and enhanced language development (Hungerford et al., 2000; NICHD Early Child Care Research Network, 2000b). In addition, type of care appears to make a difference, with some evidence suggesting that children fare best in high-quality centers (NICHD Early Child Care Research Network, 1999, 2000b) and worst in unregulated family day-care homes or in relative care (Kontos, Howes, Shinn, & Galinsky, 1995).

The NICHD Study of Early Child Care, a large-scale, 10-site, longitudinal study of the effects of infant child care on young children's development, is unique in that child-care effects are considered only in the context of family factors and in that child-care quality was studied intensively. Results do not consistently support a negative effect of nonmaternal care. Rather, in line with more complex ecological and transactional models, family factors, especially the quality of parent–child interactions, have been shown to be most central to young children's development, although quality of child care is also important. For example, contrary to the findings of Belsky and Rovine (1988), there were no main effects of child-care attendance on children's attachment security at 15 months. Infants who were either in care or at home were equally likely to be secure or insecure, and the strongest predictor of insecurity was maternal sensitivity. However, when child-care effects were found, they were found among infants whose mothers were less sensitive, suggesting an interaction between quality of care at home and aspects of the child-care experience in the first year of life. That is, infants were more likely to be insecure when *both* maternal and caregiver responsiveness was low or when children with less responsive and sensitive mothers were in unstable child care or in many hours of child care, consistent with a multiple-risk-factor model.

Children's compliance, self-regulation, peer competence, and behavior problems at 24 and 36 months were predicted by earlier family variables and quality of care, with family variables carrying much more weight than parameters of child care, including amount, type, or quality. Effects in these analyses were additive, with child-care quality adding to the variability in outcomes over and above family resources and mother–child relationship variables (NICHD Early Child Care Research Network, 1997b, 1998, 2002b). In addition, at both 54 months and kindergarten age, quality of care was predictive of better cognitive and language functioning. In contrast, hours in care also predicted caregiver ratings of problem behaviors at 54 months and both maternal and teacher ratings at kindergarten age, even after family variables and child-care quality were controlled. This suggests that children who spend long hours away from home in early childhood, especially in group settings, may engage in more structured activities that support cognitive development but may also have difficulty regulating their own behavior, especially aggression toward peers and compliance with adults. They also appear to crave more adult attention than children in fewer hours of care (NICHD Early Child Care Research Network, 2001b).

Suffice it to say that child care, whether in home or in a center, must provide children with adequate numbers of familiar, consistent, warm, and responsive caregivers who have both a genuine concern for children and some basic knowledge of child development. Unfortunately, there is a serious shortage of child care, even care of only moderate quality. Furthermore, the lack of uniform federal standards for day-care centers and the limited controls on family day-care homes mean that many settings are understaffed, must rely on untrained workers, and are plagued by high staff turnover, all of which have been shown to be detrimental to young children (Kontos et al., 1995; Phillips, 1988; Whitebook, Howes, & Phillips, 1990). The result of this child-care crisis is that those children most in need of high-quality substitute care are often those who are least likely to receive it. Rather, children from distressed or disorganized families are most likely to receive custodial care in substandard facilities rather than stimulating and nurturing care that might help them to overcome problems (Lamb, 1998; Scarr, 1998; Zigler & Gilman, 1996). This is true despite the fact that we know enough about the needs of young children to assume that higher quality care may serve a compensatory function for children at risk and may prove to be an important venue for primary prevention in the future (Ramey & Ramey, 1998).

Cultural Factors

Cultural beliefs and values about childrearing, children's roles in the family, and children's rights and responsibilities also influence parental behavior toward children and the nature of parent–child relationships (Parke & Buriel, 1998). Subgroups within North American society differ widely in beliefs about such questions as what constitutes effective and appropriate disciplinary practices. Some groups value reasoning and explanation, whereas others consider physical punishment not only acceptable but also necessary. Moreover, there is evidence that cultural and ecological factors interact with childrearing styles. For example, evidence shows that in dangerous inner city neighborhoods stricter use of limit setting and control serve as protective factors (Deater-Deckard, Dodge, Bates, & Pettit, 1996), especially when paired with high levels of warmth (McLoyd, 1998). Cultural pressures to excel intellectually differ, as do expectations for mature behavior within the family setting. The limits of acceptable behavior at different ages also vary with cultural values, for example, with regard to the expression of aggression within the family and the peer group. These and other cultural variables have an important influence on family organization, role assignments, communication patterns, childrearing strategies, and affect expression, all of which ultimately affect family climate and child development.

Clinical Implications

Several parents have called our project to seek advice about their children's difficulties in child care and at home. The similarity among these cases was striking in terms of presenting complaints, although they differed in complexity. In each instance, parents called the project after their preschool-age son was threatened with expulsion from a child-care center; complaints focused on marked aggression toward peers (including biting), noncompliance with staff, tantrums and noncompliance at home, and intense sibling conflict and jealousy over parental attention. In one instance, a boy of 3 was adjusting to a younger sibling who was becoming mobile and sociable. He and his younger sister were in a high-quality center for less than 20 hours per week. The family situation appeared stable, although his parents were confused and baffled about how to deal with the boy's aggression toward his sister and toward other children. It is noteworthy that this child was solicitous of his sister when at the child-care center; his aggression toward her was evident only when he had to share his parents with her. In this example, it appeared that the combined stress of coping with an appealing younger sibling and adjusting to a child-care setting was more than this youngster could handle, and he was expressing his upset and confusion by lashing out. He may not have been ready for out-of-home care; also, the combination of fewer hours with his mother and having to share her time and attention may have been too much for him. Suggestions were made about increasing his individual, special time with each parent and about handling the aggression and tantrums firmly and consistently.

In several other instances, however, the issues were more complex. Children's difficulties occurred in the context of high levels of family stress, including financial pressures, job stresses, marital discord, and difficulties with extended family. The quality of the mother–child relationships in these families was very poor, with mothers appearing abrupt, uninvolved, depressed, and drained. These mothers were so immersed in and overwhelmed by their own problems that they appeared unable to take their child's perspective or to recognize that 3- and 4-year-olds require individual attention, nurturance, warmth, and support from a consistent adult. These parents worked long hours in high-pressure jobs, and their preschoolers spent from 50 to 60 hours a week in center care. Despite the pressures on these mothers, their husbands were less involved than they were in child care.

When we visited these homes and observed these youngsters in our laboratory playroom, as well as in their child-care settings, we were struck by their neediness. These were young children who cooperated readily with us and their mothers during our home visit and playroom observations. They blossomed during the testing portions of the sessions, when they received the undivided attention of a friendly, supportive adult; they also reveled in the opportunity to come alone with their mothers to our playroom and even willingly cleaned up the toys at the end of the play period, something they would never willingly do at home. However, observations in their child-care settings revealed socially isolated children who were relatively ignored by peers and caregivers. In one instance, the staff at the center was clearly mishandling the child's problems, possibly exacerbating his difficulties and also indicating an extremely poor understanding of young children's emotional needs and level of cognitive development. This 3-year-old was isolated often and threatened with expulsion. Center staff were abrupt and irritated with him, even when he was behaving appropriately (and even with our observer in the center). The director suggested to this child's parents that he be banished to his room as soon as he arrived at home, in order to punish him for his misbehavior. Of course, this was just what this very needy and anxious youngster, who obviously craved time with and attention from his parents, did not require. These examples certainly do not indict all child-care settings, but they highlight the complex interactions among parenting skills and resources, family stresses, and the nature of the child-care setting. In particular, they underline the importance of well-trained, psychologically minded child-care staff who are sensitive to the meaning of young children's behavior and able to recognize that behavior problems are often a signal of unhappiness, anxiety, and distress.

SUMMARY

A number of variables associated with the development of problems in preschoolers have been reviewed in this and preceding chapters. These include child characteristics, parenting behaviors, family composition and interaction patterns, and factors in the family's wider social environment. The complex direct and indirect relationships among relevant factors were depicted in Chapter 1, Figure 1. In general, the transactions over time between child characteristics (including possible biological vulnerability, personality and temperamental dispositions, and developmental needs and competencies) and parenting factors (primarily the quality of parental affective involvement with the child and childrearing approaches) are the strongest predictors of children's social and emotional functioning. However, family climate, as indexed by the quality of the marital relationship, family composition, and parental personality and psychological well-being, also appears to affect the child's psychosocial adaptation. Family climate appears to have both a direct and an indirect impact on children, mediated through the effects of the family environment on parental availability, sensitivity, and childrearing strategies. Finally, more general aspects of the psychosocial environment, including the quality and availability of social support for parents, the nature and availability of institutional supports, and the availability of material resources, affect the child both directly and indirectly. Such factors, however, have their greatest impact on the child via their effects on parental well-being, the level of stresses within the family, and the ability of parents to carry out their parenting functions. In this context, the issue of child care was highlighted, as it has particular relevance for parents and young children.

Although all these factors appear important when problems are conceptualized in general or abstract terms, particular factors appear more relevant than others when individual children are considered. That is, although various factors converge to produce problems, the mix of relevant factors probably varies from child to child (the principle of equifinality). Thus, for the children discussed earlier, different aspects of child–family transactions seemed salient. For example, in considering Jamie's difficulties, biological vulnerabilities or personality dispositions (i.e., within-child factors) appeared most relevant, as other obvious family contributors to childhood problems were not in evidence. Moreover, it was our clinical impression that Jamie's problems were mitigated by a stable and supportive family environment in which stresses were minimal and his unique needs were respected and responded to by caring and concerned parents. Teddy's family environment was likewise positive, characterized by parental unity and mutual support. The early conflicted and negative transactions between Teddy and his parents, especially in view of their high standards and expectations for maturity and compliance, had the potential to escalate into more serious difficulties. However, it appears that parental flexibility, in tandem with developmental changes in Teddy's social understanding and behavioral control, ultimately were associated with the resolution of early difficulties.

Annie's continued problems may be interpreted to illustrate the importance of early mother–infant reciprocity and positive affective engagement, as well as the escalation of mother–child conflict over time. These problems occurred in the context of unrealistic maternal expectations and inflexible childrearing strategies that failed to accommodate to the child's emotional or developmental needs. These difficulties were compounded by limited paternal support and the possibility that there were additional problems within the family system. Finally, Robbie illustrates the complex interactions among possible biological vulnerability, parental personality problems, and chronic ongoing family disruption and turmoil. Furthermore, his problems worsened, despite an apparently warm and positive mother–child relationship.

In summary, then, multiple factors within the family and the wider social environment interact with child characteristics, and together they converge to create problems in children. However, problems in individual children probably develop from different combinations of factors, with different implications for treatment and for long-term outcome. These issues are addressed in subsequent chapters.

CHAPTER 5

Sibling Relationships and Young Children's Development

Sibling relations figure prominently in any consideration of the development of preschoolers, because many preschool-age children have to cope with the birth of a sibling, and many others must adjust to the role of being the younger brother or sister. Developmental psychologists have only begun to systematically examine the emergence of complex and affectively laden sibling relationships in the past 20 years. The interested reader is referred to several comprehensive review articles and books (Dunn, 1983, 1985; Dunn & Kendrick, 1982); much of what follows is based on these and several more recent sources. However, these early writings by Judy Dunn are still the most widely cited and authoritative sources on the development of sibling relationships in young children.

Although it is widely recognized that peer relationships play a central role in children's social development and although a huge literature exists on peer relationships (see Chapter 6), much less attention has been paid to the role that siblings play in children's socialization. Whereas relationships with peers are, by definition, relationships between relative equals, sibling interactions are characterized by complementary roles and role asymmetries, including differences in dominance and submission, that derive from the necessary age differences between nontwin sibling pairs (Hartup, 1983; Stoneman, Brody, & MacKinnon,

1984). Older siblings serve as companions, attachment figures, role models, and teachers; younger siblings are help seekers, pupils, imitators, and playmates. The emotional bond between siblings is almost always intense, and conflict between siblings tends to be the more salient aspect of the relationship in the minds of many parents, despite the many positive features of most sibling relationships. Developmental scientists are beginning to delineate the important role played by siblings and have suggested that sibling relationships provide children with quite different social experiences and serve different functions in their socialization than do relationships with peers (Hartup, 1983; Stoneman et al., 1984). Awareness is growing that children's social understanding, prosocial behavior, and moral development are influenced by relationships with siblings (Dunn, 1983, 1985; Dunn, Brown, & Maguire, 1995), in the context of the family system and parent–child relationships. Likewise, in some family contexts, young children appear to hone their aggressive and coercive strategies in sibling interactions (Garcia, Shaw, Winslow, & Yaggi, 2000; Patterson, 1984).

In our own study of parent-referred problem preschoolers, parental concerns about sibling conflicts were among the main issues leading parents to seek help. Indeed, there was a significantly higher proportion of firstborn children with younger siblings in the problem group in our first study than in the comparison group, and the presence of a sibling was associated with higher ratings of aggression at age 3. Thus, in our sample of parent-referred hard-to-manage preschoolers, the presence of a sibling appeared to exacerbate already extant parent–child conflict or to sensitize parents to concerns about their preschooler's aggressive and demanding behavior. Parents invariably described aggressive and provocative behavior toward the sibling that ranged from relatively typical and age-appropriate squabbles over toys to more premeditated and serious attempts to harm a younger child. In some instances, parents seemed to be overly fearful of their child hurting the infant, whereas in others the older child's resentment of the younger sibling was quite angry and overt. Hard-to-manage children who were the younger of two or more siblings were also involved in sibling conflicts, although parents seemed less concerned about these confrontations, feeling that the older child could take care of him- or herself.

In this chapter, I describe the typical reactions of toddlers and preschoolers to the birth of a sibling and then discuss the nature of the relationship that develops between siblings over the first few years of life.

Sibling relationships are seen as having an important influence on social cognitive development and general socialization. The role of parents in moderating sibling relationships is addressed, as is the impact of the birth of a second child on the family system. Finally, the discussion focuses on sibling relationships in families in which one child has been identified as a problem.

REACTIONS TO THE BIRTH OF A SIBLING

Rutter (1981) has suggested that the birth of a sibling is among the major stressors that young children must learn to deal with routinely. Indeed, many of the behavioral changes that parents describe following the birth of a sibling appear to reflect the typical ways in which young children respond to stress. The popular focus on "sibling rivalry" is based on the view that "dethronement" (Stewart, Mobley, Van Tuyl, & Salvador, 1987) and jealousy are the most salient aspects of the sibling relationship and that the major impact of the birth of a sibling is its effect on the mother–child relationship. Thus it is assumed that young children feel displaced and resentful and that the need to share parental attention and affection with the sibling is the primary issue to be addressed. This is undoubtedly important, as illustrated by the comments of one very bright and verbal 3-year-old we know. Shortly after his sister's birth, he poignantly expressed his fear that his sister was going to take all his mother's love and that there would not be enough left for him. However, Dunn and Kendrick (1982), as well as others (e.g., Abramovitch, Corter, & Pepler, 1980; Stewart et al., 1987), have noted the complexities inherent in sibling relationships, which can best be characterized as ambivalent. Although rivalry and jealousy are often apparent, many children also show increased maturity, concern for others, and independence after the birth of a sibling.

Several studies have documented the nature and extent of initial reactions to the birth of a sibling and the characteristics of the relationship that develops between siblings in early childhood, highlighting both positive and negative aspects (Dunn & Kendrick, 1982; Stewart et al., 1987). These authors argue that putting emphasis only on the rivalry for parental love and competition for adult attention leaves out many important features of the sibling relationship that have an impact on children's socioemotional development and on the family system.

They maintain that in addition to resentment, strong bonds of friend-ship, companionship, and affection develop between young siblings and that siblings learn a lot from each other about feelings, about handling competition constructively, and about acceptable patterns of social behavior.

Several studies that have examined the initial response of toddlers and preschoolers to the birth of a sibling show general agreement that children display a mix of reactions—positive, negative, and anxiety laden (Dunn & Kendrick, 1982; Field & Reite, 1984; Stewart et al., 1987). These include regressive behavior such as increased clinging and separation distress, toileting accidents, the desire to drink from a bottle, feeding problems, and crying. Children are also likely to become more angry, aggressive, and noncompliant, although, contrary to popular be-lief, aggression and confrontation are usually directed at parents, not at the infant sibling. Dunn and Kendrick (1982) note a dramatic increase in mother–child conflict and confrontation in the immediate postpar-tum period, especially during the times at which the mother is involved in feeding and otherwise caring for the new baby. In general, the inci-dents they describe suggest intense anger toward the mother and a des-perate attempt to gain attention from her. In addition, expressions of anxiety and social withdrawal are often apparent. Thus a mixture of re-gression, anxiety, and defiance often characterizes the reactions of young children to the birth of a sibling.

In addition to these negative behaviors, however, observers have noted increased maturity and independence, often in the same children who are showing regression or confrontation in other domains of func-tioning. Children may react with increased anger and noncompliance, but at the same time they may show increased independence in self-help skills or a surge in language development. This evidence under-lines the complexity of children's reactions, as well as the exacerbation of typical, developmentally related conflicts within the child, such as confusion over mastery and autonomy. Young children confronted with the birth of a sibling are particularly ambivalent about whether they want to maintain their dependence or become more independent. Al-most all the children observed by Dunn and Kendrick (1982), who were between 18 months and 4 years old at the birth of the sibling, reacted with some combination of behaviors reflecting this ambivalence, with younger children having more frequent toileting accidents and older children becoming more clingy. Thus there is strong evidence that tod-dlers and preschoolers react intensely to the birth of a sibling and that overtly negative reactions are directed primarily at parents rather than at the new infant.

Dunn and Kendrick (1982) also note that toddlers and preschoolers are extremely interested in and curious about the new baby; they ask questions, want to help with caretaking, express affection, and often imitate the infant's behavior. Children as young as 18 months are interested in holding the baby or helping their mothers, although these same children may express their hostility quite openly, for example, by suggesting that the mother return the infant to the hospital. Thus ambivalence is more characteristic of the feelings children have for the newborn than outright and unmitigated dislike. This initial ambivalence appears to reflect a complex process of adjustment to the reality of sharing parents and grandparents with another person who is helpless and fascinating, as well as extremely demanding of adult time, attention, and affection.

THE DEVELOPMENT OF SIBLING RELATIONSHIPS

Once older children have gotten over the initial stress of the arrival of the younger sibling, they begin to adapt to the complexities that are a natural consequence of integrating a new member into the family circle. Two longitudinal studies of adaptation to the birth of a sibling have been conducted (Dunn & Kendrick, 1982; Stewart et al., 1987). In both studies stable, two-parent families were studied prospectively from the third trimester of the mother's pregnancy with her second child through at least the first year postpartum. In both studies, firstborn children ranged in age from just under 2 years to 4 years at the time of the sibling birth. A combination of observational and interview data were collected during home visits. Dunn and Kendrick (1982) obtained detailed narrative accounts of ongoing natural interactions in the home, and these accounts provide an especially rich source of information on developmental change in parent–child and sibling relations.

Dunn and Kendrick's (1982) data indicate that although relationships between siblings remain complex and ambivalent, the intense reactions that were apparent initially had waned considerably by the end of the first month or so and appeared to represent transient stress reactions rather than a long-term pattern of adaptation. The intensity of the initial reaction was not predictive of more serious problems in adjustment to the sibling. Rather, children who responded more explosively were more likely to learn to get along with their siblings than were children who became seriously withdrawn. In addition, children who expressed interest in and affection toward their infant siblings early on were more likely to have positive relations with them in toddlerhood. Stewart et al. (1987) also report that children initially showed high rates of regression and confrontational behavior but that these reactions had waned considerably by 4 months postpartum. In addition, most firstborns expressed interest in the newborn and assisted their mothers with caretaking in some way, by holding the baby, fetching diapers or other objects, and amusing the baby. These studies document the fact that children's reactions to a sibling's birth are multifaceted.

Toddlers and preschoolers appear to use complex strategies to help them adjust to the presence of a younger sibling. Both Dunn and Kendrick (1982) and Stewart and colleagues (1987) emphasize the importance of imitation or "regression" as an adaptive strategy. They argue that asking for a bottle, reverting to baby talk, or having toileting accidents, for example, may be the child's way of maintaining or regaining parental attention. Imitation of the baby's behavior may also allow the child to work through conflicts using fantasy and role playing. Field and Reite (1984) also noted that young children increased their use of fantasy after the birth of a sibling, and they suggest that this helped the children to cope with both the temporary separation from mother and the marked changes going on in the family. Most of the children in this study, when observed during free play, engaged in fantasy play with aggressive themes. Fantasy aggression was directed both toward the mother and the new baby, with aggression toward the baby more common.

These findings may suggest that children use fantasy to express their anger and ambivalence toward the infant but that they are more likely to act out their anger and confusion about parental love and attention more directly toward their parents by becoming confrontational and by generally showing more immature behavior. The longitudinal data also suggest that parents need not be concerned that children are reverting to earlier, more primitive forms of behavior. Rather, children may be using earlier, more familiar forms of behavior as a bridge to higher level functioning (Dunn & Kendrick, 1982). In most instances, "regressive" behaviors were relatively short-lived initial reactions to the sibling's birth. As younger siblings developed, the sibling relationship changed as well.

The nature of sibling relationships obviously becomes even more complex as the younger child develops mobility and begins to explore the world of objects actively. At this point the younger child is a much more serious threat to the older child, and it is at this time that more overt physical conflict is likely to develop. As the younger child becomes more independent and more of a social being, the competition for adult attention intensifies. Squabbles over toys and territory become more intense as both members of the dyad participate in play (Dunn & Kendrick, 1982). Stewart et al. (1987) reported that confrontations with parents were common during the first few months after the sibling birth but that by the end of the first year preschool-age children were engaging in more frequent conflict with younger siblings. As younger siblings reach toddlerhood, the older children are likely to complain about intrusions into their toys and games; this seems to be a particular source of stress among same-sex dyads. In this context, the older siblings are likely to rely on their superior cognitive and linguistic skills and physical coordination in settling squabbles, thus asserting their dominance in the relationship. In response to the power tactics of their older siblings, young toddlers seek and usually get parental assistance.

By the end of the second year, however, the younger sibling is capable of retaliating with physical aggression, which often serves to escalate the encounter. Younger siblings are also able to initiate conflict, by age 2 or somewhat earlier, by teasing or otherwise provoking the older preschooler. These interactions, although upsetting to parents, teach children about dominance and power, indicate some appreciation of the other child's vulnerabilities, and ultimately lead to the development of skills in the negotiation and resolution of disputes (Dunn & Kendrick, 1982). At the same time that conflict and confrontation may be more evident in the sibling relationship, the younger sibling is also becoming more of a companion and playmate for the older child. In this way the positive bond between them may become stronger. Despite frequent conflicts over possessions, young siblings may spend much of their time in cooperative play.

SIBLING RELATIONSHIPS AND SOCIALIZATION

Dunn and Kendrick (1982) emphasize the important role sibling interactions play in facilitating socialization of both younger and older children. Children as young as 3 are capable of adjusting their speech to make it simple enough for their younger siblings to understand. They also show empathy and concern for their sibling's distress, indicating early signs of social perspective taking and prosocial behavior. Younger siblings, likewise, may comfort older siblings or express concern about their distress. In general, the mutual regulation of social behavior occurs often in the interchanges between very young sibling pairs. Pretend play, turn taking, and sharing are all facilitated by the social interaction occurring within the sibling dyad. Children also learn to negotiate to solve disputes in interaction with siblings. Finally, older children serve as models for their younger siblings, who in turn serve as pupils for their older sibling's teaching.

In a series of studies, Dunn and her colleagues have demonstrated associations between the complexity of sibling play interactions, particularly pretend play involving role enactment and other aspects of social-cognitive functioning (e.g., Dunn et al., 1995; Dunn & Kendrick, 1982; Youngblade & Dunn, 1995). For example, Youngblade and Dunn (1995) observed young sibling pairs during free play and found that 33-month-old toddlers who had older siblings who engaged them in social pretend play that involved shared scenarios and role taking performed better on a series of social-cognitive tasks at 40 months. Toddlers who engaged in more pretend play were more skilled on emotion recognition and perspective-taking tasks and on false-belief tasks that required the child to take another person's perspective and to recognize that different people can act on different information than were toddlers who rarely engaged in pretend play with older siblings. Youngblade and Dunn (1995) suggest that some of the same skills that toddlers learn during dramatic play with older siblings may also be required to succeed on tasks that rely on the ability to consider the thoughts and feelings of others and to think about their own behavior in relation to the partner. Other researchers have likewise found that children with older siblings are more advanced than children with only younger siblings on social-cognitive tasks and theory of mind tasks that require awareness of inner states and differences in perspective (e.g., Ruffman, Perner, Naito, Parkin, & Clements, 1998). In addition, Dunn et al. (1995) found that prosocial interaction with an older sibling appears to predict kindergarten children's responses to moral vignettes; children with more harmonious sibling relationships during the preschool years were more likely to show empathic concern for the victim when told stories about moral transgressions such as cheating, taking toys, and hurting a peer.

Taken together, these studies indicate that siblings, like parents, play an important role as socialization agents. The focus so far has been on young children's social awareness and prosocial behavior. Evidence also links negative peer relations to aggressive behavior. This is discussed in more detail later.

INDIVIDUAL DIFFERENCES IN SIBLING RELATIONSHIPS

Wide individual differences are seen in the character of ongoing sibling relationships (Dunn & Kendrick, 1982). Some sibling pairs are characterized primarily by positive interactions and cooperative play, despite the occasional squabble; others show a mixture of positive and negative interactions; still others engage in quite severe and continuous conflict, with few instances of cooperative play. Several variables have been examined in order to explain some of these variations in the quality of sibling relationships, including the gender composition of the sibling pair, the age differences between them, and their temperamental characteristics.

Gender Composition

The gender composition of sibling pairs has been examined in several studies as one possible determinant of the character of sibling relationships. When this factor is evaluated in terms of the gender of the older sibling, the data on this issue are contradictory. Dunn (1983) reviewed evidence suggesting that girls are more nurturant toward their younger siblings than boys are and that younger siblings seek more help and comfort from their older sisters. Some studies indicate that these sex differences in nurturance and caregiving depend on the specific behaviors observed and on the age of the children at the time of the observation. Similarly, some studies suggest that girls are more involved as teachers of younger siblings, whereas boys are more likely to become aggressive. On the other hand, both Dunn and Kendrick (1982) and Pepler, Corter, and Abramovitch (1982), who studied preschool and school-age sibling pairs, reported relatively few sex differences in prosocial behavior, imitation, or aggression when children were studied over time.

In addition to considering the effect of the gender of the older sibling, studies have compared the interactions of same-sex and opposite-sex sibling pairs. Again, the findings are not consistent. Some data suggest more conflict among same-sex dyads (Stewart et al., 1987), and some studies suggest that more imitation and prosocial behavior occur in same-sex dyads (Dunn, 1983; Pepler et al., 1982). Dunn and Kendrick (1981) examined changes in the social behavior of same-sex and opposite-sex dyads that occurred when infants were between 8 and 14 months old. In same-sex pairs, both children increased the amount of positive interaction, including vocalization, smiling, and joint play; younger siblings also became more negative, a reflection of their increased autonomy and of the more advanced social skills that permitted them to stand up for themselves as they entered toddlerhood. In opposite-sex pairs, both children became more negative over time, as reflected in increased fighting, toy taking, and protests; neither member of the dyad became more positive, suggesting that older opposite-sex siblings were not making allowances for their younger siblings' behavior. These differential results also indicate that developmental changes do not reflect merely an increase in interaction with development. Dunn and Kendrick (1981) suggest that same-sex pairs may begin to become more aware of gender similarity and identify with one another, whereas opposite-sex dyads may become more aware of the differences between them. Further, these findings may be related to differences in maternal behavior. The researchers noted that mothers paid more attention to younger children who were opposite in sex from their firstborns. As only a handful of studies have addressed questions about the effect of gender composition on the interactions among siblings, and as the few extant studies differ widely in terms of study methodology and age of participants, it is not yet possible to draw any firm conclusions about how the gender composition of sibling dyads influences the nature of interaction at one point in time or over the course of early development. The age spacing of siblings also was thought to be important, although studies find little support for this view (Dunn, 1983).

Temperament

Individual differences in child temperament as they relate to the development of sibling relationships have begun to receive some attention recently. The issue of child temperament is especially relevant to a consideration of the sibling relationships of hard-to-manage preschoolers.

According to Dunn and Kendrick's (1982) findings, children who were reported by their mothers to be difficult to manage, as indexed by negative mood and intense emotional reactions to upset, were more likely to withdraw at the time of the sibling's birth, becoming tearful, sullen, and dependent on transitional objects for comfort. Difficult boys were especially likely to show this initial reaction, and it was likely to persist. By 8 months after the sibling's birth, many of these children were worried, fearful, demanding, and irritable and had sleeping and feeding problems. Thus these findings suggest that children who are difficult to handle have a harder time adapting to the birth of a second child and establishing a positive relationship with the younger sibling.

Similar findings are reported by Brody, Stoneman, and Burke (1987a) in a study of school-age children and their same-sex, preschool-age siblings who were observed in a semistructured play interaction at home. Maternal ratings of high activity and intense emotionality were associated with high levels of conflict and quarreling between sisters, regardless of whether the younger or the older sister was seen as more active and/or intense. High levels of activity among younger brothers was associated with high levels of conflict but also with high levels of prosocial behavior, suggesting that active younger brothers engaged in more interaction, both positive and negative, with their older brothers. The older brother's activity level did not predict the quality of sibling interaction. However, when older brothers were more emotionally intense, their younger brothers engaged in more aggressive and argumentative behavior. These two studies highlight the importance of considering children's personality characteristics as potential contributors to individual differences in sibling relationships. Of course, these studies raise questions about the direction of effects, as well as about how genetic similarity between sibling pairs influences both their personality characteristics and the quality of their relationship. These are clearly fruitful areas requiring further study.

PARENTING AND SIBLING RELATIONSHIPS

Changes in the Mother–Child Relationship after the Birth of a Sibling

It seems obvious that the way parents behave toward both younger and older siblings, as well as their expectations about children's behavior toward one another, will have an effect on the interaction between siblings. Parents' initial reactions to the second child's birth and their ability to include the older child in the process of family adaptation appears to set the stage for later sibling relationships. In addition to establishing a relationship with a younger sibling, the older child must respond to decreased parental attention and modified parental expectations. Dunn and Kendrick (1982) document the marked change in mother–child interaction after the birth of a sibling. Mothers spend less time in playful interaction and in conversation with the older child and considerably more time in confrontation. Moreover, when interactions between mother and firstborn do occur, the child is more likely than before to initiate the exchange, be it playful, conversational, or confrontative. This may account for the angry responses of firstborns who had experienced a warm and positive relationship prior to the birth of the sibling. In addition, parents often expect more mature behavior from the older sibling, just when the child is particularly vulnerable and ambivalent. This pressure for greater maturity may be paired with increased time spent with substitute caregivers or with fathers, further confusing and stressing the child. Increased father involvement in child care may ultimately strengthen the father–child relationship, or the father may become involved in daily struggles for compliance that lead to increased conflict.

Initial reactions to the birth of a sibling and the quality of later sibling relationships are also related to other aspects of family functioning and the earlier parent–child relationship. In Dunn and Kendrick's (1982) study, maternal fatigue and depression were associated with more withdrawal, sadness, and anxiety on the part of the firstborn, presumably in response to depressed maternal mood and consequent decreases in caretaking and sensitivity to the older child's emotional needs. When mothers and their firstborns had previously had a positive relationship characterized by much joint play and cooperation, the negative reaction to the birth of the sibling tended to be particularly intense, and the firstborn child, especially a firstborn girl, was likely to be more hostile and aggressive toward the sibling 14 months later. This probably reflects the older child's resentment and jealousy of the sibling and the yearning for undivided maternal attention. Further, Dunn and Kendrick (1981) reported that mothers spent more time playing with second-born children who were opposite in gender from their firstborns. As already noted, this may account, in part, for the increased conflict that developed between opposite-sex sibling pairs between 8 and 14 months.

However, maternal behavior toward both the firstborn and the younger sibling can also have a positive effect on the quality of the sibling relationship. Older siblings in the Dunn and Kendrick (1981) study appeared to develop more empathy toward and engage in more positive interaction with their younger siblings if mothers involved them in caretaking as a shared experience from very early on and also discussed and modeled respect for the baby as a person with distinct needs and feelings. This approach seems to encourage prosocial behavior and greater understanding of the infant, facilitating the development of empathy, at the same time that it minimizes feelings of being shut out by the close mother–infant bond. In addition, high levels of paternal involvement with the child often served to ameliorate the negative reaction to the sibling birth. This probably is best interpreted as both a direct effect of increased father–child contact on the firstborn child and as an indirect effect of the quality of the marital relationship on the older sibling and on the mother's ability to provide nurturance to both children.

Attachment Security and Sibling Relationships

Sibling relationships and attachment security have been examined in a few studies that focused on either attachments between younger and older siblings or on how attachment security in older siblings is related to their relations with younger siblings. Stewart and Marvin (1984) reported that when 3- and 4-year-olds were left alone with their younger siblings in a waiting room, over half responded to their younger sibling's distress by providing reassurance and comfort, for example, by hugging the infant and explaining that their mother would eventually return. In addition, the younger siblings displayed attachment behaviors toward their older siblings, seeking proximity and contact with them and using them as a secure base for play. However, not all preschoolers sought to comfort their distressed younger siblings, and not all younger siblings reached out toward their older brothers or sisters. Older siblings who showed more advanced social-cognitive development, as reflected in their ability to take the perspective of another, were more likely to comfort and reassure younger siblings; those younger siblings who had experienced nurturance and caregiving from more cognitively mature siblings were more likely to seek comfort from them when distressed, suggesting that these mutually regulated attachment and caregiving behaviors were part of their ongoing relationship. Finally, it is interesting to note that mothers were more likely to ask the more cognitively mature older siblings to take care of the younger sibling in their absence than was the case with non-perspective-taking older siblings. This may suggest that maternal socialization played a role in the development of children's sensitivity to the needs of their younger siblings or that mothers were more likely to make such requests of more socially mature children. It may also suggest something about the attachment security of the older siblings.

Three recent studies have asked whether attachment security is associated with the children's adaptation to the birth of a sibling or with the quality of the sibling relationship. Teti, Sakin, Kucera, Korns, and Das Eiden (1996) examined changes in attachment security in firstborns after the birth of a sibling. They found that Q-sort security scores declined after the birth of a sibling, and especially so for older toddlers (over 24 months). In addition, more maternal involvement with the firstborn both before and after the sibling birth and higher levels of marital harmony predicted higher levels of security after the birth of the sibling, suggesting that qualities of the earlier mother–child relationship helped the firstborn deal with the presence of a newborn in the family. When mothers remained emotionally engaged with the firstborn, security did not decline, once more underlining the importance of family processes and maternal support in children's adjustment to normal stressful transitions.

Attachment security also appears to be directly related to the quality of sibling relations. Teti and Ablard (1989) observed mothers and both older and younger siblings in the laboratory during separations and reunions, as well as during play; less secure older siblings (mean age = 4 years) were less likely to respond to younger siblings' distress in mothers' absence than were secure older siblings, who were more likely to try to comfort younger siblings. Secure infants with secure older siblings were also less distressed during separation from mother. When mothers were directed to play with one or the other sibling, jealousy and aggression were less common when infants and preschoolers were both secure.

Volling and Belsky (1992) examined attachment security in infancy, mother–child interaction in the preschool period, and mother–child conflict at age 6 in firstborns who were observed in home visits interacting during free play with toddler siblings. Relations between siblings were more conflict ridden and aggressive when the older sibling had been insecurely attached in infancy, when mothers had been intrusive and controlling with the child at age 3, and when mother–child conflict was also high when the child was 6. Moreover, attachment security and earlier mother–child interaction predicted the level of sibling conflict even with concurrent mother–child conflict controlled, suggesting that the early mother–child relationship and ongoing family climate set the stage for sibling interactions later on. These investigators also included fathers. Although attachment to father did not predict the quality of the sibling relationship, when the father–child relationship was more positive, older children were more prosocial with younger siblings.

These findings highlight an important aspect of the positive and supportive relationship between young siblings, as well as of the interrelationships among child, sibling, maternal, and paternal behaviors and expectations. They suggest that when older siblings have experienced involved and responsive parenting, their internal working models of relationships and their ability to empathize with distressed younger siblings are reflected in more active caregiving and nurturance and that the sibling relationship is characterized by more positive affective involvement as well. Thus, consistent with the findings of Sroufe and Fleeson (1986), positive relationships between parents and older siblings appear to be carried forward to new relationships within the family system. In contrast, insecurity and family conflict appear to predict less harmonious, engaged, and positive relationships not only between parents and children but also between siblings, even in early childhood, underscoring the importance of considering relationships within the family context.

Styles of Childrearing and Sibling Relationships

The studies of attachment and sibling relationships also support the proposition that the nature of childrearing strategies will influence the quality of sibling relationships more generally. Families that are child centered and warm are more likely to foster both positive parent–child and sibling relationships. Brody et al. (1987a) suggest that consistent use of nonpunitive childrearing strategies and responsiveness to children's needs are associated with less aggressive and conflicted sibling interaction and a more positive relationship. This is consistent with the general view of childrearing and socialization explicated in Chapter 4. Other aspects of parenting have also been hypothesized to relate to the nature of sibling relations. For example, differential maternal behavior that unfairly favors one child over another has been hypothesized to lead to problems between siblings, particularly to more aggressive and conflicted interactions (Brody et al., 1987a; Dunn, 1983). Brody et al. (1987a) specifically examined this issue in their sample of same-sex sibling pairs. Mothers and siblings were observed in a semistructured play interaction at home that included a construction activity and a board game. Mothers directed significantly more prosocial behavior, as well as negative and controlling behavior, toward the younger siblings, but differential maternal behavior was unrelated to the quality of the sibling interactions observed in a similar situation on a different occasion. Brody et al. (1987a) suggest that the older siblings understood that their younger siblings required more help and direction completing the play activities. In addition, it is worth noting that mothers addressed both more positive and more negative comments to the younger children, so that the differential behavior was not just in the direction of more positive or affectionate interactions. In the Volling and Belsky (1992) study, differential treatment interacted with attachment security, such that firstborns who had been secure were not less positive with their siblings despite differential treatment. The authors suggest that secure children are less concerned about parent availability and less threatened by differential treatment than are insecure children.

Several other studies have suggested that mothers behave differently with firstborns than with second borns, whereas still others do not document clear differential treatment (see Dunn, 1983). Moreover, findings depend on context and on the age of the children. For instance, there is evidence that mothers attend more to younger children when both children are present but that firstborns receive more individual attention. However, few studies have actually examined the relationship between differential treatment and sibling interaction, making this an important issue for further research. The studies that have examined differential maternal behavior, by necessity, confound maternal behavior with age differences between siblings. Thus maternal behavior toward siblings might be similar at various developmental points, although differences are apparent when mothers are observed interacting with two children who are at different developmental stages. Dunn and her colleagues (Dunn, Plomin, & Nettles, 1985) examined this question as part of a longitudinal study of within-family environmental influences. Mothers and each of two siblings were observed at home during feeding and play when each infant was 12 months old. Measures of maternal positive affection, verbal interaction, and negative control showed surprisingly high consistency from the first baby to the second, and consistency held for both same-sex and opposite-sex sibling pairs. Similar results were obtained by Moore, Cohn, and Campbell (1997), who observed mothers interacting with first- and second-borns at 2 months postpartum during feeding and play. These data suggest a relatively enduring maternal behavioral style that is fairly independent of the specific eliciting characteristics of the infant. Additional work will need to be conducted to replicate and extend these interesting findings.

Other contextual factors also appear to influence the quality of sibling interactions. Both Brody et al. (1987a) and Corter, Abramovitch, and Pepler (1983) assessed the influence of maternal presence versus absence on the nature of sibling interactions. In the Brody et al. (1987a) study, siblings and their mothers were observed at home during a semistructured play session, with the experimenter providing the materials. Corter et al. (1983) observed naturally occurring interactions in the home. Despite these differences in procedure, both studies revealed a marked decrease in sibling interaction when mothers were present, with a particularly dramatic drop in cooperative and prosocial behavior. The absolute amount of aggressive behavior also dropped in mothers' presence, although the relative proportion of aggressive acts increased in the Corter et al. (1983) study. This may reflect attention-seeking behavior or, as this was an unstructured home observation, the fact that mothers may be more likely to make their presence known when they think a conflict is about to begin or to escalate. Parents frequently voice concerns about the ability of their children to cooperate. The findings from these two studies are interesting in that they indicate that children do quite well on their own and that prosocial interactions predominate. This may suggest that, at least with many school-age children and their preschool-age siblings, parents need not monitor their interactions too closely or feel the need to intervene whenever a conflict ensues. As is the case with peer relations, children need to learn to solve problems and resolve disputes on their own without too much adult intrusion.

Dunn and Munn (1985, 1986) specifically examined the nature of sibling conflicts and how children resolved them. They also assessed how mothers dealt with quarrels between the preschool- and toddler-age children in their sibling sample and what the consequences of maternal interventions were. It is worth noting that sibling pairs engaged in some form of conflict about eight times per hour. Preschool-age older siblings aggressed physically roughly one-fourth of the time, but they also used relatively mature means of conflict resolution, including distracting the younger child, justifying their actions with a reason or rule, and making conciliatory gestures or statements. By 24 months of age, a number of younger siblings were likewise using these more mature strategies on occasion, highlighting the important role that sibling interaction can play in socialization. Furthermore, cross-age correlations suggest that younger siblings may learn specific strategies, such as justifying their actions and referring to rules, from their older brothers and sisters.

Mothers intervened in just over half the disputes observed. Moreover, children sought maternal intervention when they were aggressed against but not when they were the aggressors. Mothers responded differently to their younger and older children in the context of sibling quarrels. They were more likely to attempt to distract the younger child, but they also were more likely to prohibit the older sibling and then to teach explicit principles about social conventions and other peoples' feelings, not unlike the behavior described by Zahn-Waxler et al. (1979) in response to children's transgressions in other contexts. Thus mothers referred to the younger child's feelings, explained the reasons for the younger child's actions, and suggested conciliatory behaviors to deescalate the conflict. When younger siblings were 24 months old, mothers stated social rules equally often to both children in response to disputes between them. Maternal interventions were associated with younger children's use of both more mature strategies and physical aggression. For example, children whose mothers suggested conciliatory behaviors were more likely both to resolve some disputes peacefully and to hit during others. Overall, maternal involvement in sibling quarrels was related to both more frequent conflict and physical aggression between siblings, as well as to use of more mature strategies of conflict resolution. Maternal involvement may provide young children with a larger repertoire of behaviors suitable for resolving disputes, or these findings may indicate that when children engage in more frequent conflict, mothers are more likely to intervene with an array of responses. These maternal interventions involved teaching children about appro-

priate rules and social behaviors, and children showed increased awareness of social rules and of the effect of their behavior on their siblings,
apparently as a result of this maternal teaching. It is noteworthy that, although Dunn and Munn (1985, 1986) coded maternal strategies such
as punishment and physical intervention, these occurred too infre-
quently to be analyzed.

Several more recent studies also have examined how parents intervene in sibling disputes. Perlman and Ross (1997) reported that maternal interventions in quarrels between sibling pairs who were 2 and 4
years old, respectively, were associated with fewer power struggles and
less aggression. Kramer, Perozynski, and Chung (1999) studied preschool-age children and their older siblings, as well as the types of
interventions engaged in separately by mothers and fathers. Disputes
were most often verbal and rarely physical, and parents generally
tended not to intervene. The frequency and intensity of sibling conflict
did not vary by parent, but fathers used more controlling interventions
with younger sibling pairs and mothers were more passive when siblings were older. When parents did intervene, disputes tended to be
more prolonged but were resolved; more frequent conflict episodes ensued when parents ignored the dispute. This suggests that parental intervention, especially child-centered interventions that helped children
settle the dispute amicably, led to more peaceful interactions, whereas
disputes that were not resolved flared up again. These data, paired with
those of other investigators (Dunn & Munn, 1986), suggest that parents
are being helpful when they intervene in a teaching role to help young
siblings learn to settle disputes.

There is no doubt that the birth of a sibling leads to many changes
within the family system that are likely to have an impact on the marital
relationship and on the relationship of each parent to the older child.
Some of the many changes in the mother's relationship with the older
child have been discussed. In addition, it has been suggested that paternal involvement in parenting can help ameliorate some of the stress on
the mother, whereas father's involvement with the older child may further cement their relationship and help the child to cope with the loss
of undivided maternal attention. The nature of the marital relationship
may also change with the additional responsibilities of a second child.
Both parents may feel more stressed and have less time to devote to
their own relationship, leading to increased strains in the marriage. This
too will feed back to affect the older sibling's feelings of security and

willingness to cooperate with parental wishes. In addition, marital distress and overt marital conflict witnessed by the children has been found to be associated with more sibling conflict (Brody, Stoneman, & Burke, 1987b). This finding may reflect the direct effects of modeling, the anxiety and upset caused by a tense family environment, and/or the indirect effects of marital distress on parenting, including the provision of inadequate guidelines for the resolution of conflict (Davies & Cummings, 1994). On the other hand, an increase in paternal involvement in family activities usually would be expected to have a positive effect on the family system.

SIBLING RELATIONSHIPS IN FAMILIES WITH HARD-TO-MANAGE CHILDREN

Very few studies have examined the sibling interactions of hard-to-manage preschoolers, although it is safe to assume that they are problematic. For example, Richman et al. (1982) found that sibling conflict at ages 3 and 4 was predictive of continuing problems at age 8. This finding may reflect the aggressive behavior of the target child, as well as ongoing family discord and disruption. However, it is also possible that continuing conflict between siblings contributes to maternal concerns about aggressive and coercive behaviors that are reasonably typical. Mash and Johnston (1983) examined the interactions of clinically diagnosed hyperactive boys and their brothers in comparison with nonclinical pairs of brothers of comparable age. Dyads were observed interacting during free play and structured tasks. Few significant differences were found within sibling pairs. However, hyperactive boys and their nonhyperactive brothers engaged in more reciprocal conflict than comparison dyads. High rates of negative behavior in the hyperactive and nonhyperactive brother pairs were associated with maternal reports of less skill and knowledge of parenting, suggesting that sibling conflict might have contributed to mothers' negative self-evaluations or that these mothers may have been less adept at helping their children resolve disputes. These observations are consistent with maternal reports of high rates of sibling conflict among children with externalizing problems. The role of the hyperactive child in initiating and maintaining the conflict is not clear from this study, and probably varies with the relative age of the diagnosed child and his brother. For example, it is reasonable to suppose that older hyperactive boys will be more aggressive and more likely to bully their younger brothers, whereas younger hyperactive boys will be more likely to irritate, provoke, and tease their older siblings.

Patterson (1980, 1984) has noted that in families with aggressive children, both target children and their siblings initiate conflict and contribute to its escalation into high-intensity encounters. He considers coercive family processes, with their origins in the parent–child relationship, as important training grounds for sibling conflict, which in turn spills out to the school setting and the wider community. Both modeling and negative reinforcement play a role in maintaining high levels of dyadic conflict in certain family contexts. Few studies, however, have examined whether sibling conflict predicts behavior problems over and above negative parenting. It may be that sibling conflict serves as a marker of coercive family interaction patterns or that sibling conflict may contribute even further to poor self-regulatory and negotiation skills that predict problems outside the family system. Garcia et al. (2000) examined this issue in a sample of high-risk inner-city boys living in relative poverty. Observed sibling conflict that was destructive and highly negative was associated with maternal ratings of externalizing problems at school entry, after controlling for earlier problem behavior and rejecting parenting (observed at age 2 in the laboratory). Most important, however, the interaction between sibling conflict and earlier rejecting parenting predicted both teacher and mother ratings of aggressive behavior at age 6. Consistent with a dual-risk model, when children had negative relations with both their mothers and their siblings, they were especially likely to be seen as aggressive across home and school contexts. These findings are also consistent with attachment-theory and emotional-security perspectives in suggesting the importance of early harmonious relationships for later functioning and underscoring the potential negative sequelae of coercive, ongoing negative family processes.

Clinical Implications

The families in our study, with a hard-to-manage preschooler already creating conflicts in the marriage or taxing parental resources, were severely stressed by the birth of a second child. In addition, because many of the second children were born shortly after the firstborns' second birthdays, the older children were often about to start preschool just as the younger siblings were entering toddlerhood and becoming more active and demanding rivals for parental attention. Some children reacted to this dual threat to their relationship with their mothers by showing intense separation distress in nursery school and/or increased anger and defiance at home. In addition, many mothers in our study described conflict and ambivalence between their children.

In a typical example, Jamie L.'s younger brother was born when Jamie was about 2½ years old. His mother described initial tantrum behavior and moodiness, along with a tendency to ignore his baby brother. By the time his brother was 10 months old, Jamie showed extreme shifts in behavior, showering his brother with love and attention one minute and becoming hostile and aggressive the next. When Jamie was followed up 1 year later, his mother commented on the frequent conflict between Jamie and his brother Jeffrey, who was nearing his second birthday. Although Jamie often became upset and angry when Jeffrey entered his room or wanted to play with his toys, Jeffrey also instigated fights by teasing and provoking Jamie and then crying when Jamie responded. Mrs. L. noted that Jeffrey set Jamie up to get into trouble, and vice versa. Despite this, the two were able to play together quietly from time to time, and their relationship was not a totally negative one.

Several mothers of especially aggressive and noncompliant boys with younger sisters worried about leaving their children together out of sight. They felt the need to supervise their sons constantly for fear that they would intentionally harm their baby sisters. Indeed, one mother of a 42-month-old boy, among the most aggressive, angry, and noncompliant in our sample, expressed concern about his extreme jealousy and animosity toward his 18-month-old sister. As with Jamie, this youngster's problems were apparent from very early infancy, but they tended to escalate after his sister's birth. Although he expressed some interest in his baby sister in early infancy, his handling of her tended to be rough, and as she got older, he became increasingly more aggressive, often expressing anger and annoyance at her social initiations. At the 6-year follow-up interview, this child's mother commented on her daughter's patience and devotion to her older brother, who either ignored her or harassed her and was rarely pleasant or affectionate toward her.

Similarly, the mother of one 29-month-old boy called the project shortly after the birth of her daughter. Although her son, too, had been an extremely difficult child since early infancy, his intensely angry reaction to the birth of his baby sister precipitated her call. She described her relationship with her son as one of constant conflict and was at a loss about how to cope with the increase in noncompliance, tantrums, and separation distress that accompanied the sibling birth. Although tantrums had been frequent, occurring as often as three or four times weekly, they had risen to as many as five a day and were occurring in response to almost any request. He had also become exceedingly clingy, refused to visit peers, wanted to drink from a bottle, and requested a pacifier. Consistent with the descriptions presented by Dunn and Kendrick (1982), however, his relationship with his sister was characterized by ambivalence rather than by outright rejection. He did show some curiosity about her, was interested in holding her, and did express affection toward her, caressing and kissing her. However, the day before his mother called the project, he had spit on his sister, and his mother was afraid that his caresses sometimes bordered on aggression, another rather explicit indication of his ambivalence.

These observations suggest that the initial reactions of hard-to-manage children are more extreme than usual, although similar in type to those described by Dunn and Kendrick (1982). Furthermore, it appears that the problems that are exacerbated by the birth of a sibling are less transient in children with preexisting problems. Rather, they appear to exaggerate a pattern of maladaptation that was apparent before the sibling birth and to increase mother–child conflict still further. Several of the mothers in our project expressed worry about rejecting their problem children in their efforts to curtail aggressive behavior and to protect the more vulnerable younger children. These mothers were intensely upset by the negative behavior their problem youngsters showed toward their siblings, and, although they were sensitive to the needs of both children, they were uncertain about how best to handle this complex situation.

On the other hand, not all children identified as problems by their parents had troubled relationships with their siblings, although their initial reactions may have involved ambivalence. Annie J. was nearly 5 when her sister was born, and she was extremely interested in helping her mother to care for the baby. She reacted initially with some bedwetting. When the baby was 6 months old, Annie started kindergarten. Although Annie had loved going to nursery school, the transition to kindergarten was quite stressful for her, and she had several episodes of school refusal. This may have partly reflected the excessive anxiety she felt at leaving her mother and sister home alone for prolonged periods of time at the stage in which her sister was becoming more socially responsive and engaging. Given the intensely conflict-ridden relationship between Annie and her mother, the prospects of leaving home for several hours each day may have intensified her anxiety about additional displacement and rejection by her mother. On the other hand, as her baby sister got older, Annie was involved increasingly in caregiving and also in playing with her sister and keeping her amused. It appeared, overall, that her relationship with her sister was very positive and close, and this may have helped to fill the emotional void left by her relatively poor relationship with her mother. Dunn and Kendrick (1982) also note that especially warm sibling relationships may sometimes compensate for confrontational mother–child relationships.

Problem children with older siblings were less likely to become engaged in constant sibling battles, or at least in battles that were serious concern to parents. Both Teddy M. and Robbie S. had older siblings who, by the time we saw them, were able to cope with their little brothers' annoying and intrusive behavior. Arguments and tattling were more frequent than overt physical confrontations, and as the older siblings entered elementary school, they more easily escaped to their rooms or the homes of peers, thus avoiding conflicts some of the time. Robbie's older sister was basically positive and supportive of her difficult younger brother, although she also resented the attention that he demanded from their mother and the fact that family outings were sometimes spoiled or curtailed because of his uncooperative or provocative behavior. Teddy often tagged along after his older brother, but they played quite well together, and their parents considered them good friends.

However, older siblings did not always cope this well. In another family, in which the younger brother was a behavior problem and the baby sister had a chronic physical illness, the 7-year-old sister became depressed and withdrawn. She was defiant at home, and her school performance deteriorated. It seemed clear that she was feeling quite neglected by her parents, who were preoccupied with the problems presented by their younger children and did not have the time or resources left to meet her needs adequately. Other older sisters were confused by their younger brothers' annoying behavior and the attention it elicited from those around them. One 5-year-old sister of a problem youngster commented wistfully to the home visitor, "My brother is weird. He always takes my toys." It is also worth noting in this context that most of the siblings of our hard-to-manage children were doing reasonably well, despite the difficulties evident with the target child and/or more generally in patterns of interaction within the family.

SUMMARY

In summary, preschool children typically react with a range of problem behaviors when they must adapt to the birth of a sibling. In most families, these behaviors represent relatively brief and transient stress reactions rather than long-term patterns of maladjustment. In children not identified as having behavior problems, sibling relationships appear to range from quite positive and warm to quite hostile, although most sibling relationships reflect a blend of positive and negative features. The ability of children to adapt to the birth of a sibling is partly related to aspects of parenting and the family climate, as well as to the children's personalities and more typical style of responding to stress and environmental change. Not surprisingly, children considered to be difficult before the birth of a second child have a particularly hard time dealing with the sibling birth and adapting to the attendant changes in the family system. This difficulty may be ameliorated by parental sensitivity to the older child's feelings and by continued involvement with him or her, both alone and as a helper in taking care of the younger child. However, the older child's hostility and frustration, whether directed at the parent or the younger sibling, may also serve to exacerbate mother–child conflict as the mother may rebuke the older child and seek to protect the younger one from harm. Fathers may play a central role here in easing these conflicts. As younger siblings mature, relations between older and younger children become more complex. Although conflicts over toys and attention are often salient, siblings also socialize each other, and a sibling may help to fill the void created by a troubled or rejecting mother–child relationship. Over time, siblings often become not only rivals but also companions and friends.

CHAPTER 6

Peer Relationships and Young Children's Development

PEER BEHAVIORS IN PRESCHOOL CHILDREN

Jeremy and Jonathan, both 30 months old, are standing at the water table in the preschool classroom. Jonathan is filling a plastic container with water and spilling it out, watching the water splash down the drain. Jeremy watches and then goes to get another container. He, too, begins to fill his container with water and spill it out. The two boys stand side by side, both emptying and refilling their plastic pails, glancing at each other and exchanging a few words. They continue playing like this for several minutes until Jonathan drops his pail and runs off to ride the tricycle. Soon after, Jeremy, too, loses interest in this activity and finds something else to do.

This is a classic example of the parallel play typical of young preschoolers, who spend a good deal of their time watching, imitating, and learning from each others' play. Parallel play is marked by the similarity of the participants' actions and by their awareness of each other, despite relatively little direct verbal exchange or turn taking. It appears that by engaging in parallel play, children begin to learn about the synchrony of behavior that is necessary for more sustained bouts of cooperative interaction. Parallel play represents an early form of social interactive play that occupies a proportion of children's social activities across the pre-school years, although the types of parallel activities that preschoolers select increase in complexity with age (Hartup, 1983; Rubin, Bukowski, & Parker, 1998). In the interaction just described, the children are engaged in an exploratory activity; with increasing age and cognitive sophistication, basic exploration gives way to more complex construction activities, in which children may engage in parallel fashion (Rubin et al., 1998). This vignette also illustrates the transient nature of young children's play encounters (Corsaro, 1981).

> Four-year-olds Ian and Mike are building in the block corner, making a huge rambling structure. They are talking animatedly as they work, discussing the placement of the blocks and whether the building should be a garage or a castle. Mike adds some blocks to the foundation; then he steps back and watches while Ian adds some more blocks that jut out from the main structure. They continue to build, working together, taking turns, and talking as they play, engrossed in what they are doing. Zach comes along, picks up a block, and tries to add it to the building. Both Ian and Mike shout, "No!" and Ian says, "Don't! You can't build here!" Zach persists in trying to put the block on; Ian continues to protest and pushes Zach. The teacher intervenes.

This example illustrates a number of typical features of preschool peer interactions. First, turn taking, social and task-oriented conversation, and cooperation toward a goal become increasingly important components of play in older preschoolers. This complex sequence of interactions indicates that the two boys are able to regulate their own behavior in order to take turns and work together. This vignette also suggests that Ian and Mike have some ability to share and to take the other person's point of view into account. Further, the differentiation of self from other is needed before two individuals can coordinate their activities in such a fine-tuned and mutually regulated way. In addition, this type of cooperative activity requires some degree of means–end thinking, the ability to plan and work toward a goal. Finally, young children are capable of establishing strong bonds of friendship with others, and this may be reflected in prolonged bouts of joint play and cooperation. The cooperative play between Ian and Mike is an example of the marked strides that are made from roughly 30 months to 48 months in the development of preschoolers' social competencies. At the same time, possessiveness, lack of sharing, and conflict also characterize social interactions among preschoolers (Shantz, 1987). Conflicts over space, toys, and activities are common occurrences in preschool classrooms, although, like the episode just described, they are usually short-lived. In this instance, Ian and Mike did not want to share their ongoing activity with Zach; possibly they also did not want an outsider intruding into their relationship, either because their play had reached a level of mutually satisfying, though precarious, cooperation that could easily be destroyed by the addition of a third child or because of a special bond between them that led to exclusivity in choice of play partners (Corsaro, 1981). Like possession struggles, the entry of a newcomer into an ongoing activity is often the source of conflict (see Corsaro, 1981; Shantz, 1987). In this instance, protecting one's turf, be it space, materials, or partner, becomes the overriding goal, and children do not take the feelings of the newcomer into account as they reject his bids outright. At this stage of development, too, there is a tendency to lash out physically and to protest verbally rather than to negotiate a mutually agreeable compromise solution to the impasse.

> Jill and Julie are in the playhouse, deciding whose turn it is to be the baby, when Sam, a younger child, comes along. They grab him by the hand in a playful manner, and Jill says, "Sam, you be the baby. I'll be the mommy." The discussion then ensues about what role Julie should take, the daddy or the big sister. Finally, they agree that she should be the daddy, so she goes off to the dress-up corner to get a hat.

Although it is often difficult for new children to enter an ongoing activity, at other times, children's groups form and reform spontaneously. Furthermore, research has shown that girls are more likely to incorporate boys into an ongoing activity than vice versa (Corsaro, 1981). In this instance, a younger child was brought into the play and given the role of the baby, suggesting a certain reality-based assignment of roles, despite the decision that Julie should be the daddy. This example also illustrates the opportunity for sex-role learning, symbolic thinking, and perspective taking afforded by young children's sociodramatic play. Finally, Jill and Julie avoided a conflict on role assignment by incorporating a younger child into the game, one who complied with their wishes that he be the baby. They also successfully negotiated what Julie's role in the play should be.

Peter, age 4½, is running around the preschool classroom making believe he is a dragon. He is giggling and laughing and is quite excited, and he is unconcerned about where he is going. He runs right through the block corner, knocking down other children's buildings, pretending that he is the biggest dragon in the world. He runs up to other children in playful attack, making a ferocious face and growling at them, then bursting into laughter. The other children are not amused by this, however. One boy pushes Peter out of the way; another shouts, "Dumb-dumb, you're knocking down my house!" A third begins to cry and goes to tell the teacher.

In this example, a slightly older child is engaged in fairly complex fantasy play that involves adopting the role of an imaginary creature. This suggests a certain degree of flexible and creative thinking, as well as some conception of hypothetical roles (Rubin et al., 1998). On the other hand, Peter is so engrossed in his own activity that he is unable to appreciate the impact of his rather boisterous play on others. Although his affect indicates that this is a game and that he is being playful, other children find him provocative and annoying and respond with varying types of protest: They respond physically and verbally and seek adult intervention. This overexcited role playing of a quasi-aggressive sort may escalate to a full-blown aggressive incident between the child who is overly active and rambunctious and others who are engaged in more quiet problem-solving activities. Or other children may join in, leading to an energetic chase or to playful wrestling. Such interchanges may help children learn to stop just short of real aggression, or they may deteriorate into a fight, depending on the degree of self-control exhibited by the participants.

These vignettes were meant to illustrate the enormous changes in children's social development that are apparent from the early to the late preschool period. The ability to engage in sequences of cooperative play in the context of complicated constructive and fantasy activities depends on a number of gains in social abilities that are thought to derive from transitions in cognitive processes. Social exchanges that incorporate turn taking, mutual regulation and negotiation of goals, conversation, and role enactment suggest changes in self-control, representational and means–end thinking, perspective taking, rudimentary understanding of intentionality, memory, and language ability. When such exchanges also include joint planning toward a goal, they also imply some understanding of events beyond the here and now. They rely, as well, on the ability to attend to the partner's behavior and to respond appropriately in terms of affective tone, verbal content, and ongoing motor activity. Thus a good deal of synchronization must occur if the playful interaction is to be prolonged beyond the one or two turns characteristic of toddlers, because inappropriate behavior from the partner is likely to lead either to conflict or to the termination of the interaction (Hartup, Laursen, Stewart, & Eastenson, 1988). Finally, these peer encounters depend on the ability of play partners to regulate the expression of negative emotion, so that potential areas of conflict do not escalate into fights or arguments Shantz, 1987).

THE DEVELOPMENTAL IMPORTANCE OF PEERS

As should be evident from these vignettes, peer relations, like relations with parents, siblings, and other family members, play a crucial role in young children's development (Hartup, 1983; Rubin et al., 1998; Shantz, 1987). Although early social relations develop in the context of the family, as children move into toddlerhood and enter preschool, they spend increasingly more time in the company of other children. Further, as more and more children enter child-care settings with age-mates during infancy and toddlerhood, they are exposed to other children for prolonged periods of time at earlier ages than was true even 10 years ago. These experiences with relative equals complement those with adults, who have greater authority and hence ability to control children's behavior than do peers. Piaget (1932) argued that experiences with age-mates are necessary if children are to move beyond an egocentric orientation and begin to take the views of others into account. Because interactions with peers are reciprocal and not based on the constraints imposed by either socially sanctioned authority or necessary dependency, children are in a better position to engage in negotiation and compromise (Hartup, 1983; Shantz, 1987). Of course, children are often in situations in which power relations are not entirely equal. For example, one child may dominate in decision making or allocation of resources by virtue of age, size, knowledge of the situation, or personality style. However, social interactions with peers are more equal than those with adults. As such, they force the child to give greater consideration to the wishes, feelings, and viewpoints of others and to take more responsibility for maintaining the interaction if mutually satisfying and cooperative relationships are to ensue. Thus the social skills that are learned in the course of early peer relations are seen as complementary to those learned with adults and as necessary for future social relations (see also Sullivan, 1953).

Although research demonstrates that rudimentary perspective-taking skills develop within the family context and are evident in the prosocial behaviors even of toddlers (Eisenberg & Fabes, 1998; Zahn-Waxler et al., 1979), it is also clear that children learn much about the rules of social exchange in the peer group. Turn taking, sharing, control of aggression, empathy, helping, sex-role learning, role taking, strategies of conflict resolution, and moral reasoning all develop within the peer group, as well as within the family, and appear to be central components of the ability to establish reciprocal friendships and maintain relationships with others in the larger peer group (Rubin et al., 1998). Thus it is generally agreed that social competence has its roots in the quality of early family relationships (e.g., Eisenberg & Fabes, 1998; Hartup, 1983; Sroufe, 1983; Thompson, 1998). At the same time, as children's social networks widen during the toddler and preschool years and their interest in contacts with other children becomes pronounced, the nature and complexity of their social reasoning and their social behavior with peers show profound changes that signal a new phase of developmental organization.

At a general level, Brownell (1986) has discussed the convergence of social and cognitive development that occurs during the second year of life. She argues that as children's symbolic reasoning develops—reflected in rapid strides in language ability, early causal reasoning, awareness of basic social routines, and the emergence of rudimentary perspective taking—parallel cognitive, social-cognitive, and social developmental advances occur. Cognitive-developmental reorganizations appear to underlie these changes. In the social domain, for example, the object-mediated play of the 1-year-old is replaced by the more complex play of the toddler that includes more communication over a distance and longer sequences of turn taking, both of which require some awareness of the partner as a separate person (Brownell, 1986). In the preschool period, advances in self-other differentiation and in role-taking skills are associated with the emergence of sustained bouts of cooperative play and pretending. The complexity of this play can likewise be related to changes in these and other underlying cognitive competencies. Conversely, children's social experiences with peers clearly influence their ability to make sense of and reason about the events going on around them (e.g., Corsaro, 1981), suggesting reciprocal relationships among cognitive development, social cognition, and social behavior. The emergence of prerequisite cognitive abilities and the experience of age-appropriate interactions with other children combine to lead to a fairly predictable sequence of development in children's social skills and social reasoning abilities.

Normative Conflict

Study of the social interactions of preschoolers highlights the importance of conflict and its resolution and the development of prosocial behaviors, as well as gains in cognitive skills. Shantz (1987) has suggested that conflict, defined as incompatible goals or behaviors between individuals, is central to change and developmental progression. She argues that conflict over toys, activities, role assignments, appropriate responses, and so on in the preschool setting sets the stage for numerous prosocial, as well as agonistic, interactions. Further, through conflict and its resolution, children learn to regulate their behavior in the peer group, as they practice and internalize appropriate rules of social exchange. Although much of the research on preschoolers' interactions has focused on aggressive encounters, Shantz concludes, from a review of the literature, that low-level conflicts are more common and that they are usually solved before an outright aggressive interchange erupts. Furthermore, she notes that the content of children's conflicted interactions shows developmental change. Toddlers and young preschoolers are more likely to argue over possessions and space, whereas older preschoolers are more likely to have disputes about appropriate behaviors, classroom rules, ideas, or the way a fantasy role should be played. In this context, children learn to share, to take turns, to negotiate, and to compromise. They also learn about moral rules and conventions, as well as about others' feelings and perceptions.

Normative Prosocial Behavior

Despite the importance of conflict and its resolution and the focus on aggressive encounters, a much larger proportion of children's interactions tend to be prosocial. Cooperative and parallel play activities predominate among preschoolers (Rubin et al, 1998; Shantz, 1987).

Young children also demonstrate the ability to show sympathy and concern for others; they help one another and comfort those who are distressed (Eisenberg & Fabes, 1998). Such prosocial behaviors are in evidence in the direct interactions among children, and they are rehearsed during sociodramatic play episodes. Although Piaget argued that the egocentrism of preschoolers precluded the development of such prosocial behaviors, much current research indicates that young children, although still concrete in their thinking, are capable of some degree of decentration; that their activities, thoughts, and feelings are not totally focused on themselves, and that Piaget underestimated the cognitive and social capacities of preschool children (see, e.g., Gottman & Parkhurst, 1980; Rubin et al., 1983, 1998; Shantz, 1987; Zahn-Waxler et al., 1979). Preschoolers engage in a good deal of prosocial behavior that is reflected in the quality of their play and their concern for others.

Group Entry

Preschool children are also capable of showing a lack of concern for the rights and feelings of others, and this is evident from their responses to the social overtures of others, as well as in the relative frequency of possession struggles and conflicts over toys. Corsaro (1981) conducted a detailed ethnographic study of the attempts made by preschoolers to enter ongoing social groups. He noted that roughly half of the group entry attempts he observed met with initial resistance. Children were likely to claim ownership of the toys or space, to say that the area was overcrowded or that there were not enough toys for new members, to deny that the newcomer was a friend, to cite arbitrary rules about the groups' needs, or to issue a blanket refusal. Children who approached a group in an aggressive manner or who tried to take over were less likely to be accepted than those who used a more subtle approach that involved parallel play. Corsaro (1981) suggests that the high level of unsuccessful bids to join ongoing play groups may reflect the fact that the newcomer disrupts the tenuous balance of the game or activity.

Friendship

Friendship and familiarity also play a role in children's choices of playmates and in their willingness to let others join their ongoing activities.

There is evidence that preschoolers have preferred playmates and even "best friends" with whom they band together and exclude others (Corsaro, 1981). Children also tend to prefer familiar to unfamiliar peers and are more likely to engage in prosocial behaviors such as sharing with children they know (Rubin et al, 1998). Prior peer experiences also appear to influence the quality of children's play. Children engage in more frequent and more elaborate fantasy play with familiar than unfamiliar peers (Gottman & Parkhurst, 1980). Harper and Huie (1985) reported that both prior experience with peers and familiarity with classmates were associated with children's participation in interactive play, whereas children without prior peer group experience were more likely to spend time in solitary activities. Preschool friends spend more time together and, therefore, are also more likely to engage in conflict. However, they tend to resolve disputes more amicably, for example, by negotiating a solution or by stopping the conflict, presumably because they do not want to jeopardize the relationship (Hartup et al., 1988). In addition, there is evidence that the presence of familiar preschool peers in the same classroom facilitates the transition to kindergarten (Ladd & Price, 1987), possibly because familiar playmates serve a supportive function for each other in a new environment. Although it has been argued by some (e.g., Selman, 1981) that preschool children's egocentrism precludes the development of affective bonds of friendship that move beyond the momentary here and now, studies clearly indicate that this characterization underestimates the ability of preschoolers to develop intense and mutually supportive bonds with age-mates (see Corsaro, 1981; Gottman & Parkhurst, 1980; Rubin et al., 1998). Preschoolers establish specific emotional connections with special friends whom they favor as playmates, express affection toward, show concern for, and miss when they are absent.

Normative Gender Differences

Gender also influences the nature and quality of peer interactions. Same-sex friendships are more common across the preschool and elementary school years, with children often actively avoiding opposite-sex playmates. The favored activities of boys' and girls' groups also differ markedly (Hartup, 1983; Maccoby, 1988, 1990; Martin & Fabes, 2001). For example, boys tend to engage in more active and rough-and-tumble play than girls, who tend to spend more time in dramatic play and construction activities. Boys also become involved in more frequent aggressive interactions, including property conflicts (Maccoby, 1988; Parke & Slaby, 1983), whereas girls are likely to avoid the rough, aggressive, and active play of boys (Martin & Fabes, 2001). Corsaro's (1981) observations in preschools indicate that boys have an easier time than girls gaining entry into mixed-gender play groups and that boys are also more likely to be accepted by an all-girls group than vice versa. Despite the predominance of separation by sex, there is evidence that opposite-sex peers sometimes develop strong attachments during the preschool years (Gottman & Parkhurst, 1980). However, it is not clear what happens to such friendships in the early elementary school years, when children's groups become even more strongly segregated by gender (Maccoby, 1990).

INDIVIDUAL DIFFERENCES IN BEHAVIOR WITH PEERS

Despite this relatively predictable developmental progression, children vary widely in their social behaviors and in their appreciation of their social worlds. Individual differences in children's peer experiences and the quality of their relationships with peers have been studied in terms of social behavior in the peer group, peer acceptance or rejection, and friendship relations (Rubin et al., 1998). In addition, there is a growing interest in peer victimization and in differing manifestations of aggression toward other children, including aggression that is reactive to provocations (reactive), aggression that is controlling and bullying (proactive), and aggression that inflicts emotional harm on others' self-esteem and on their relationships with peers (relational aggression; see Coie & Dodge, 1998; Crick & Grotpeter, 1995; Schwartz, Dodge, & Coie, 1993). The social-cognitive processes that underlie these different patterns of aggressive and prosocial behavior are also of interest, but they are difficult to study in young children. Research is just beginning to delineate the child characteristics and socialization processes that may partly account for individual differences in these various aspects of prosocial and aggressive behavior with other children (e.g., Fabes et al., 1999; Schwartz, Dodge, Pettit, & Bates, 1997; Schwartz, Dodge, Pettit, Bates, & the Conduct Problems Prevention Research Group, 2000). In addition, the longer term consequences of these variations in aggressive and prosocial behavior, especially aggressive and antagonistic behavior, and of victimization by peers are of interest because there is growing evidence that children who experience stable difficulties with peers that begin in the preschool or kindergarten years are at risk for problems in adjustment in elementary school and adolescence (e.g., Brendgen, Vitaro, Bukowski, Doyle, & Markiewicz, 2001; Schwartz, McFadyen-Ketchum, Dodge, Pettit, & Bates, 1999).

Children differ widely in their tendency to be sociable, shy, or aggressive; they also differ widely in the quality of their play. Moreover, these individual differences are thought to be important predictors of later development, partly because of their effects on other children. Even in preschool, children are very much aware of which children are the leaders and which are the troublemakers. Children who are more positive, cooperative, sociable, and concerned about the rights of others are more likely to be sought out as playmates, and this is likely to enhance their opportunities to interact with others, thereby developing their competence with peers even further. The ability to respond appropriately and reciprocally is also likely to be related to peer popularity: Children who are more adept socially are more likely to be chosen as attractive partners.

Conversely, children who are disruptive, provocative, aggressive, and predominantly negative in affect are more likely to elicit negative responses from others and to be rejected by peers. Children whose play is aggressive and disorganized or those who lack the skills to engage in mutual turn taking, sharing, listening, and responding appropriately in the context of the ongoing activity are likely to be avoided as playmates (Hart, DeWolf, Wozniak, & Burts, 1992; Ladd & Burgess, 1999; Ladd & Price, 1987; Milich, Landau, Kilby, & Whitten, 1982). Furthermore, Ladd and Price (1987) found that time spent in cooperative play and extensiveness of positive social contacts in preschool were not only related to concurrent measures of peer popularity but also predicted peer status at the beginning and end of kindergarten. Similarly, aggressive and negative interactions in preschool were associated with a concurrent measure of peer rejection, and they predicted peer rejection in kindergarten. This relationship was especially strong for boys, who were more likely to be both aggressive and rejected. Moreover, evidence from this study and others suggests that aggression may persist in children who are intensely and inappropriately aggressive in preschool, possibly fueling a cycle of peer rejection that predicts continued inappropriate behavior with peers (Coie & Dodge, 1998; Ladd & Burgess, 1999). On the other hand, children who are somewhat shy and withdrawn, although they may not be considered popular, are likely to have reciprocal friendships and not to be rejected (Ladd & Burgess, 1999). However, the combination of withdrawn behavior and aggression bodes particularly poorly for later development (Coie & Dodge, 1998).

Recent research has attempted to examine more fine-grained differences in the negative and asocial behaviors of children beyond just a focus on "aggression." Distinctions have been made between children who are picked on and bullied by others and who then either retaliate or withdraw (e.g., Schwartz et al., 1999, 2000). Children who are both victimized and victimizers, not surprisingly, have the worst adjustment. However, it is not clear that stable patterns of victimization or bullying are established before school entry, although it is likely that the small group of highly aggressive children who are identified early as showing severe problems with peers and at home are also the children who end up being bullies and victims in middle childhood. Still, large-scale longitudinal studies that track children from preschool age to middle childhood and that also examine peer social status and competence in the peer group are only beginning to appear.

Sociable children, then, do well with peers, and aggressive children tend to be rejected, despite their interest in playing with others. However, it is also clear that not all aggressive children are rejected. Whether or not rejection is a concomitant of aggressive behavior appears to depend partly on the nature of the aggression and on whether the aggressive child can also be prosocial (Coie & Dodge, 1998). Evidence also indicates that some children do not seek out play partners but tend to stay off by themselves on the sidelines. Some of these children may be neglected by peers, but they tend not to be actively rejected in the same way that aggressive children are. For example, Rubin (1982) observed the social interaction patterns of a group of preschoolers. Children classified as socially isolated spent more free play time unoccupied or watching the activities of others and less time in social conversation than their classmates, who had been classified as normally sociable or highly sociable. Socially withdrawn children not only initiated less interaction themselves but also received fewer interaction bids from others. When isolated preschoolers were involved in play, it was more likely to be a relatively immature form of exploratory activity. Their decreased social involvement was also reflected in less sociodramatic play with others, play that is seen as an important avenue of socialization and social-cognitive development. Even when paired with another child during free play, isolated children talked to themselves more and their partners less than their more sociable peers in comparison groups. Children who seem "tuned out" and socially withdrawn are more likely to be ignored by classmates (Peery, 1979), providing them with fewer opportunities to engage in those social activities thought to enhance social competence.

Studies of children with behavior disorders indicate that difficulties with peers is a pervasive and continuing problem (Campbell, 1990; Hinshaw, 1994). The few studies that have examined the social interactions of young children with externalizing behavior problems have found, not surprisingly, that they were more aggressive with peers than controls when observed in preschool (e.g., Campbell & Cluss, 1982), although they were not found to be less sociable with peers. Cohen and her colleagues (Cohen, Sullivan, Minde, Novak, & Helwig, 1981) found that hyperactive kindergartners were more likely to disrupt peers' play and to engage in solitary activities than their nonhyperactive classmates. Leach (1972) reported that 3-year-olds with marked separation problems in preschool were less competent with peers and that their tendency to avoid interaction and to give in to peer conflict persisted over the first several months of school. These few studies point to the poor social skills evidenced by preschoolers with varying types of behavioral disturbances and underline the need for additional research on the correlates and consequences of problematic peer skills. Although peer research has burgeoned in recent years, clinically diagnosed preschool children with behavior problems have been studied only rarely in the peer group; instead, research has focused on community samples of young children (e.g., Ladd & Burgess, 1999; Schwartz et al., 2000).

The evidence from nonreferred samples of preschool children suggests that both aggressive children and hyperactive–impulsive children are likely to be rejected by peers. Studies of school-age children confirm that clinically referred aggressive and overactive children are less popular with peers and are more likely to be overtly rejected by classmates than to be merely ignored (e.g., Dodge, 1983; Pelham & Bender, 1982). Furthermore, measures of peer rejection show relative stability over time (Brendgen et al., 2001; Dodge, 1983; Ladd & Price, 1987): Rejected children who enter new peer groups are likely to display negative, annoying, and provocative behavior very early in the acquaintanceship process, and this behavior appears to lead to further rejection, even in a new group (e.g., Dodge, 1983; Pelham & Bender, 1982). In line with a transactional model, this suggests a cyclical pattern of influences between the rejected child's social status and his or her poor social skills. Inappropriate and annoying behavior initially leads to peer rejection, which, in turn, leads the rejected youngster to increase the intensity of his or her futile attempts to gain acceptance, leading to further rejection. Furthermore, persistent rejection by peers is likely to have an effect on a child's self-esteem and social expectations of others, and these in turn may exacerbate social problems and contribute to other difficulties as well. Follow-up studies of children with behavior problems indicate that difficulties with peers tend to persist and to become more severe as children get older (see Chapter 8).

SOCIAL REASONING

In addition to directly studying children's peer relations by examining the quality of children's play in preschools and other group settings, theorists and researchers have focused on children's understanding of social rules and social relations. Selman (1980) and other theorists (e.g., Damon, 1977) have suggested that children's reasoning about the social world develops in sequential fashion, with children going through stages of social-cognitive development that parallel Piaget's stages of reasoning about the physical world. These ideas are related to more recent interest in children's "theory of mind," that is, their awareness of their own and others' inner states and cognitive processes (see Bjorklund, 2000). According to this model, the first level, the "egocentric or undifferentiated" perspective, is apparent in young preschoolers and is reflected in a lack of distinction between the child's perspective (including perceptions, thoughts, feelings) and those of others. Children at this level do not recognize that others can interpret experiences differently from the way they do; they also tend to confuse physical and psychological aspects of the social world. For example, young children may define a playmate as "nice" if he gives them candy or a toy rather than in terms of a psychological characteristic, such as concern for others. The second level, the subjective or differentiated perspective, is defined by the child's growing ability to understand that someone else's viewpoint may be different from his or her own. Children are beginning to be aware of psychological characteristics and the fact that different individuals may perceive events differently. However, they are unable, at this stage, to coordinate their own views with the views of others or to understand the reasons for differences in perspective. Children reach these stages at different ages, although, consistent with a Piagetian framework, all children go through all stages in the same sequence. Selman (1980, 1981) believes that most preschoolers are able to function only at the first level, although some older preschoolers reach the second level, which is more characteristic of elementary school children.

In the context of peer relationships, Selman (1980, 1981) and others (e.g., Damon, 1977) have tested this theory by examining children's developing concepts of friendship. Selman's general theory of sequential stages of social development is confirmed by his work, as well as by the work of others (reviewed in Selman, 1981). He calls the first level of children's friendship conceptions "momentary physical playmate," a term that denotes that the child's view of friendship is determined by proximity and frequency of contact. According to Selman (1980, 1981), the child does not think in terms of an enduring relationship or seek playmates based on psychological characteristics. Rather, friends are playmates, and when children disagree, they are no longer friends. Furthermore, conflicts and fights occur over space and activities, rather than over other, less tangible issues. Because the basis for friendship is physical rather than psychological, the thoughts, feelings, and desires of others are not relevant. Although a child may be aware that another child wants the same toy, at this level of social reasoning any sharing that occurs is most likely to be a function of dominance and submission, prior possession, or adult intervention and not due to the child's reasoning about how the other child feels when unable to have access to the coveted toy. Conflicts are resolved by physical fighting or by leaving the scene.

At the second level of friendship reasoning, children are beginning to take psychological characteristics into account. This stage is termed "one-way assistance" by Selman (1981), who notes that these children define a friend as someone who does what one wants (e.g., lets you play with his toys). A friend is also someone "you like" and someone "you know" better than other children. Conflict is also seen as a one-way street: It is caused by the actions of one person toward another (e.g., not sharing toys). Thus conflict can be resolved by one person's actions, such as giving up a toy. However, feelings are recognized. Children are friends with those they like and not friends with those they do not like.

Furthermore, at this stage children recognize that one person's actions can influence how another person is feeling (you feel bad when someone won't let you play with him or his toys).

Although research interviews confirm relatively concrete thinking among preschoolers, as well as limited ability to empathize with others or to conceptualize relationships as existing beyond the here and now, behavioral observations and children's conversations with one another indicate that children's social interactions with peers actually involve more complex social reasoning (e.g., Corsaro, 1981; Gottman & Parkhurst, 1980). Thus, as already noted, young children demonstrate some empathy, perspective taking, and concern for others when observed interacting with playmates, although they may not be able to articulate what they or others are feeling when asked directly or when required to imagine how they would feel in a hypothetical situation. Similarly, when asked about conflict resolution, young children may report that they would fight or tell the teacher, although observational studies of children's behavior suggest that they have a broader repertoire of situationally appropriate problem-solving strategies (e.g., Hartup et al., 1988). For example, toy struggles may lead to fights, but they may also result in some form of negotiation, sharing, or reasoning about why one child should play with the toy first.

Similarly, Selman's (1980, 1981) model of friendship concepts suggests that preschoolers rarely form meaningful friendships with other children that involve concern, caring, sharing, or awareness of the other child's absence or that involve a more long-term bond. However, observations in preschools and of children interacting at home indicate that this is not the case (e.g., Corsaro, 1981; Gottman & Parkhurst, 1980; Rubin et al., 1998). Young children clearly establish close relationships with other children that involve spontaneous sharing of toys, as well as of thoughts and feelings, albeit at a different level than one would expect from school-age children. Young children are capable of expressing worry and concern for the welfare of friends and of missing them in their absence, clearly an indication of some appreciation of a relationship that goes beyond the here and now. Children's ability to negotiate to solve disputes also suggests somewhat greater social reasoning ability than is implied by Selman's model (Hartup et al., 1988; Shantz, 1987). Furthermore, analyses of young children's conversations indicate awareness of the listener's needs and characteristics, as well as more conversational reciprocity than is implied by theories that emphasize the egocentrism of preschoolers (e.g, see Gottman & Parkhurst, 1980; Shantz, 1987; Shatz, 1983, for discussions of this and related issues). Finally, the data on preschool children's perceptions of classmates indicate that they are relatively accurate in identifying children who behave inappropriately and aggressively, as well as those who are socially adept. This finding suggests that young children possess at least some rudimentary awareness of the behavioral characteristics of peers. They are also aware of which behaviors contribute to liking and which behaviors are aversive and cause children to be avoided by peers. Research on school-age children has also focused on social expectations, attributions of intent, and reputation as potentially influencing social status and behavior with peers (Coie & Dodge, 1998). Because of methodological constraints, research on social cognition has emphasized school-age children, rather than preschoolers.

In summary, the rapid changes that occur in young children's social abilities with peers have been well documented. From toddlerhood to the preschool period, children master the basic rules of reciprocity that are necessary for successful social interaction and social conversation as they establish relationships with children outside the family circle. These experiences with peers parallel and complement experiences in the family; experiences with others also influence and are influenced by changes in children's reasoning about their social world. However, children also show wide variations in sociability and the ability to deal with conflict, which appear to affect their acceptability as play partners. The long-term impact of children's early experiences with peers remains a topic of current interest and debate, a topic to which I return later in this chapter.

FAMILY PREDICTORS OF INDIVIDUAL DIFFERENCES IN CHILDREN'S PEER RELATIONS

It is generally agreed that individual differences in children's social behavior, both in the peer group and in close dyadic friendship relationships, are shaped in part by earlier and concurrent experiences in the family. Most explanations that link family and peer relationships have emphasized associations between the quality of parent–child interactions and children's social competence with peers. These include explanations derived from attachment theory, from more general considerations of the quality of parenting and the parent–child relationship, and from specific aspects of discipline and limit setting.

From an attachment-theory perspective, the quality of the early attachment relationship should predict preschoolers' ability to play cooperatively with peers, their tendency to be aggressive or withdrawn, their attractiveness as play partners, their overall popularity in the peer group, and their ability to sustain friendships with specific children (e.g., Coie & Dodge, 1998; Rubin et al., 1998). Sroufe and colleagues (Carlson & Sroufe, 1995; Sroufe, 1983; Sroufe & Fleeson, 1986) emphasize the effect of early attachment security on the development of feelings of self-esteem and self-efficacy. That is, children who feel more competent and self-assured by virtue of their positive early experiences with nurturant and responsive caregivers and their secure attachments will be better able to reach out to others; their relationship history will carry over to their ability to form positive relationships in the peer group and to establish meaningful, reciprocal friendships. According to this view, characteristic ways of relating to others, as well as attitudes toward and expectations of others' availability in relationships, develop out of early experiences with caregivers and ultimately influence children's friendship choices and their general social behavior. For example, several studies suggest that securely attached children are more likely to be socially competent in the peer group as preschoolers, whereas their anxious–insecure counterparts are more likely to experience difficulties with peers (e.g., Booth, Rose-Krasnor, & Rubin, 1991; Sroufe, 1983). Thus the association between secure attachment and competence in the peer group may reflect children's positive expectations about reciprocity in relationships and a positive sense of self (Rubin et al., 1998).

From a broader perspective on parenting behavior, mothers who are sensitive and responsive to their children are also more likely to engender social understanding and self-awareness by providing explanations, discussing feelings, and modeling positive behavior toward others (e.g., Dunn, Brown, & Beardsall, 1991; Eisenberg & Fabes, 1998; Thompson, 1998). This situation should also have implications for links between parent–child relations and preschool children's social behavior with peers and peer acceptance. A large body of research on childrearing patterns and children's behavior in the peer group suggests that involved and nurturant parents who also set high standards for their children's behavior and use reasoning and explanations when enforcing limits have children who are more socially competent and prosocial with peers (Eisenberg & Fabes, 1998; Rubin et al., 1998).

Maccoby and Martin (1983) have suggested that the nature of maternal control strategies and the affective tone of the relationship between mother and child will set the stage for more general attitudes toward cooperation and positive interactions with others, whereas a more negative relationship may be modeled in more aggressive and negative encounters with peers (e.g., Strassberg, Dodge, Pettit, & Bates, 1994). Children's general "willingness to comply" with parents also may be apparent in the peer group, in which more compliant and agreeable children are better able to play cooperatively with others (see Eisenberg & Fabes, 1998; Kochanska, 1997). This finding suggests that parents' characteristic manner of handling social encounters and resolving conflicts in the home teaches children prosocial strategies and appropriate methods of conflict resolution that facilitate positive social exchange in the peer group and in dyadic friendships; in contrast, high levels of family conflict exposes them to less mature strategies that impede the development of social cooperative skills and are reflected in negative, demanding, or coercive behaviors. In addition, family interactions appear to influence children's ability to regulate the expression of negative affect and their interpretations of social interactions with other children (e.g., Davies & Cummings, 1994; Dodge, Pettit, & Bates, 1994; Eisenberg & Fabes, 1998). Children who have difficulty either expressing positive affect or inhibiting the inappropriate expression of negative affect will be more likely to have difficulties playing cooperatively with other children, will be more likely to be rejected or victimized by peers, and will be less likely to have close, reciprocal friendships.

Studies also have found an association between parent–child relationships, children's prosocial behavior, and peer popularity in young children. For example, Hart et al. (1992) examined the association between parental disciplinary styles, preschoolers' behavior on the playground, and peer popularity. Parents who used more proactive, inductive, and positive forms of limit setting that included explanations and reasoning had preschool children who engaged in fewer disruptive encounters on the playground; girls and older preschoolers with inductive mothers were more prosocial. In addition, these children were more popular with peers, according to both teacher and child nominations. Moreover, the link between disciplinary style and children's popularity with peers was accounted for by children's disruptive and prosocial behavior, consistent with a modeling perspective. That is, these and other studies suggest that when children have learned positive and prosocial ways of relating to others in the family context, they are more likely to be valued as playmates. Conversely, children whose parents engage in harsh discipline, which in turn is likely to be modeled in aggressive play, will be more likely to be rejected by other children, even in preschool.

In this way, studies demonstrate that the use of positive proactive controls and explanations and parental warmth are reflected in better cooperation at home and in the peer group and that negative discipline strategies are associated with more negative interactions with peers and lower peer popularity. Parents who are rejecting, uninvolved, and often angry and who frequently employ physical punishment to enforce limits are more likely to have children who are aggressive with peers (Coie & Dodge, 1998). Some evidence also suggests that certain types of parental deviance, such as psychopathology (particularly depression) and poor parental self-control (as reflected in high levels of family conflict and in child abuse), are each associated with young children's poorer control of aggression toward peers (Coie & Dodge, 1998; Dodge et al., 1994; Strassberg et al., 1994; Zahn-Waxler, Cummings, McKnew, & Radke-Yarrow, 1984).

For example, Dodge et al. (1994) recruited a large representative sample of children at the time they preregistered for kindergarten and followed them longitudinally from kindergarten to fourth grade. Children who were disciplined severely in early childhood (through age 5), including discipline characterized as probable or definite physical abuse, were more likely to be rejected by peers across the early elementary school years than were nonmaltreated children, even when socioeconomic status was controlled. Teachers also rated these children as less popular with peers at each assessment, and mothers saw them as more socially withdrawn. Using this same data set, Strassberg et al. (1994) found a linear relationship between parents' use of physical punishment (none, spanking, more violent methods including hitting child with an object) and children's reactive aggression and bullying. Children who were the victims of severe maternal physical punishment were most likely to bully peers on the playground and to respond to other children's provocations (real or imagined) with angry aggression; children who were spanked were also more likely than children who did not receive physical punishment to engage in reactive aggression toward peers. Boys were especially likely to engage in reactive aggression and bullying when spanked by their fathers. Moreover, disciplinary styles tended to aggregate across parents, so that if one parent used physical discipline, the other parent was also more likely to do so; spanking by both parents was most common. Children in families in which neither parent used physical punishment were by far the least aggressive with peers. These relationships between harsh physical punishment, children's aggression, and peer rejection appear to be partly a function of children's negative expectations about peers' behaviors and intentions, expectations that appear to be learned in the family context and that are associated with reactive aggression (Dodge et al., 1994).

The links between family and parenting characteristics and children's behavior with peers are undoubtedly complex. In part, they are likely to reflect children's general temperamental or personality style—that is, children who are positive and cooperative at home may also be that way with peers, whereas some children who are negative and noncompliant at home may also be more likely to behave that way with peers. In addition, as Bell (1968) has suggested, children not only react to but also elicit certain childrearing practices by virtue of their temperament and their initial responsiveness to attempts at parental control. For example, children who are cooperative and compliant are likely to elicit reasoning, compromise, and negotiation from parents that may carry over to encounters with peers; whereas children who tend to be defiant and uncooperative will be more likely to elicit harsh and angry parental responses that may influence the way they cope with conflicts in the peer group. Similarities in parent–child interaction (cooperation and reasoning or harsh discipline and defiance) also partly reflect genetic similarities between parents and their children in relevant personality characteristics related to mood, reactivity, and regulation (Rothbart & Bates, 1998), which in turn are expressed as individual differences in the expression and regulation of negative affect and as differences in prosocial behavior and positive mood.

In keeping with a transactional model of development, it would also be logical to hypothesize that experiences with peers also feed back, in reciprocal fashion, to influence the quality of parent–child relationships, as well as relationships with siblings. Few parents of adolescents would be likely to quarrel with this statement, but its application to preschoolers may be less obvious. However, it is likely that parents' perceptions of their children will be influenced by their observations of their children's social behavior with peers. These perceptions may, in turn, have an effect on parental limit setting, on parents' interest in facilitating contact with peers, and on the degree of independence permitted in play settings with other children. For example, parents' willingness to step back and let children settle their own disputes might be expected to have an effect on children's learning to negotiate, share, and compromise. However, when parents perceive their children as excessively aggressive, they may be more likely to jump in prematurely to enforce the nonviolent settlement of squabbles between peers, thereby depriving their children of important learning opportunities. Parental perceptions of their children's peer relationships probably also influence their willingness to seek out peer experiences for their children, either by enrolling them in preschool or group child care or by inviting other children over to play. In this way parental attitudes and expectations might be expected to interact in a reciprocal fashion with children's social competence.

In general, then, current research and theory converge to suggest that family experiences influence the nature of social development and directly and indirectly shape children's social experiences with peers. Consistent with a transactional model of development, the relations between child characteristics and parents' strategies of childrearing are reciprocal, reflecting both biological/genetic and social factors that, in turn, predict the opportunities that young children have to socialize with peers, as well as the quality of their relationships with friends and in the peer group. Research and theory also point to a number of family processes that may account for socialization influences beyond genetics, including children's tendency to model parental behavior, affect, and negotiating strategies; children's expectations and attributions learned in the family about whether responses from others will generally be positive and accepting or hostile and rejecting; positive affective qualities of the parent–child relationship that predict feelings of self-worth and self-efficacy and that may in turn be related to empathy and concern for others; and children's sensitivity to conflict and negative emotional arousal learned in the context of dispute resolution. In addition, children with particular temperamental or personality characteristics will be more susceptible to these family processes (see Bates et al., 1998; Belsky et al., 1998; Kochanska, 1995). Conversely, parents with certain personality attributes and attitudes will be more likely to model particular behaviors and to use more positive and proactive childrearing strategies or more negative and controlling ones. Taken together, these examples make it clear why Hartup (1983) has talked about the "synergy" between the family and peer social systems.

THE CLINICAL IMPLICATIONS OF PEER PROBLEMS

Wide agreement exists in the research indicating that difficulties in the peer group are frequently a concomitant of both internalizing and externalizing behavioral disturbances in young children (Coie & Dodge, 1998; Rubin et al., 1998). However, it is less clear whether peer problems should be viewed as a correlate, cause, or consequence of other difficulties (Parker & Asher, 1987). The prognostic significance of peer problems also has been the subject of much discussion and speculation (see Coie & Dodge, 1998). A number of short-term longitudinal studies of nonclinical samples suggest that both aggressive behavior toward peers and social withdrawal show some stability across the preschool years and into early elementary school (e.g., Buss, Block, & Block, 1980; Kohn, 1977; Ladd & Price, 1987). Indeed, longitudinal studies of aggression in both referred and nonreferred samples also indicate quite marked long-term stability, a finding that has led Olweus (1979) to suggest that aggression may be as stable as IQ. Furthermore, there is evidence that aggression shows continuity across generations (Eron & Huesmann, 1990). In general, these longer term studies have been conducted with children who were identified as aggressive at school age, so it is unclear how generalizable these results are to preschoolers. However, recent research on high-risk community samples suggests that in a small proportion of young children, especially those with high levels of family disruption and stress, aggression and other problems are quite stable (see Campbell et al., 2000, for a review). This small group of stably aggressive and noncompliant children undoubtedly have difficulties in the peer group (Campbell et al., 1994; Coie & Dodge, 1998).

The data on the persistence of externalizing problems are much clearer than the findings on social withdrawal, which tend to be more equivocal. Some studies have found that shy, withdrawn children continue to function more poorly, both academically and socially, than their more sociable peers (Rubin et al., 1998). Rubin et al. (1998) suggest that seriously withdrawn children, especially those who are temperamentally inhibited from early infancy and whose parents are either unresponsive or overprotective, may be at risk for problems in the peer group. This is because their unassertive and wary behavior with other children may foster social isolation, both because they are not chosen as play partners and because they do not seek out peer contacts. Lack of peer experiences may further exacerbate peer problems at school entry, reflecting lower peer competence and continued reticence with other children. Although this theoretical perspective is compelling, there are few data to support the long-term implications of early social withdrawal. It is generally agreed that children who are shy and withdrawn in one group may be accepted in another (Asher, 1983) and that internalizing problems in general are not likely to persist in preschoolers or kindergarten children (Fischer, Rolf, Hasazi, & Cummings, 1984; Ladd & Burgess, 1999). Indeed, Ladd and Burgess (1999) found that socially withdrawn children who were studied longitudinally from kindergarten entry to the end of second grade were not less likely to have mutual friends nor more likely to be rejected by peers. This finding highlights the potential protective role of friendships, even for children who are shy and unassertive or who may be victimized in larger play groups (Schwartz et al., 2000).

Thus problems with peers in preschool, especially isolated or short-lived problems, may be a sign of a difficult developmental transition, for example, into preschool or group child care and may be of limited predictive significance for long-term adjustment. The young child who goes through a period of frequent toy struggles or who has some difficulties playing cooperatively with others, in the absence of other problems in social or cognitive development, is likely to outgrow these behaviors, especially with support and limit setting from significant adults. On the other hand, severe peer problems in preschool may signal the need for intervention. Aggressive and bullying behavior in the peer group, especially in the context of high levels of poorly regulated angry affect, may serve as a marker or correlate of a range of other externalizing problems, including tantrums, noncompliance, and poor impulse control with parents and other adults that may persist (e.g., Campbell al., 1996; Fischer et al., 1984; Pierce et al., 1999; Richman et al., 1982). The studies that have examined this question are discussed in more detail in Chapter 8.

The mechanisms that mediate the relationships between peer competence and outcome remain to be explicated. As noted earlier, peer difficulties may be one important indicator of problem severity. The abilities to establish friendships and to function adequately in the peer group are among the major developmental tasks of early childhood. Children who are having difficulties negotiating a range of developmental transitions that include separation from mother, the development of autonomy and a sense of self, the establishment of reasonable internal controls over impulses and emotions, and the ability to cooperate with age-mates are clearly at higher risk for continued problems in adaptation than children who cope with these developmental tasks more easily. Thus peer difficulties may be a correlate of problem severity and, therefore, associated with poor outcome. However, from the perspective of a transactional model of development, persistent peer problems are probably also both a cause and a consequence of poor outcome at each developmental transition point. Poor peer relations might be expected to influence a young child's self-esteem and feelings of self-efficacy and thereby exacerbate symptoms. At the same time, difficulties with impulse control, immature social reasoning, or frequent expressions of anger and defiance will influence the quality of a child's relationships with peers, with such children being less desirable play partners and friends. Furthermore, as already noted throughout this book, the expression of symptomatic behavior, including problems getting along with other children, is often related to ongoing stresses within the family. In an attempt to illustrate some of these complex issues further, I return to the descriptions of our prototypic study children.

ILLUSTRATIONS FROM HARD-TO-MANAGE CHILDREN

The children from our longitudinal study who were described in Chapter 3 varied greatly in the quality of their relationships with peers, both at the initial interview and over the course of their early development. However, severe initial peer problems and peer relationships that worsened with development tended to be associated with poorer outcomes at age 9. Other children, despite problems in the family, appeared to function well with peers and to derive a good deal of support from the peer group.

Jamie L.'s parents initially contacted the project partly because of their concern with Jamie's peer relationships. Even as a 3-year-old, Jamie was exceedingly aggressive with peers. His parents and preschool teacher agreed that he tended to become overexcited when around other children. Jamie's parents described him as aggressive and wild; he tended to disrupt the play of other children in nursery school and to provoke fights by running up to others and grabbing toys or interfering in their activities. As a result of this behavior, other children did not want to play with him, and Jamie spent much of his time in solitary activities. Despite this, he very much wanted to play with others. However, when he did approach other children, he tended to be rough and forceful, attempting to dominate their play, and the interaction almost invariably ended in a fight. This outcome served to increase Jamie's isolation even further, as children actively avoided him. Not only was Jamie rejected by his preschool classmates, but he was also avoided by other children in his neighborhood; further, other children's parents were reluctant to invite Jamie over to play or to have their children visit him. These problems were still in evidence at age 4.

Jamie's difficulties with peers have remained a continuing theme throughout his development. At the age 6 follow-up, both his mother and his first-grade teacher commented on his poor ability to get along with other children. Jamie's mother noted that, although he was generally less aggressive with other children than he had been, Jamie occasionally became involved in fights with peers, presumably in response to frustration, what Coie and Dodge (1998) term "reactive aggression." Whereas school-age children rarely engage in physical fights with peers but instead rely on verbal aggression (Hartup, 1983; Shantz, 1987), Jamie continued to get into physical fights with other boys in his class. In addition, Jamie evidenced more subtle but annoying behaviors such as those found to lead to rejection from classmates (Dodge, 1983; Pelham & Bender, 1982). He was described by his teacher as disturbing others, interrupting ongoing classroom activities, and clowning. These behaviors may have represented inappropriate attempts to gain peer attention and acceptance.

Peer problems continued to be serious at the age 9 follow-up. Jamie's mother described him as having no close friends, although she also noted that he wanted friends very badly and worried a good deal about not having friends. Despite his desire for friends, Jamie was still getting into fights with others, acting provocative and disruptive in school, and behaving in ways guaranteed to lead to rejection. His mother saw him as unable to compromise or follow games with rules, as socially immature, and as a bully. The few children with whom he did play tended to be younger than he, children he could boss around and control. Jamie's difficulties in the peer group appeared both chronic and severe. Even though he had reached the age at which boys' peer contacts tend to be extensive, he still could not play cooperatively with others. Thus Jamie appeared to be at continuing risk for poor interpersonal relations. In addition, it should be emphasized that Jamie had been afforded numerous opportunities to spend time with other children. He attended structured after-school activities with other children, such as Boy Scouts, but these experiences are uniformly negative for him.

Thus, throughout development, Jamie's relationships with peers have been poor, characterized by excessive aggression, an inability to compromise or share, and difficulties in reflecting on the effect his behavior has on others and in anticipating the consequences of his aggressive outbursts. These inappropriate behaviors appeared to be one manifestation of Jamie's persistent and severe difficulties with self-control and frustration tolerance, and they appeared to have contributed to his history of rejection by peers, something that persisted from preschool to middle childhood, both in school and in his neighborhood. The peer rejection that Jamie has experienced may, in turn, not only interfere with the acquisition of more appropriate social behaviors by depriving him of the typical experiences with peers that facilitate socialization but may also exacerbate peer problems, as Jamie's fruitless attempts to make friends become increasingly desperate, further undermining his self-esteem. In this instance, then, early peer problems may be interpreted as contributing, in a sort of snowball effect, to the persistence of general difficulties at school and at home.

In contrast, Annie J. has consistently gotten along well with her peers, and it may be that her good peer relationships have, in part, compensated for her chronically troubled relationship with her mother. When Annie was first seen in the project, she had had only very limited experiences with other children. At the age 4 follow-up, despite her mother's reports of continuing problems at home, Annie was doing well in preschool, as reflected in her cooperative play with classmates. Similarly, at age 6, although her mother continued to see Annie as overactive, inattentive, and uncooperative at home, Mrs. J. reported that Annie played well with other children. Indeed, Annie's teacher saw this as a particular strength, and she commented spontaneously on Annie's sociability and good relationships with her classmates. This same pattern was in evidence at the age 9 follow-up. Although Mrs. J. still reported that Annie was overactive, distractible, argumentative, and a worrier, she also reported that Annie had a number of stable friendships with girls in the neighborhood and that she played well with other children, was concerned about the welfare of her friends, and got a good deal of satisfaction from playing with others. In addition, Annie was involved in several extracurricular activities with other children, and she excelled at these. Again, consistent with reports since preschool, her third-grade teacher reported that she was doing well socially, as well as academically.

Despite the evidence discussed earlier linking the quality of parent–child relationships to success in the peer group, Annie was doing well in this domain. This may reflect her relatively more positive relationship with her father and sister that have served to compensate somewhat for her relatively impaired relationship with her mother. Annie's success with peers, paired with her good academic performance and her excellence at ballet, may all contribute to the feelings of competence and self-worth that have permitted her to focus some of her energies on more adaptive pursuits outside the mother–child relationship. Further, her early successes in the peer group may have contributed to feelings of self-esteem that helped her to achieve success outside the home. In addition, there is a good deal of evidence indicating that some resilient children are able to overcome problems in the home environment that place other children at risk and that girls are more resilient than boys (Masten & Coatsworth, 1998). Another, less optimistic possibility is that Annie's good functioning in middle childhood will change as she reaches adolescence or young adulthood, when problems in interpersonal relationships beyond the mother–child dyad may surface.

Robbie S. has shown a less consistent pattern of relationships with peers. No peer problems were noted when his mother was first interviewed, although Robbie had been in day care from a very early age and, therefore, had had extensive contact with other children. When he was observed in preschool at 3 years of age, the school observer specifically commented on his cooperative play with other children, despite the fact that he was the youngest child in the class. His preschool teacher likewise reported that Robbie was doing well; she saw him as highly sociable and not at all aggressive or provocative with others. Similarly, Robbie was continuing to do well with peers at the age 4 follow-up.

However, as family problems worsened and as Robbie became embroiled in his parents' divorce proceedings, his peer relationships deteriorated as well. In kindergarten, he was described as very aggressive with peers. His teacher was especially concerned because he seemed to lash out at others without provocation, for example, by throwing things at them, apparently out of frustration. Similarly, at the age 6 follow-up, Robbie continued to evidence problems with peers in school. His first-grade teacher described him as aggressive and disruptive; he tended to bully other children and often got into physical fights at recess. Even during 30-minute classroom observations conducted during structured, teacher-directed activities, Robbie was observed to get into several alter-cations with children sitting near him. Because of his aggression with peers and his poor behavioral control in general, Robbie was ultimately placed in a special class for children with behavior problems. On the other hand, Mrs. S. also noted that Robbie had friends in the neighbor-hood, including a "best" friend who lived up the street; she reported that they could play together for hours without incident.

By the age 9 follow-up, his family situation had settled down some-what, and Robbie was seen as somewhat improved, although he was still getting into the occasional fight, particularly at recess. Both his mother and teacher were more concerned with Robbie's inattention and need for adult direction than with his peer relationships. He continued to have the same friends in his neighborhood with whom he was de-scribed as playing well. Robbie's peer problems, then, seemed to occur against a background of stable friendships that have lasted from early childhood. He had a history of good peer relationships from early child-hood, as well as a positive and warm relationship with his mother. Thus, it appeared that Robbie had a number of strengths that bode well for future interpersonal relationships and that his aggressive outbursts were related rather directly to ongoing stresses within the family rather than to an inability to relate to other children.

Finally, Teddy M. was first seen at just under 2½ years. At that time, peer problems were not a particular concern, although Mrs. M. described Teddy as prone to get quite excited around other children. She also, quite appropriately, attributed this to his age and his relative lack of experiences with age-mates. Teddy started preschool when he was 3½ and did well socially. By the age 6 follow-up, however, Mrs. M. was somewhat concerned about Teddy's shyness with other children. He preferred to stay at home to play with his brother rather than go to visit friends. Although Mrs. M. noted that Teddy had friends with whom he played at school, he tended not to initiate play with them; rather, he waited for them to invite him over. Even then, however, he was often reluctant to go without his brother. On the other hand, Teddy's first-grade teacher commented on his good social skills and noted that he was well-liked by other children. Because of Teddy's shyness and what his parents saw as his social immaturity, he was retained in first grade. When seen at age 9, his teacher reported that he was doing well in second grade. His mother remained concerned about his shyness and failure to initiate play with others. Although Mrs. M. reported that Teddy did not have any close friends, she did note that he had several friends with whom he had played for several years. Overall, then, it appeared that Teddy may be less outgoing than many children his age, relying a good deal on his older brother for companionship, but he did not seem to have impaired relationships with other children. Rather, he seemed to be functioning reasonably well in the peer group as elsewhere, despite some unevenness in his development.

SUMMARY

In this chapter peer relationships have been discussed with a focus on the developmental importance of experiences with age-mates. The interplay among family influences, peer experiences, and social-cognitive functioning has been emphasized. In particular, the quality of parent–child relationships is seen as having an effect on the quality of children's relationships with peers, mediated by the impact of childrearing strategies and attachment security on children's early social skills, feelings of self-efficacy, and prosocial behavior. Children appear to learn prosocial behavior patterns, conflict resolution strategies, and awareness of the feelings of others in the family setting, and these social skills have an effect on their acceptance in the peer group. Experiences in the peer group, in turn, facilitate social development by giving children a range of experiences with sharing, role taking, affect regulation, and control of aggression, among other things, experiences that are unique when they involve age-mates rather than adults.

Typical patterns of peer interaction in the preschool setting were also described in order to illustrate some of the major developmental changes observed in the preschool years. Early peer interactions consist of interest in and curiosity about the peer and what he or she is doing, and this curiosity develops into imitation, as reflected in the parallel play of young preschoolers. Children then begin to engage in more reciprocal exchanges that involve turn taking and sharing. With further development, the peer encounters of preschoolers can include rather elaborate games and socio-dramatic play bouts that include role assignments, the negotiation of joint goals, shifts in roles, and successful attempts at conflict resolution that appear to influence and be influenced by changes in underlying cognitive structures. Observations of peer interactions may provide a window into the development of some social-cognitive processes. However, observational studies of social behavior and interview studies of children's reasoning lead to somewhat different conclusions about the relative sophistication of young children in the social domain. Social-reasoning studies suggest that children are more limited in their social skills than do observations of their actual behavior or their conversations with playmates. It appears that children may "know" how to behave in socially appropriate and sensitive ways but be unable to describe the process or their underlying motivations when asked about them directly.

Individual differences in patterns of behavior in the peer group may also be important. Patterns of aggression and social withdrawal may be a signal of developing problems. Furthermore, aggressive and shy children are more likely than their more skilled counterparts to be avoided or ignored by playmates. This may give them fewer opportunities to learn to behave appropriately with other children and further exacerbate peer problems. There also is some evidence to suggest that peer problems may be of prognostic significance, particularly when they occur in the context of a number of other problems in social development that seem to have an impact on the quality of interpersonal relationships in the family and beyond.

CHAPTER 7

Prevention and Treatment of Behavior Problems in Young Children

So far I have discussed the nature of relatively common behavior problems manifest in the preschool period and have examined the complex relationships between family interaction patterns and child behavior. I also have discussed typical patterns of social development and contrasted them with atypical or problematic social behavior in the peer group and the family. The onset and early course of children's problems were traced in illustrative descriptions. Although allusions were made to a variety of interventions, none was discussed in detail. In this chapter, the major empirically supported approaches to treating problem behavior in preschool children are discussed and evaluated.

In addition, important distinctions need to be made between prevention and treatment, as well as between universal and targeted prevention programs (see Coie et al., 1993; Cummings et al., 2000, for more extensive discussions of these issues). Targeted prevention, and to some extent early intervention, generally refer to programs that are provided to children deemed at risk to develop problems in social and/or cognitive functioning, with the goal of stopping problems either from developing at all or, once identified, from becoming more serious with development. Head Start is the prime example of a prevention/early intervention program targeted to a specifically defined group of low-income preschool children presumed to be at risk because of demographic characteristics. Universal prevention programs are those provided to all children; some obvious examples include immunizations and educational programs for pregnant women about the risks of using alcohol, drugs, or tobacco during pregnancy. Regrettably, there are few examples of such programs for preschool children that focus on social and emotional development (see Offord, Kraener, Kazdin, Jensen, & Harrington, 1998). Treatment, in contrast, refers to interventions provided to children and families after a problem has been identified and diagnosed. To some degree these distinctions between prevention and treatment are theoretical, because many children attending programs such as Head Start already have clearly identifiable problems. Conversely, more financially secure families may seek treatment in the absence of a clearly diagnosable problem in hopes of preventing problems later. At a practical level, however, different funding streams often support prevention and treatment programs. Thus many prevention and early intervention programs are considered early or compensatory education, whereas treatment programs are generally included under the rubric of mental health services. The growing awareness of the complexity of early development and the need for comprehensive programs that cut across government bureaucracies and funding sources may pave the way for more integration of educational, pediatric, and mental health programming (Offord et al., 1998; Shonkoff, Lippitt, & Cavanaugh, 2000; Shonkoff & Phillips, 2000).

The available literature on intervention with children of preschool age focuses primarily on prevention programs such as Head Start that emphasize promoting school readiness in children living in poverty rather than on studies of treatment outcome for behavioral and emotional problems. Two exceptions stand out in the prevention area; these are programs that are targeted at children who show aggression and oppositional behavior in kindergarten such as Fast Track (Conduct Problems Prevention Research Group, 1992) and the Montreal prevention trial (Vitaro, Brendgen, & Tremblay, 1999). Most descriptions of both the prevention and treatment of behavior problems emphasize school-age children, and studies that have evaluated the efficacy of traditional psychological treatments have concentrated almost exclusively on children of school age or older (e.g., see reviews by Lonigan, Elbert, & Johnson, 1998;Weisz & Hawley, 1998; Pelham, Wheeler, & Chronis, 1998; Weisz & Weiss, 1993), except in cases in which the focus is on severely impaired children such as those with autistic spectrum disorders (e.g., Rogers, 1998). In general, research on intervention in early childhood emerges from three distinct traditions. Targeted prevention programs for children deemed at risk that emphasize social and emotional development and compensatory education programs that attempt to enhance cognitive and preacademic skills frequently focus on preschoolers and their parents. These programs aim to prevent the onset of problems or to ameliorate problems that are apparent in early childhood (Shonkoff & Phillips, 2000). Standard parent management training programs, with and without other components, are sometimes tailored specifically for parents of preschool and kindergarten children, especially children showing oppositional behavior and symptoms of ADHD (e.g., Barkley et al., 2000; Eyberg, Boggs, & Algina, 1995). More recently, several investigators have attempted to intervene at the level of the mother–toddler relationship and the family system in order to promote secure child–mother attachment and better family functioning, with the ultimate goal of enhancing socioemotional and cognitive development in young children (e.g., Lieberman, Silverman, & Pawl, 2000; McDonough, 2000).

These distinct strands in the treatment outcome literature reflect a number of trends, including referral patterns, the types of problems recognized and considered significant at different ages, and the recent emphasis on empirically supported treatments for children. Given that the focus of this book is on what we *know* about problems in young children and what we can *do* about them, I emphasize empirically supported treatments and newly emerging treatments that have at least some research support, as well as their implications for both changing the developmental trajectories of young children at risk and informing theoretical models of etiology. The range of therapeutic preschool programs and psychodynamic treatments that have not been carefully evaluated are not discussed.

Regardless, children such as Jamie and Annie, who were described in previous chapters, have tended to fall through the cracks. They come from intact and relatively well-functioning families with adequate financial resources and the wherewithal to seek appropriate treatment, making them ineligible and inappropriate for many programs geared to young children at severe psychosocial risk. Furthermore, surprisingly little has been published about what to do for such children or families; nor are there many resources available. Treatment programs that focus on the behavior problems of preschoolers from a broad perspective that includes family relationships are not readily available, especially if the preschooler is developing well intellectually. Thus much of what we suggested to parents and much of what we discuss in this chapter is based on common sense, on knowledge of developmental processes and the developmental needs of young children, and on prior experience with school-age children and their families.

As pointed out by Kovacs and Paulauskas (1986), psychological treatment with children usually involves some combination of interventions that may include traditional psychotherapy, behavioral or cognitive-behavioral interventions, family therapy, and/or drug therapy. The choice of specific modality or modalities is determined primarily by the discipline and theoretical orientation of the clinician conducting the assessment, the nature of the setting (e.g., private practitioner, mental health clinic, pediatric setting), and the financial resources and motivation of the parents. A related issue is which family member or members are the focus of treatment. In traditional approaches, the child receives therapy on a weekly or twice-weekly basis, with parent guidance seen as an adjunct to the main treatment with the child; the problem is conceptualized as residing primarily within the child or reflecting the child's inability to cope with environmental stress. Behavioral parent training, on the other hand, emphasizes work with the parents, who are taught to change their ways of interacting with their child in order to change the child's behavior in the natural environment. In this framework, the parents' ways of handling the child are identified as the target of change, and in many cases, the child may not even be seen. When children are included, it is usually to observe patterns of parent–child interaction in order to provide feedback to parents and to assess outcome rather than to include children as direct targets of intervention. In contrast, family approaches usually focus on the entire family system as the unit requiring change. In some instances, the marital dyad may be the target of intervention, even though the presenting complaints may emphasize problems in a child. It should be obvious that these piecemeal approaches are not consistent with the more comprehensive developmental psychopathology perspective espoused in this book.

In this chapter, the most commonly used treatment approaches are discussed briefly, with an emphasis on work with preschoolers and their families. The focus is on parent training, compensatory education, and parent–child psychotherapy, the latter geared to enhancing the parent–child relationship. Parent training programs are discussed in detail, because there is a good deal of information available on the efficacy of such programs with parents of young children. Primary prevention and compensatory education programs are examined, because they have been carefully evaluated and because mental health workers who deal with families that do not fit into the category of "high risk" in the traditional sense have much to learn from the approaches used in some of these programs. The few studies that have examined parent–child psychotherapy are also discussed. Finally, I return to our descriptions of prototypic children to highlight the various combinations of treatment approaches that may appear warranted in a particular instance and to evaluate efficacy from a clinical perspective.

ISSUES IN INTERVENTION WITH PRESCHOOL CHILDREN

From both a clinical and a research perspective, it is important to consider a number of issues when making recommendations for treatment and when evaluating the relative merits of various treatment approaches. It is not meaningful merely to ask whether or not treatment with children is effective. Rather, one must start with the basic assumption that treatment can enhance development for some children under some circumstances. Thus it is necessary to evaluate the relative effectiveness of specific treatments for particular problems in children of a given age, with a number of contextual factors considered simultaneously. Among the more obvious factors to consider are the developmental status of the child, the nature of the problem, the age of onset and severity of the problem, and existing family resources (Kovacs & Paulauskas, 1986). A number of variables identified in previous chapters, such as family intactness, parental mental health, the quality of the marital relationship, and parental motivation, as well as material resources, are important in determining whether therapy will be tried, what approach is deemed most appropriate, and whether the intervention will lead to change. Furthermore, as pointed out in Chapter 3, the diagnostician must make a clinical decision about whether the difficulties that led to referral are simply age-appropriate, normal variations in behavior; problems that are likely to reflect no more than a difficult developmental transition or transitory reaction to stress in an otherwise well-functioning child; or problems that appear to be more serious and likely either to persist or to lead to other problems as development proceeds. In addition, even if the problems are deemed to be age-appropriate or transitory manifestations of a stressful developmental transition, assessment may suggest that work with the family is in order. For example, in some instances, it may seem necessary to educate parents about development in order to help them understand the likely reasons for their child's age-appropriate but upsetting behavior; in others, it may seem important to modify parents' expectations and strategies of child-rearing; in some instances, it may be necessary to deal with hidden issues, such as marital distress, that may have led to dysfunctional family relationships and family conflict, with the focus inappropriately on the child's problems.

Treatment recommendations for parents and preschoolers must make the child's developmental level and immediate psychological needs a central consideration, while also taking into account longer term developmental issues. Thus treatment modalities that deal with the child in the here and now, that are relatively structured and goal oriented, and that emphasize the child's problems within a family and social context seem most appropriate for work with preschool children and their families. Because preschool children are so dependent on family members and other caregivers, treatments focused only on the child seem misdirected; changes in the caretaking environment often will be necessary to bring about changes in the child, especially changes that will be maintained over time.

An appreciation of the cognitive developmental level of young children also has implications for treatment. Harter (1983) has conducted a theoretical analysis of the cognitive-developmental limitations of preschoolers, suggesting a number of reasons that traditional psychodynamic approaches to treatment seem inappropriate. Taking a Piagetian perspective, she argues that the cognitive-developmental functioning of preschoolers is characterized by relatively concrete, egocentric, and nonreflective thought (see also Selman, 1980). Furthermore, because preschoolers have only a limited recognition of the range of human emotions, more abstract, insight-oriented and cognitive techniques would not be expected to be effective with this age group. For example, if preschoolers have not yet developed the self-consciousness or self-reflective capacities to be able to recognize their own problem behavior, to identify and label complex emotions in themselves or others, or to understand and reason about their own motivations, it would not be reasonable to assume that therapeutic techniques that rely on self-reflection and the understanding of the meaning and consequences of one's own behavior would be successful. Harter (1983) also proposes that egocentric thinking and prelogical thought interfere with the ability of preschoolers to comprehend interpretations, because they have difficulty accepting the therapist's view of events and are unable to make the complex links necessary to integrate the therapist's interpretation of events with happenings in their daily lives.

Harter's (1983) work also suggests that young children have difficulty recognizing the simultaneous presence of two emotions, particularly contradictory ones, thus making it difficult for them to deal with ambivalent feelings toward others. She proposes that emotion recognition in self and others develops through a sequence of levels from concrete and egocentric to more complex, abstract, and other-oriented, similar to levels proposed by Selman (1980, 1981) in his discussion of the development of friendship concepts and interpersonal understanding. Similarly, according to this view, young children have difficulty conceptualizing latent or hidden feelings, and they do not clearly differentiate between their own feelings and those of parents during the preschool years. In addition, preschoolers do not yet have a clearly developed sense of self or of self-esteem, as they tend to think in terms of concrete characteristics of persons such as gender or size rather than in terms of abstract psychological attributes. Finally, preschoolers cannot grasp the notion of a therapeutic relationship because they do not conceptualize helping and trust in the same way that adults or older children do (Kovacs & Paulauskas, 1986).

Much of this analysis makes sense, but it also may underestimate the capabilities of young children, at least insofar as their ability to identify some salient emotions and to have some rudimentary notions of their causes. Furthermore, it is important to distinguish between the capacities that young children exhibit in social interaction and their abilities to step back and reflect on their behavior and its meaning. Although preschoolers can engage in only limited metacognition (thinking about mental processes, "theory of mind") and although they do not engage in recursive thinking (thinking about other people's thoughts about themselves), it is not known which, if any, of these cognitive capacities is a necessary ingredient of therapeutic change. Indeed, many adults probably never develop to Selman's higher levels of social reasoning. The relationship between these levels of reasoning and the ability of individuals of any age to profit from a therapeutic relationship requires study in its own right. Support and respect from a caring adult may have an impact on a child's sense of self-esteem (e.g., Bretherton, 1985), independent of more sophisticated analyses of relationships. Thus a cognitive-developmental analysis of the limitations of dynamic therapies raises many of the same issues that confront the developmentalist in trying to integrate children's overt behavior with their verbal understanding of internal cognitive and affective processes, as well as interpersonal relationships. This is clearly an area worthy of further research.

Cognitive-behavioral techniques that have as their goal cognitive restructuring or training in problem-solving strategies also are probably beyond the grasp of most preschoolers (Cohen et al., 1981), given these children's limited tendency to reflect spontaneously on their thought processes, their decision-making style, or the effect of their behavior on themselves or others. However, independent of these potential cognitive-developmental limitations, the importance of interventions that include other members of the family and/or the wider social environment appears obvious. The extant literature suggests that structured techniques that modify parenting strategies and provide parents with improved management skills and information about children's developmental needs appear to have promise. Before discussing these approaches, I briefly describe several common approaches to intervention.

THERAPEUTIC MODELS AND LEVELS OF ANALYSIS

Therapeutic approaches have been classified by Alexander and Malouf (1983) in terms of etiological formulations, the goals of intervention, and the level at which intervention occurs. Thus they distinguish among biological models, intrapsychic and cognitive processing models that emphasize individual internal (conscious and/or unconscious) processes, learning theory models that focus on overt behaviors, interactional or family-systems models that stress relationships, and sociocultural models that focus on broader social forces. This seems a useful scheme for conceptualizing major approaches, although those that appear to have the most promise for work with preschool children and their families tend to cut across these levels of analysis or to target several levels simultaneously.

Until recently, only the traditional psychodynamic approaches had anything resembling a developmental perspective (Alexander & Malouf,

1983). Whereas the orthodox Freudian focus on unconscious conflicts, psychosexual development, and fixation and regression (e.g., Klein, 1932) is not in synchrony with recent advances in developmental theory, ego-analytic and object relations theories have had an important impact on developmental formulations of attachment and peer relations (e.g., Bowlby, 1969; Mahler, 1968; Sullivan, 1953). Although these theories have not spawned systematic interventions for preschool children that have been evaluated empirically, some of these ideas have been incorporated into relatively eclectic dynamic interventions (e.g., Fraiberg, 1980; Lieberman et al., 2000). Biological approaches to treatment recognize maturational influences on development, but psychosocial developmental factors and their interaction with biological processes tend to be ignored. Family-systems theories include notions of family development, but individual needs and developmental trajectories do not figure prominently, at least in any explicit manner, although therapeutic interventions are generally tailored to be consistent with children's developmental levels and competencies. Behavioral parent training programs have recently been broadened to incorporate a more developmentally informed view (Eyberg et al., 1995) and to consider bidirectional influences (Barkley, 1997). Factors in the wider social environment (Dumas & Wahler, 1985; Kazdin, 1997) must also be taken into account when designing programs and evaluating outcome.

Biological Approaches

At the most basic level, biological models of psychopathology rest on the assumption that genetic predispositions underlie many behavior disorders, and much recent interest focuses on genetic factors and on the balance among neurotransmitters (e.g., Rutter, Silberg, O'Connor, & Simonoff, 1999). One logical extension of this perspective is the search for treatments that alter underlying biological mechanisms. Despite the appeal of this assumption, however, the actual "disease process" that underlies most behavior disorders is not known. The pharmacotherapy revolution reflects the current biological trend in psychiatry. In the child mental health field, virtually hundreds of studies have examined the use of various psychotropic medications with school-age children and adolescents diagnosed as showing ADHD, depression, anxiety, and a range of other problems in psychosocial adjustment (Swanson, McBurnett, Christian, & Wigal, 1995). Although the effectiveness of particular medications, most notably the impact of stimulants on hyperactive children, has been well documented, little is understood about the nature of drug effects, their modes of action, or their long-term effect on biological functioning or psychological development. Thus, although some practitioners believe that stimulant medication is the treatment of choice for hyperactive children, the use of behavior modifying drugs with very young children has recently generated controversy (Coyle, 2000; Marshall, 2000).

In a recent article, Zito et al. (2000) reported an upsurge in the use of medication for children between the ages of 2 and 4 enrolled in both government and privately funded managed care organizations, with stimulants, especially methylphenidate, prescribed most frequently, followed by antidepressants (selective serotonin reuptake inhibitors, or SSRIs). Over the period from 1991 through 1995, the use of stimulants with preschool children enrolled in these medical services increased threefold. More important, all of these medications are "off label" for young children, meaning that they have not been approved for use with children under 6. These alarming findings have prompted a call for research on the use of medication with young children because of their unknown effects on neurological, sensory, and cognitive development (Coyle, 2000). Use of medication with young children is also a cause for concern, given the difficulties in accurately diagnosing ADHD and other disorders in preschool children and the fact that medication is often used as a substitute rather than as an adjunct to psychosocial treatment. The National Institute of Mental Health (NIMH) is in the process of designing and launching a double-blind trial of stimulants with very young children The ethics of this decision remain controversial, but appropriate precautions for this study may be in place because only families who do not benefit from an initial trial of parent management training will be enrolled in the drug trial. This may protect the particular families enrolled in this research project, because they will be provided with appropriate monitoring of drug effects and with human-subjects protection. But the negative implications of drug trials for young children seen in general clinical practice in an era of rising health care costs and calls for belt tightening cannot be ignored. Should the results indicate that the medication is effective, we can expect an even sharper increase in prescriptions for very young children, in the absence of careful drug monitoring and accompanying psychosocial interventions for the family. Moreover, only long-term follow-up studies will provide unequivocal data on the impact of medication usage on the neurological and psychological development of young children. Short-term clinical trials will not indicate whether or not there are sleeper effects or other sequelae from the early use of psychotropic medication. Medication may have a role to play in the treatment of seriously impaired preschool children with behavior problems, but it is likely that it will be widely prescribed for a range of problems, from the terrible 2's to bona fide psychopathology. Although arguments may be made by responsible people in favor of such a drug trial, the potential negative impact of this decision needs to be carefully weighed as well.

Several small-scale studies have examined the use of methylphenidate (Ritalin) with hyperactive preschool children; early studies suggested that negative side effects outweighed positive changes in behavior (see Campbell, 1985, for a review). In a recent study, Musten, Firestone, Pisterman, Bennett, and Mercer (1997) studied 31 4- to 6-year-olds with diagnoses of ADHD using a triple-blind design, with each child receiving placebo and two dosages of methylphenidate. Most children also met criteria for co-occurring oppositional defiant disorder. Of note in this study is the high rate of parent refusal (of the original 109 eligible families, only 31 actually completed the drug trial). Medication, however, did lead to improved performance on measures of sustained attention, focused attention, and delay, as well as on parent ratings of symptoms. In addition, side effects were in evidence, especially at the higher dosage (0.5 mg/kg). This small-scale study provides suggestive evidence, but given the small and biased sample and the lack of long-term follow-up data, it is difficult to draw strong conclusions on efficacy. Moreover, the lack of data from teachers is a serious shortcoming of the study. Clearly, we must await the NIMH study results to more clearly evaluate this question. Other medications have not been studied systematically in young children.

Intrapsychic and Cognitive Processing Approaches

Intrapsychic or traditional psychodynamic approaches to treatment focus on changing personality organization, resolving unconscious conflicts, or otherwise changing intraindividual mental processes that are not observable or easily operationalized. Although in the 1980s most practicing child clinical psychologists identified themselves as psychodynamic in orientation (Tuma, 1989), as already noted, there is very little in the way of systematic research that evaluates the efficacy of the many approaches that fall under this rubric. The few studies that do exist are poorly designed and do not meet basic standards for empirical research on therapy outcome (see Kovacs & Paulauskas, 1986, for discussions of these issues, which are beyond the scope of this chapter). In addition, studies have not considered the effectiveness of therapy for children under 6. Furthermore, the relevance of these approaches to the problems of young children can be questioned, as noted earlier.

Because, as discussed earlier, it is unclear to what degree preschoolers can conceptualize problem behavior, verbalize directly about problems or concerns, or understand the meaning of a therapeutic relationship, traditional psychodynamic and child-centered therapeutic approaches tend to rely on play as the medium of expression that is most natural and comfortable for young children. Although the therapeutic relationship is seen as central, as is the establishment of an accepting environment in which conflicts, concerns, and worries can be expressed, the therapist facilitates the child's expression through play, either as playmate or participant observer, and intervenes little in the child's life beyond the protected environment of the playroom. This is in contrast to behavioral and family approaches in which the therapist intervenes directly in the child's family environment, either with specific suggestions about changes in parental behavior or with more subtle attempts to change parental attitudes. Play therapy approaches run the gamut from nondirective play therapy as exemplified in the work of Virginia Axline (1969), in which the supportive environment is seen as facilitating development and helping the child to reach his or her potential through the expression of feelings and the resolution of conflicts, to more psychoanalytic approaches in which interpretation of the play is seen as central to change (e.g., Klein, 1932). Despite the intuitive appeal and wide use of play techniques, controlled studies on the effectiveness of play therapy with clinically identified preschoolers are lacking (Russ, 1995).

Although a variety of cognitive-behavioral treatments have been developed for use with children and show some promise for problems such as depression and anxiety (Kaslow & Thompson, 1998; Ollendick & King, 1998), these approaches have proven less effective with disruptive children (Hinshaw, 1994). Moreover, they are appropriate only for school-age children and adolescents. These increasingly popular interventions focus on the rational, thinking side of the personality and attempt to influence the way people interpret events and react to them, giving them some cognitive control over thoughts and feelings. Young children, however, appear to be less amenable to these techniques, given their level of cognitive development. In particular, the cognitive approaches used with children involve reflecting on their own cognitive processes (e.g., attention, impulse control, decision making), as well as on the impact of their behavior on others (consequential thinking). Preschoolers appear to have difficulty stepping back to think about these internal processes. Also, although preschoolers begin to become more aware of the effects of their behavior on others as their perspective-taking abilities develop, it is unlikely that specific training in cognitive restructuring or in the reinterpretation of ongoing events will generalize to influence their behavior in the natural environment.

Modifying Overt Behavior

Behavioral approaches that target and attempt to change overt behaviors have been utilized with children of all ages for the past 30 years. Scores of studies have demonstrated that learning principles can be employed to change children's behavior. Thus it has been demonstrated that such troublesome behaviors as tantrums, aggression toward peers, noncompliance with requests, and social withdrawal can be modified when rewards (either social or tangible) are given for appropriate behavior and withheld for inappropriate behavior (e.g., time-out, withdrawal of privileges) or when appropriate behavior is modeled and reinforced. Methods such as time-out, giving contingent praise, and offering tangible rewards such as toys or treats for good behavior are used almost routinely in many preschool and day care centers, and many parents, across a range of educational levels, employ behavioral approaches when disciplining their children (Barkley, 1997; Eyberg et al., 1995).

Much of the empirical work in this area has focused on training parents to be more effective in setting consistent and predictable limits on their children's behavior. Earlier outcome studies, based on strict operant conditioning procedures, indicated that formal treatments showed short-term effectiveness with behavior-disordered preschoolers but that gains did not automatically generalize to other behaviors or were not maintained consistently after treatment ended (Eyberg, 1987; Kazdin, 1997). This early work derived from a strict learning theory view in which behavior change was conceptualized in mechanistic terms and was seen as deriving solely from the child's learning history defined in terms of environmental contingencies. Such a unidirectional view is inconsistent with most current thinking in the field of child development or child psychopathology. Furthermore, the developmental level of the child was not considered routinely, so that the meaning of the parent-identified behavior was not placed in a developmental context. As a result exploratory behavior ("getting into everything"), age-appropriate defiance and testing, or bed-wetting might have been targeted for change if the behavior was annoying to the parent who sought treatment, even though the behavior in question might well have been developmentally appropriate or even an important expression of a developmental issue.

In line with recent theoretical advances, the focus of many parent training programs has been narrowed to emphasize a particular age range and broadened to consider the behavior from a developmental point of view (Eyberg, 1987; Eyberg, Schuhmann, & Rey, 1998). Programs also have been expanded to incorporate a systems view of the family and, therefore, to address more general family interaction processes that may influence the ability of parents to appropriately implement and follow through on behavior management programs for noncompliant and aggressive children (Brody & Forehand, 1985; Dadds, Schwartz, & Sanders, 1987; Eyberg et al., 1995; Webster-Stratton, 1984, 1985). In addition, parent training programs also include more focus on constructive problem solving and anger management (Conduct Problems Prevention Research Group, 1992). Some therapists have attempted to build in experiences to promote generalization across settings; still others have added educational components aimed at improving parents' understanding of normal developmental processes in an attempt to change parents' cognitions about the meaning of a particular behavior at a specific developmental period. Programs may focus on the parent–child relationship by teaching parents more appropriate and responsive ways of interacting with their preschooler (Eyberg, 1987; Eyberg et al., 1995). Thus behavioral parent training programs now are likely to include both didactic information about the use of rewards and punishments and components that are more characteristic of relational and/or cognitive restructuring approaches to treatment. Several of these are discussed in detail later in this chapter.

Interactional or Family-Systems Models

Whereas family-systems models run the gamut, from those that emphasize symbolic processes to those that stress overt behavior patterns, family-interactional or -systems models all focus on interpersonal rather than intrapsychic processes. Although one family member, most often a child, may be identified as the problem, from this perspective the problem lies within the family, and the child's symptoms have functional significance for the family as a whole. Family therapists examine, among other issues, intergenerational boundaries, family alliances, the structure and nature of relationships within the family, whether particular family members are isolates, how power is distributed, and how decisions are made. From a systems perspective, symptoms are seen as maintaining some form of equilibrium within the family, even though it may be dysfunctional. For instance, an oppositional and defiant preschooler may be seen as removing the focus from marital problems and, thereby, allowing the parents to avoid dealing with a more threatening problem; or anger toward a spouse may be expressed primarily through disagreements over childrearing that are then reflected in inconsistent limit setting and in child misbehavior. Children's problems also may serve to keep extended family members such as grandparents involved in child care or other aspects of family functioning, leading to blurred boundaries across generations and often placing decision making in the hands of nonnuclear family members (see Alexander & Malouf, 1983; Haley, 1976). Parents may successfully avoid interaction and intimacy by focusing all their attention and energy on a difficult preschooler, or a mother who is overinvolved with her child may use problem behaviors as a rationale to avoid the separation experiences associated with preschool entry. In each of these examples, the child's behavior serves other needs within the family system. Indeed, although a particular child in the family may be identified as the problem member, there is evidence that parent-referred children do not always differ from nonreferred siblings (Patterson, 1980) or from unrelated controls. Furthermore, from a family-systems view, it may be argued that behavioral approaches that merely attempt to modify the symptomatic behavior in the problem child are likely to fail if other aspects of the family system are not also considered during treatment. In fact, some family-systems theorists (e.g., Framo, 1975) argue that child behavior problems are inevitably associated with marital dysfunction, although studies indicate that this is not the case (Dadds et al., 1987).

Family-systems approaches appear promising, and evidence is accumulating of their efficacy with school-age and adolescent children and their families (Alexander & Malouf, 1983), although the effectiveness of only the more behaviorally oriented family treatment techniques has been evaluated systematically. I did not locate any controlled studies examining the efficacy of family therapy when the referral problem focuses on preschool children's behavior difficulties. It seems clear from the cases of some of the children described earlier that family problems are indeed an important component of the child's ongoing difficulties. More work in this area is clearly warranted.

Sociocultural or Community Interventions

The approaches discussed so far focus on children and/or families. However, efforts also have been directed at larger units, including communities or particular groups within the population. In general, these programs fall under the rubric either of primary prevention or early intervention rather than treatment in the traditional sense. These programs tend to be tied more closely to political viewpoints and the social policy initiatives than to the mental health community, although mental health institutions such as community mental health centers derive from the prevention focus (Winett, 1998) that grew out of the Great Society programs of the 1960s and 1970s. Prevention efforts emphasize enhancing development in young children (Coie et al., 1993; Ramey & Ramey, 1998). Thus community intervention or prevention programs are based on the premise that the well-being of children and families can be improved through a range of programs that target health, nutrition, work and living conditions, and family life, as well as cognitive and social development (Winett, 1998). Community programs tend to focus on enhancing competencies and adaptive functioning while deemphasizing psychopathology. Rather, it is assumed that appropriate interventions, timed at crucial periods of development or provided to particular groups who may be at risk, will serve to prevent problems and thus limit the need for more costly treatments that are focused on psychological maladaptation.

Interventions as diverse as the federally funded Women, Infants, and Children (WIC) program's nutritional supplements for low-income families, the TV program *Sesame Street*, and vaccinations all are based on notions of prevention, although they target different levels of functioning and different subgroups of the population. In general, community prevention programs occur at the level of a social system, such as the preschool or day care center, the community clinic, or the neighborhood, and they are focused on large numbers of children rather than on a few who are specifically referred once a problem has been identified. On the other hand, early intervention programs such as Head Start identify high-risk groups who are then eligible for the program. Thus, although all or most 3- and 4-year-olds may benefit from preschool attendance, the specialized curricula designed for children living in poverty are not necessary for middle-class children living with educated parents in stable families. Although Head Start and other compensatory education programs for low-income children have been criticized as hastily conceived, inadequate, and costly (Scarr, 1998), convincing evidence shows that many of these programs have a positive impact on cognitive and social development, and some long-term follow-up studies suggest that a range of gains in social and academic functioning are maintained (e.g., Lazar & Darlington, 1982; Reynolds, Temple, Robertson, & Mann, 2001; Shonkoff & Phillips, 2000). Several early intervention and primary prevention programs for preschoolers are discussed in more detail subsequently.

THERAPEUTIC APPROACHES FOR BEHAVIOR PROBLEMS IN PRESCHOOL CHILDREN

Although it appears useful to examine treatments from the perspective of models and levels of analysis, as already noted, the lines between these various treatment approaches are becoming increasingly blurred. As models of development become more complex and as more and more data underline the importance of family and social context variables in understanding children's development, both normal and abnormal, therapeutic approaches have become less doctrinaire and more eclectic. The therapeutic preschool programs, parent training approaches, and primary prevention programs discussed in this section focus on the child and family from more than one perspective. For example, they may combine behavior management with educational intervention or family treatment. Furthermore, some systematic attempt is made to evaluate outcome using objective measures of behavior change.

Parent Training Programs for Oppositional Children

As noted earlier, parent training programs are among the most widely used and intensively studied interventions for behavior problems in preschoolers. In general, these programs have been evaluated most thoroughly with children considered oppositional and defiant, whether or not other symptoms such as inattention, impulsivity, and overactivity, are also present. The reason is partly that young children with oppositional problems usually are also impulsive and overactive; moreover, ADHD, when diagnosed in young children, rarely occurs in the absence of oppositional and defiant behavior (e.g., Lavigne et al., 1996). Most recent reviews of child-focused treatment are relatively enthusiastic about the effectiveness of parent training in modifying a variety of behavior problems, especially aggression and noncompliance in children across a wide age range (Brestan & Eyberg, 1998; Kazdin, 1997), although these authors and others also note inconsistencies in the literature. For example, Weisz, Weiss, Alicke, and Klotz (1987) conclude that behavioral parent training programs tend to be more effective and long-lasting with younger than with older children. However, Eyberg (1987) is the only author to address the effect of parent training programs on behavior problems in preschoolers specifically, and she concludes that all programs are not equally effective. Eyberg (1987), Kazdin (1997), and others (e.g., Dadds et al., 1987) emphasize both program characteristics and family factors that are associated with treatment follow-through, treatment efficacy, and maintenance of treatment effects. Programs with the most general effects on parent–child interaction and the most long-term efficacy, assessed specifically in samples of preschoolers, go beyond strict reinforcement contingencies and the use of time-out in order to deal with other aspects of family functioning. These successful programs all teach parents to use contingent and descriptive praise, to ignore annoying behaviors, to decrease criticism and vague commands, and to use time-out for destructive, aggressive, and noncompliant behavior (e.g., Dadds et al., 1987; Eyberg et al., 1995; Webster-Stratton, 1985). However, they vary on several dimensions, including group versus individual administration, the presence or absence of the child during treatment sessions, the length of treatment, paternal involvement, and the use of other treatments in addition to the behavior management training.

An interesting approach to parent training was developed by Sanders and Christensen (1985) for oppositional preschool children and their parents. They compared the effectiveness of a regular parent training program conducted in the home with parent training combined with planned-activities training. All parents were taught typical child management skills, including the use of praise for appropriate behavior, providing clear instructions and commands, ignoring irritating behavior, and using time-out for aggression and noncompliance. Parents were observed with their children at home and given feedback on their own behavior. Parents in the planned-activities condition were also given a generalized set of problem-solving strategies to use in situations such as shopping trips, birthday parties, visits, and car rides—situations that are often stressful for families with preschool children. Parents learned how to prepare children for upcoming events, to plan activities meant to avoid conflict, and to state expectations for good behavior explicitly beforehand. These skills were modeled by the therapist, role-played by parents, and coached. Both the parent training and the planned-activities treatments were effective, as indexed by observations obtained at home during breakfast and structured parent–child play, at bathtime, and at bedtime. Moreover, at a 3-month follow-up, therapy gains were maintained. Indeed, children and their parents did not differ from a nonreferred comparison group. The observations, modeling, and feedback appear to be attractive features of this program, as is the selection of situations about which parents complain frequently.

Webster-Stratton (1984) and Eyberg et al. (1995) combine training in child management methods as outlined previously with training in more general ways of interacting sensitively and positively. Eyberg et al. (1995) emphasize the impact of treatment on interaction patterns within the family, termed parent–child interaction therapy. Their treatment program, also designed primarily for parents with young oppositional children, suggests that strengthening the parent–child relationship leads to broader and more long-term effects on family functioning. The relationship-enhancing portion of treatment includes teaching the parents active listening, as well as appropriate responsiveness to their children's initiations and verbalizations; the ability to follow their children's lead in a nondirective play situation; and the provision of emotional support. This phase is followed by training in more typical child management skills, including contingent and consistent praise, ignoring and not criticizing, and the use of time-out. Evaluations of parent–child interaction therapy indicate improvements in oppositional and noncompliant behavior at the completion of treatment, as indexed by both parent reports and observational measures.

Such a combined treatment approach makes sense from several vantage points. Research on children's socialization indicates that qualitative features of the mother–child relationship and of day-to-day interaction, particularly positivity and warmth, are associated with general compliance and a willingness to comply (see Chapter 4). Mutual expectations and the relationship history appear central. Thus it may not be very helpful to modify specific disciplinary practices if more general qualitative aspects of the mother–child relationship are not changed as well. In the absence of a positive and mutually rewarding relationship, children may not have adequate incentives to be cooperative, except possibly to receive tangible rewards. In general, however, tangible rewards are unlikely to facilitate the internalization of standards, values, or independent self-regulation. In addition, research by Dumas and Wahler (1985) indicates that in troubled mother–preschool-child dyads, mothers often respond indiscriminately to children's behavior, with positive, negative, or neutral responses appearing to be independent of the child's antecedent behavior. Moreover, these mothers exhibit high rates of negative and unsupportive behavior, which may then exacerbate child noncompliance and attention seeking. It appears that a poor relationship has developed in these dyads and that the children have learned that interaction with their mothers is basically unrewarding. This formulation of parent training, which targets both specific parenting behaviors and more qualitative aspects of the relationship, is congruent with clinical experience and the formulation of the problems of many young children, as illustrated by Annie and her mother, who were described earlier.

The role of father involvement in treatment was examined by Webster-Stratton (1985) using this approach. Parents and their young oppositional children participated in treatment. One group consisted of two-parent families (including boyfriends or stepfathers; all fathers or father surrogates were involved in child care and attended most treatment sessions), and the other group consisted of father-absent families. Although both groups of mothers made significant changes and although gains were maintained at a 1-year follow-up, women whose spouses or boyfriends participated in treatment were more positive with their children, who in turn were more compliant. Moreover, significantly more two-parent families were classified as responders based on their overall response to treatment, whereas single mothers were more likely to be nonresponders. These findings underline the importance of support from a close family member in facilitating changes in parenting practices. However, it is unclear from this study (1) whether father involvement directly influenced child behavior because fathers changed their childrearing strategies and/or increased their involvement in childrearing, (2) whether fathers' presence in treatment served to encourage mothers to modify their behavior toward their children, (3) father presence had a more general and indirect, but supportive, effect on mothers that facilitated change, or (4) whether some combination of these factors accounts for the findings.

The role of father involvement in treatment may also be related to the quality of the marital relationship, as it has been suggested that marital discord may interfere with successful parent training. Persistent conflict between parents would be expected to undermine the ability of parents to work together and provide consistent limits on and rewards for child behavior. This belief is in line with clinical impression and with the literature on the relationship between child conduct disorders and marital problems (Emery, 1999; see also Chapter 4, this volume). Dadds et al. (1987) assessed the combined effects of parent management training and partner support training in couples having a preschool child who showed oppositional behavior. Half the couples had reported that they were satisfied with their marriages, and half reported significant levels of marital distress. Half the maritally distressed couples and half the maritally satisfied couples were randomly assigned to parent management training alone; the remaining couples received parent management training paired with partner support. Parent training included instruction in the home in using contingent praise and timeout, as well as the training in generalization to stressful situations such as bedtime, shopping, and so forth that was described earlier. Couples in the partner-support treatment also learned to work together to solve problems and to provide each other with mutual support. Although parents in all groups were more effective with their children posttreatment, the maritally distressed group who did not receive partner-support training did not maintain these gains at a 6-month follow-up. Dadds et al. (1987) note that aversive interaction between parents is associated with concurrent child misbehavior. Furthermore, fathers in the partner-support training were more likely to participate in child care. This suggests mutual and bidirectional influences of improved parent communication, decreased stress and resentment, and improved parenting skills. However, more research is required before the active ingredients of these programs and their mutual interactions can be delineated. It is worth emphasizing that these authors point out that their marital intervention is designed only as an adjunct to parent training and that in more severely distressed couples more intense systems therapy may be indicated.

Taken together, these studies indicate that broad-based parent training approaches that take into account other aspects of family relationships and also involve direct observations of parent–child interaction, or that at least include role playing, coaching, and feedback, have the most obvious effect on the oppositional and defiant child and are most likely to lead to changes in the family that are maintained at follow-up. It is unclear whether parent training is effective with young children with ADHD symptoms; a few small-scale studies suggest that these programs are (Sonuga-Barke, Daley, Thompson, Laver-Bradbury, & Weeks, 2001), but these findings remain to be replicated in a larger sample. In addition, it appears that families living under more stressful conditions or parents who feel less supported socially and emotionally either may be less able to follow through with treatment initially or less able to maintain gains once treatment is over. This was true for the single mothers in the Webster-Stratton (1985) study and for the maritally discordant families studied by Dadds et al. (1987). Other studies likewise indicate that factors outside the parent–child dyad influence willingness to seek treatment and treatment response. These include family composition (Webster-Stratton, 1985), father involvement and support for treatment, social support, and maternal depression (Dadds et al., 1987; Dumas & Wahler, 1983; Wahler, 1980; Webster-Stratton, 1985). These data highlight the fact that those families most in need of treatment are often the ones without the emotional resources or instrumental supports (such as transportation or child care) to allow them to make use of available services.

Primary Prevention and Early Intervention

Most early intervention programs for preschoolers have focused primarily on academic skills, although they have differed widely in the degree of structure, the nature and amount of parent involvement, the age of entry, the length of the program, the nature of the curriculum (e.g., drill vs. discovery learning, language vs. concept development), and the relative emphasis on cognitive and language development as opposed to building social competence (Ramey & Ramey, 1998; Shonkoff & Phillips, 2000). Most of these intervention programs have focused almost exclusively on poor children living in highly stressed (usually single-mother, minority) families, with the goals of improving cognitive skills, school readiness, and social functioning in order to facilitate adjustment to elementary school and enhance academic achievement. Some programs appeared to merely prevent deterioration in treated children relative to controls, whereas others appear to have led to more long-term gains in academic functioning and behavioral adjustment (Lazar & Darlington, 1982; Ramey & Ramey, 1998; Shonkoff & Phillips, 2000). In general, parent involvement, length and intensity of program, and structured content appear to be some of the parameters associated with more obvious gains in cognitive and social functioning. Ramey and Ramey (1998) note that the most successful programs begin early in the child's life and are intensive, comprehensive, and structured. Programs that deal with both children's needs and family needs appear to be most successful.

Lazar and Darlington (1982) examined the long-term efficacy of 12 independently designed infant and preschool early intervention programs. Although programs differed on a range of factors, all emphasized cognitive development using structured curricula and intense treatment with low adult–child ratios. Overall, findings after follow-up intervals ranging from 5 to 10 years indicated that low-income children who had participated in comprehensive early intervention programs were less likely to repeat a grade and to be in special classes than untreated controls, even when initial background factors were controlled statistically. Although gains in IQ scores were not maintained beyond a 2-year follow-up across programs, children's views of their own competence and parents' aspirations for their children were positively influenced by early program attendance. Lazar and Darlington (1982) conclude that "high quality programs with careful design and supervision, using a variety of strategies can be effective for different types of low-income children" (p. 65). Other outcome assessments of early intervention programs for low-income infants and preschoolers likewise document changes in cognitive and social functioning, as well as mother–child interaction (e.g., Andrews et al., 1982; Lee, Brooks-Gunn, & Schnur, 1988; Ramey & Ramey, 1998; Shonkoff & Phillips, 2000; Slaughter, 1983).

The early programs reviewed by Andrews et al. (1982) were among the more comprehensive and ambitious because they incorporated simultaneous programs for mothers and infants followed into preschool. Thus a detailed curriculum on childrearing and child development, home management, child health, and community resources was paired with learning experiences for the children and support for mothers. The program was based on the rationale that changes in mothers' attitudes and knowledge, parenting strategies, ability to utilize existing resources, and self-esteem would be more likely to have a lasting impact on the child's environment than preschool experience alone. Posttest data revealed changes in children's cognitive functioning and in a variety of mother–child interaction measures. For example, program mothers were more positive, more sensitive, less restrictive, and more effective in their use of language and teaching strategies; children were more positive and verbal in interaction with their mothers. Some gains were maintained at a 1-year follow-up.

The findings from the programs reviewed by Lazar and Darlington (1982) and Andrews et al. (1982) indicate that intensive interventions that have a multidimensional focus on children and their parents, that employ structured curricula, and that provide a range of services over time are most likely to be effective. On the other hand, gains are often not maintained once the intervention ends. The early criticisms of Head Start and other early intervention programs (e.g., Jensen, 1969) were based on the misguided assumption that preschool experience per se should lead to long-term gains and ameliorate a range of deficits in cognitive and social functioning. As noted by Lazar and Darlington (1982) and others (e.g., Zigler & Valentine, 1979) the initial expectations for these programs were unrealistic. A year of preschool experience was expected to bridge the gap in cognitive, language, and social development between children reared in poverty and middle class children, despite massive differences in early experience, ongoing environmental input, and support for academic and social competence. More recent evaluations of comprehensive interventions, however, highlight the need to modify the family environment and to provide additional resources to help parents support their children's development (Ramey & Ramey, 1998; Shonkoff & Phillips, 2000).

For example, recent reports from the Abecedarian Project (F. Campbell & Ramey, 1994; F. Campbell et al., 2001), one of the more intense preventive intervention efforts for children living in poverty, provide evidence of long-term effects of early intervention. Shortly after birth, 111 infants were randomly assigned to treatment and control groups. Children in the treated group received high-quality child care beginning at about 4 months of age for 40 hours per week, 50 weeks per year. Quality of care was high, as reflected in a low ratio of caregivers to children, low staff turnover, and high levels of teacher training and support. In this setting, children were provided with adequate nutrition, as well as age-appropriate cognitive, linguistic, and social stimulation. In the preschool period, extra resources were directed toward language development and literacy skills. Children attended the child-care center until they entered kindergarten, and half of the treated children also received additional follow-up in elementary school. Children in the control group received nutritional supplements and social work services but attended only child care that was available in the community. Cognitive and academic differences between groups were evident from early childhood through young adulthood, despite some decline over time in both groups. Moreover, the gains in the treatment group were both more dramatic and more sustained than was true in other early intervention programs that began in the preschool period and that were less intense than the Abecedarian intervention. In addition to these gains in cognitive functioning, children in the treatment group were better adjusted and had higher self-esteem; they were also less likely to use special education services and to repeat a grade. Finally, they were less likely to drop out of school or to get into trouble. These data indicate that intensive early intervention for high-risk infants and their mothers can be effective both initially and over the long term.

Results like these from the Abecedarian Project have obvious implications for programming in the mental health arena as well. Intensive programs that focus on providing parent training and family intervention, as well as structured, therapeutic preschool experiences for young children with behavioral and emotional problems, are sorely needed. As Kazdin (1997) has argued, only intensive treatments that provide a range of services over time can be expected to have a long-lasting effect on disturbed children and their families. The theoretical framework espoused at the start of this book emphasized the importance of understanding children's development from a dynamic, transactional, family-systems perspective in which aspects of the family's social context are seen as having both direct and indirect effects on the child. Thus it is not surprising that treatment approaches that are compatible with this view and that focus on preschool children and their families in a wider social context are the ones most likely to lead to positive change.

Despite the lessons learned from early intervention studies, few comprehensive prevention programs have been implemented for young children at risk for behavior problems, except in the context of poverty. The one exception to this is Fast Track, a multifaceted, multisite prevention program for children who are screened at the end of kindergarten for cross-situational aggressive and noncompliant behavior. The goal of this long-term and intense program is the ultimate prevention of conduct problems in middle childhood and adolescence. Children considered at high risk were rated as disruptive and aggressive at home and in school, according to both maternal and teacher reports. High-risk children were randomly assigned to treatment and control groups based on school attendance (i.e., schools were considered either treatment schools or control schools, because some components of the program were implemented in all first-grade classrooms; Conduct Problems Prevention Research Group, 1992, 1999, 2002). Treated children received a range of services meant to enhance social, emotional, cognitive, and academic skills, including peer competence, emotion regulation, social awareness, and social understanding, as well as school achievement. Intervention components were carried out at school, at home, and in the community, with parents, teachers, and peers participating in different facets of the program. For example, parents participated in parent training, anger management, and child tutoring programs in both group and individual settings; target children received extra help with reading, as well as a range of classroom-wide, peer group, and dyadic interventions meant to facilitate self-regulation, social competence, and dyadic friendship skills.

At the end of first grade, modest treatment–control differences were obtained across several domains of outcomes that included parent and teacher ratings of social competence, observed parent–child interaction, observed child behavior at school, self-reported parenting behavior, peer ratings, and academic behavior. Despite improvements in some behaviors thought to mediate outcomes, such as improved parent–child interaction and better social problem-solving skills, treatment and control groups did not differ in rates of externalizing problems, as reported by parents and teachers at the end of first grade. Continued intervention through fifth grade is planned in this ambitious study, and only longer term follow-up will indicate whether this carefully designed and theoretically driven prevention program will succeed in lowering rates of conduct problems in these hard-to-manage kindergarten children.

Barkley and colleagues (Barkley et al., 2000) also mounted an ambitious early intervention program for young children who were screened for elevated levels of parent-reported inattentive, impulsive, hyperactive, and oppositional symptoms prior to kindergarten entry. Children and families were randomly assigned to parent training; to a special therapeutic kindergarten that combined behavior management and social skills training provided by expert teachers in classes of 15 children; to a combined parent training and kindergarten intervention; or to a no-treatment control group. Posttreatment assessment on a wide range of measures revealed modest improvements in behavioral control for the children attending the therapeutic classrooms but no change as a function of parent management training. Barkley et al. (2000) discuss the problems they faced with parental attendance, follow-through, and motivation and suggest that parents who are screened for prevention, as opposed to those who actively seek treatment, may be less invested in program participation. When children were followed up at the end of first grade, the positive effects of the kindergarten intervention had washed out as well (Shelton et al., 2000), although consultation with first-grade teachers was built in to facilitate generalization. Still, many first-grade teachers felt overwhelmed and were not interested in implementing behavior management or other techniques in their classrooms. Thus, once these children were confronted with the increasing demands of first grade in a large class without the additional supports they had received in the therapeutic kindergarten, their earlier improvements in behavioral control could not be maintained. These disappointing results underscore the importance of longer term interventions for children with serious problems (Ramey & Ramey, 1998), as detailed in the early studies of Head Start, and also raise questions about the limited scope of the parent training package. The lack of attention to other aspects of family functioning may also play a role.

Two other prevention programs targeting kindergarten children merit discussion. Tremblay and colleagues (Tremblay, Pagani-Kurtz, Masse, Vitaro, & Pihl, 1995; Vitaro & Tremblay, 1994; Vitaro et al., 1999) obtained ratings of aggression and hyperactivity on a representative sample of kindergarten boys in Montreal. Those who were rated above the 70th percentile were invited to participate in the research and randomly assigned to treatment and control groups. Treatment included an intensive parent training package similar to the one used in Fast Track that included training in behavior management, problem-solving, and negotiation strategies during first grade. In the second and third grades, target children received social skills and problem-solving interventions that took place in the school setting and included both high-risk children and prosocial peers. Tremblay and colleagues have reported positive effects of this intervention on parent–child relations, peer relations, and behavior problems. One important component of this program is the inclusion of high-risk children together with prosocial peers. The prosocial peers were included to serve as role models and to prevent stigmatizing the aggressive–hyperactive boys. Several analyses of mediators of treatment effects suggest that this strategy was effective. Aggressive boys who had prosocial friends were less likely to get into trouble in middle childhood and early adolescence (Vitaro et al., 1999).

Cunningham, Bremner, and Boyle (1995) also screened a large number of children attending prekindergarten in Hamilton, Ontario, Canada, for disruptive and hyperactive behavior. Families were randomly assigned to individual parent training in a clinic setting, to group parent training in a community setting, or to a waiting-list control group. Treatment involved a 12-week parent training package in behavior management that included videotaped modeling, role playing, and discussion of parenting strategies meant to promote positive parenting and feelings of competence in the parenting role. Modest gains in parenting skills, parents' sense of competence, and children's disruptive behavior were reported at posttest and at 6-month follow-up. Cunningham et al.(1995) note that immigrant parents and parents with lower educational levels were more likely to comply when the treatment was offered in a group setting in the community than in a mental health clinic; parents with lower educational levels and poorer family functioning were also more comfortable participating in a community-based group program. This raises issues of stigmatization and attributions that are rarely considered in research on intervention. Parent perceptions of whether their child's problem was really serious also influenced their willingness to participate in the program, raising motivational issues as well. Finally, Cunningham and colleagues (1995) note that it was much less costly to mount group parent training in the community, suggesting the benefits of providing such programs in the context of the developmental needs of children and families rather than under the rubric of mental health.

These studies all raise interesting issues about the extent to which even ambitious programs such as Fast Track can modify the long-term course of child and family functioning in an effort to prevent the emergence or stabilization of behavior problems in young children. Complex issues such as parental motivation, perceptions of and attributions about problem behavior in young children, and parents' own implicit theories about the causes and developmental course of these behaviors will inevitably influence their willingness first to enroll in prevention or early intervention trials and then to follow through with program requirements. Similar issues have been raised in studies of treatment (e.g., Kazdin, 1997), but these potential barriers to intervention are even stronger when parents themselves have not sought treatment but rather have been recruited on the basis of community screening. It seems logical that often busy and stressed parents will not have the resources to participate in complex and time-consuming programs, especially if they do not themselves perceive their children's problems as sufficiently serious to merit intervention. These issues clearly require further thought and systematic study if prevention trials are to be successful, both in recruiting the most needy participants and in keeping parents, especially those with the most problems, engaged in the program and able to make use of the parenting and interpersonal skills that are thought to be the crux of program effectiveness. It is also important to note that all of these programs began when children were 5 to 6 years old, and they included children with a mix of symptoms of oppositional defiant disorder and ADHD. If, as already noted, problems evident in preschool are already fairly stable by school entry, this may be late for intervention to change the nature of the parent–child relationship, parental disciplinary strategies, and children's behavior. Thus, Shaw, Dishion, and Gardner (Shaw, personal communication, March 30, 2001) are now embarking on an ambitious study to screen high-risk behavior-problem children in toddlerhood and to provide a brief but intense home visiting program that focuses on parent–child relations and disciplinary strategies. It remains to be seen whether this earlier focus on behavior management and relationship quality will prove more effective in the long term in preventing early onset behavior problems from escalating. Other studies have focused on even younger children and emphasized the quality of the mother–infant relationship, with similar goals but quite different strategies.

Treatments That Focus on the Early Mother–Child Relationship

Several therapeutic approaches also have been developed that focus on early parent–child relationships, with the goals of changing negative parental perceptions and attributions of infant and toddler behavior, as

well as enhancing parental (usually maternal) sensitivity and responsiveness (e.g., Cohen et al., 1999; Fraiberg, 1980; Lieberman et al.,
2000; van den Boom, 1994). These various approaches are primarily
based on a combination of psychodynamic and attachment theory. For
example, Lieberman et al. (2000) discuss how a mother's own experiences in early childhood and later in life can influence her perceptions
of her infant's needs, intentions, communications, and behaviors. Often,
these involve marked distortions and lack of knowledge of normal development, and the case studies presented by Lieberman et al. (2000)
suggest quite severe parental psychopathology in families at extremely
high risk. That said, several recently developed treatment approaches
for a range of mother–infant or mother–toddler dyads with different
presenting complaints have emphasized attempts to enhance the ability
of mothers to accurately read and appropriately respond to infant social
signals as a way of increasing maternal sensitivity and responsiveness.
This approach, it is hoped, will alter both the mother's internal representations of the mother–infant relationship and her actual behavior
toward her baby, ultimately modifying the quality of the attachment relationship (Cohen et al., 1999; Lieberman et al., 2000; van den Boom,
1994).

Approaches to mother–child psychotherapy have similar goals of
modifying negative aspects of the mother–child relationship and/or
making mothers more sensitive to infant cues. Nevertheless, they vary
in terms of how didactic they are, how much they rely on feedback and
structured activities, how much they focus on the mother and her past
experiences as explaining the present problems, and how much they include the infant as the focus of treatment (see Cohen et al., 1999). However, there is general agreement among most researchers and theorists
in this area that "the 'identified patient' is the child–parent relationship"
(Lieberman et al., 2000, p. 472) and that it is not meaningful to consider the problems of very young children (except in cases of autism or
clear developmental delay or other illness) in the absence of parenting
and the relationship itself. Thus, whereas Cohen et al. (1999) discuss
"infant-led" treatment in which the mother is explicitly helped to read
and respond to infant signals, Lieberman and colleagues (2000) use observations of mother–infant play as a window into the mother's conflicts
and concerns about the mothering role. These differences in emphasis
are associated with differences in technique and with some preliminary

evidence suggesting that the infant-led psychotherapy ("watch, wait, wonder") may be superior in fostering infant affect regulation and cognitive development, as well as more organized attachment strategies. Other approaches involve a family-systems framework and cognitive-behavioral methods (McDonough, 2000), but the goals are essentially the same.

Interventions aimed at the mother–child relationship have been evaluated only rarely in well-designed studies. The Cohen et al. (1999) study compared the effectiveness of Lieberman's parent–infant psychotherapy with the "watch, wait, and wonder" approach, randomly assigning 67 clinically referred infants and toddlers (10–30 months at referral) to treatment groups. Referral problems focused on relationship issues, behavioral regulation, eating and sleeping problems, and concerns about parenting. Both groups showed improvements after a 5-month treatment regimen. Thus mothers in both groups reported that the presenting symptoms had decreased and that they felt more comfortable handling the initial problem. Observations of mother–infant play revealed more reciprocity, less intrusiveness, and less conflict in both groups. However, infants in the infant-led group scored higher on the Bayley Scales of Infant Development and were rated as better regulated during testing than infants in the infant–parent psychotherapy group; they also were less likely to show disorganized attachment, and their mothers reported a decline in depressive symptoms relative to mothers in the comparison group. However, at a 6-month follow-up, there were no differences between groups, although both had maintained treatment gains (Cohen, Lojkasek, Muir, Muir, & Parker, 2002). This is one of the few studies to compare two different treatment strategies with referred infants and their mothers.

Several attempts have also been made to intervene with depressed mothers and their young children in an effort to both modify maternal depression and prevent the emergence of problems in their offspring. These efforts have met with mixed success. For example, Gelfand, Teti, Seiner, and Jameson (1996) utilized a nurse home-visiting program, focused on helping mothers to read infant signals and providing age-appropriate stimulation, to supplement regular treatment for depression. There were few effects on child outcome measures or on the mother–infant relationship. In contrast, Cicchetti, Rogosch, and Toth (2000) utilized parent–toddler psychotherapy, based on Lieberman's model, with a

sample of depressed mothers and their children. They report more secure attachments and better cognitive functioning in treated children
than in controls.

Cooper and Murray (1997) were also concerned with the impact of
depression on the mother–infant relationship and on infant outcome.
They compared the effectiveness of several treatments for postpartum
women with elevated depression scores. Treatments were delivered during home visits for 10 weeks, and families were assessed at posttreatment and again 9 and 18 months after the completion of treatment.
Treatments included cognitive-behavioral therapy focused on the mother–
infant relationship and on managing the infant, nondirective parent
counseling, psychodynamic therapy focused on the mother–infant relationship and similar to Lieberman's approach, and a no-treatment control condition. All treatment groups showed improvements in maternal
mood posttreatment, and all groups maintained gains at follow-up,
although group differences were not maintained; of note, even the untreated group showed marked improvements in mood by 18-month
follow-up. Surprisingly, there was no effect of any of the treatments on
the observed quality of mother–infant interaction, although treated
women in all three groups reported fewer relationship problems at
follow-up. These disappointing results, in concert with those reported
by Gelfand et al. (1996), suggest that brief home-based interventions
may not be adequate to effect change in the quality of the mother–infant
relationship when mothers are depressed. The role of the father and/or
other significant adults in the family is not addressed in these studies
and may be an important but overlooked aspect of treatment.

Other studies have utilized attachment theory and focused on the
importance of early interaction in an attempt to alter the quality of the
mother–infant relationship even earlier, as a means of establishing secure attachment in infants deemed at risk for insecurity. The most
widely cited of these prevention studies was conducted by van den
Boom (1994) in the Netherlands. She screened firstborn neonates from
low-SES families for high levels of irritability. She then selected 100 irritable infants and randomly assigned mother–infant dyads to either intervention or control conditions. For ethical reasons, mothers were not
told that their infants were seen as "irritable"; instead they were offered
a chance to talk with staff about their concerns about childrearing. The
intervention group received three 2-hour home visits during the 6- to 9-
month period that were specifically aimed at helping mothers read,

interpret, and respond to infant signals. At the completion of the intervention, treated infants were less irritable and more exploratory, and their mothers were more appropriately responsive. At 12 months of age, when attachment was assessed, infants in the treated group were more likely to be securely attached than infants in the control group.

Moreover, when mother–infant dyads were followed up at 18, 24, and 36 months, gains were maintained among the treated group (van den Boom, 1995). Children in the treated group were more likely to be securely attached in toddlerhood, more cooperative when observed with their mothers at 24 months, and more positive in interactions with peers. Their mothers continued to be rated as more cooperative, accessible, accepting, and sensitive than mothers of difficult infants who did not receive the intervention. It is also of interest that fathers in intervention families were also observed to be more responsive with their toddlers. Van den Boom (1995) notes both direct effects of the intervention on maternal behavior and indirect effects on child behavior and other relationships mediated by attachment security. This work highlights the possibility that even a brief and very focused intervention can have lasting effects if it targets groups at only moderate risk and provides training in specific skills and principles that can be generalized across situations and developmental levels. Although these results are promising, it will be important to replicate these findings with larger samples and to determine whether the treatment is appropriate for moderate-risk mothers in other cultures or for families living under more adverse circumstances. Clearly more research is needed on the implementation and effectiveness of this brief intervention into attachment-related parenting processes.

Taken together, these treatments suggest promising avenues for early intervention into the mother–child relationship that are aimed at enhancing attachment security and the quality of maternal affective involvement and sensitivity to infant communications. Other interventions are also under way that bridge the gap between attachment theory and behavior management, both teaching parents relationship-based skills and providing them with specific management strategies meant to lessen conflict in toddlerhood, when limit setting becomes a central concern of parents of young children (Hopkins, personal communication, 2001; Greenberg et al., 1993). Continued, systematic research is required to establish whether or not these various interventions are effective, and, if so, what mechanisms may account for changes in parent–child relationships and children's adjustment.

ILLUSTRATIONS FROM THE LONGITUDINAL STUDY

By the time they were 6 years old, the children in our longitudinal study had received a range of different treatments. In fact, 38% of the children whose parents had considered them hard to manage in late toddlerhood and the early preschool years had been referred for some form of psychological or educational help by the time they were in kindergarten or first grade. These treatments were in addition to the parent training groups that were offered to study parents when they entered the project. These additional treatments ranged from speech therapy or remedial reading programs at school through special class placement to more intensive family interventions that often included a combination of family therapy or parent counseling and a behavior management program. In some cases, help with marital communication and support was combined with behavior management, similar to the treatment described by Dadds et al. (1987). Several children were also in play therapy, and two had been given a trial of medication to control aggression and/or attentional deficits. Other parents (13%) sought advice from pediatricians, school principals, or classroom teachers but did not enter into formal treatment programs. Thus parents of 51% of the initial problem group sought some form of advice or formal help by the time of school entry. In contrast, only one child (4%) in the control group was in any formal program (speech therapy). Another 15% of comparison parents sought advice from their pediatricians about problems such as bedwetting, nail biting, and finicky eating habits, but not about major problems in undercontrolled or overcontrolled behavior.

Two of the children described in detail in Chapter 3 were in some form of treatment program when followed up at age 6, whereas parents of two children did not seek help beyond that provided in the parent groups offered to all study families. Teddy, who we initially saw as showing only age-appropriate activity and exploration and who was progressing well, had not received any form of additional help when followed up at age 6. This seemed appropriate, given his stable family situation and his satisfactory development. Teddy's parents had attended a parent group at which they received information about appropriate developmental expectations and the developmental needs of toddlers and preschoolers. They also listened to the concerns of other parents, some of whom had children who were far more difficult to control than Teddy. This helped Mr. and Mrs. M. to place Teddy's age-appropriate exuberance into a more realistic developmental perspective. It also helped them to set priorities, deciding which behaviors clearly required firm limits and which behaviors could be overlooked or tolerated as typical for that developmental period.

On the other hand, Annie and her family clearly could have benefitted from treatment beyond that provided in the parent group. Both Mr. and Mrs. J. attended the group regularly, and they improved their child management skills somewhat. They were encouraged to provide Annie more contingent praise and positive attention and to be less critical. They were also helped to establish more reasonable and age-appropriate expectations for Annie and not to let conflicts over toilet training and eating escalate. However, we were less successful in helping Mr. and Mrs. J. to understand Annie's emotional needs or to modify Mrs. J.'s negative perceptions of Annie. This was beyond the scope of the group, except in a superficial way. Work on these issues with the J.'s would have required a more intensive individual and/or family approach, possibly one aimed at helping them to understand the underlying dynamics of their family interactions, as well as to improve the mother–daughter relationship. Annie's parents, however, saw the problem as Annie's difficult behavior and were resistant to our suggestion that they might require additional help. As Annie entered school and was home less and less, and as Mrs. J. became involved with her younger daughter, her concerns about Annie abated. Mrs. J. did not seem motivated to change her conflict-ridden relationship with her older daughter. Throughout, she continued to see the problems she identified as inherent in Annie rather than as a reflection of dysfunctional relationships within the family system.

Jamie's parents likewise attended a parent training group, and they worked hard at implementing our suggestions for limit setting, use of time-out, and so forth. However, we had little to teach them, because they were already doing most of the things that we suggested. Mr. and Mrs. L. focused their efforts on trying to improve Jamie's self-control and his relationships with other children, and they did benefit from the support they received from the therapists and the other parents. Although they viewed Jamie's behavior as slightly improved at the completion of the group sessions and they felt more in control of the situation, problems did continue. At the end of kindergarten, Jamie was assessed by the school psychologist because of problems with self-control in the classroom and on the playground. He tended to get wound up and overexcited—in the classroom, Jamie often called out inappropriately or disrupted the activities of other children; on the playground, he frequently provoked fights with peers. As a result, he was on a behavioral program at school that included time-outs, special rewards for good behavior, and all-too-frequent visits to the principal's office when time-outs were inadequate. Jamie's parents worked closely with the school to monitor his progress and to make sure that there was consistency between the expectations voiced at home and at school. In addition, Jamie had regular meetings with the school guidance counselor, who worked with him on self-control and peer relations, trying to help Jamie to prevent his peer conflicts from getting out of hand. These seemed to be appropriate interventions, because Jamie's difficulties did not appear to reflect other problems in the family and because his parents appeared to be handling his problems with considerable skill, patience, and sensitivity. Jamie made some strides, and his behavior problems were under somewhat better control as he entered first grade.

Robbie's mother, Mrs. S., also attended a parent group. Mr. S. did not accompany her, because he attributed Robbie's difficulties to his wife's inadequate parenting skills. As noted in previous chapters, lack of paternal involvement and interparental blame and hostility are often correlates of behavior problems in children. Although Mrs. S. was extremely responsive to our suggestions and followed through, setting appropriate limits and providing Robbie with a good deal of positive feedback and emotional support, his problems persisted, as would be expected, given the tense and conflict-ridden home environment. In the group, Mrs. S. focused specifically on Robbie's difficulties with self-control and compliance. At the completion of the group sessions, Mrs. S. felt that she was in better control of Robbie's behavior and more consistent in her limit setting. However, it was obvious that family conflicts were contributing to Robbie's difficulties. Therefore, we also suggested that Mr. and Mrs. S. might benefit from treatment elsewhere that would focus on broader marital and family issues. Unfortunately, Mr. S. was not interested in pursuing this. As noted in Chapter 3, Robbie's parents separated when he was 4. Robbie experienced considerable upset as a result of the separation. His mother sought counseling in order to be better able to help Robbie cope with the separation, and he was eventually referred for play therapy. In addition, his mother received parent counseling and supportive therapy in an effort to help her deal with Robbie's difficult adjustment, as well as with her own anger and depression. In regard to Robbie's adjustment to the separation, Mrs. S. needed help ensuring a stable, predictable, and supportive environment for Robbie, preparing him for the changes in his living situation, and helping him to cope with the turmoil associated with visitation arrangements. She also needed support and advice about limit setting, because, in view of her own distress, it was sometimes difficult for her to continue to set sufficiently firm, consistent, and appropriate limits on Robbie's behavior. In play therapy, Robbie had an opportunity to express his confusion, anxiety about abandonment, anger at his parents, and concerns about the future, and he appeared to establish an excellent relationship with his male therapist. Although Robbie coped well in preschool and weathered the initial separation, continued interparental conflict and unstable visiting arrangements seemed to undermine his ability to cope. In kindergarten, he became seriously aggressive with other children and noncompliant with the teacher, and a behavior management program was instituted. Robbie and his mother have continued in various forms of treatment over the years. These have included special class placement and individual psychotherapy for Robbie; Mrs. S. also has sought advice from time to time about managing Robbie's behavior effectively or about helping him to weather a stressful life change.

SUMMARY

In this chapter, the various treatment modalities used most frequently with young children were reviewed. Developmental considerations in treatment selection were touched on briefly, and it was concluded that more structured and didactic treatments that focus on parenting skills and family relationships appear most appropriate for preschoolers and their families. Furthermore, these more structured treatments have been subjected to at least some degree of empirical scrutiny. The effects of traditional forms of psychotherapy (play therapy) or of more contemporary family therapy approaches on preschoolers and their families have not been evaluated systematically. Certainly, family approaches have much promise, especially when combined with interventions that focus on parenting behavior. In addition, intensive preschool programs that help young children learn to control aggression with peers and to function more cooperatively and prosocially in the peer group also may hold promise, although systematic interventions of this sort are rare for children with behavior problems who are not also developmentally delayed or at risk for other reasons.

There is evidence from early intervention and primary prevention programs suggesting that intensive, long-term, structured programs that also include parents can help young children overcome some early deficits in cognitive and social functioning. There is reason to believe that this model of comprehensive early intervention also is applicable to children and their families who are at risk because of parental psychopathology, family disruption, or poor parenting skills or for children and families in which the childhood behavior problems are not clearly associated with one of these family risk factors. It is surprising that so little empirical work has been conducted on treatments for preschoolers with more typical behavioral difficulties, such as overactivity, noncompliance, and aggression. The evidence to date suggests that parent training is relatively effective for parents with oppositional and defiant children, but it is unclear whether these treatments are also effective with children diagnosed early with ADHD.

Finally, the range of treatments used by children in our longitudinal study was discussed. Children and their families were seen in many different treatments that focused on the children's academic and social skills, parenting skills, and family relationships. Further, it was quite common for children and their families to be seen in several forms of treatment, either simultaneously or successively. This may suggest that our ability to help troubled families with the techniques currently available is limited, or it may underline the resourcefulness of some families who were willing to try different approaches. What seems clear from this review is the need for more integrated treatment programs that can help families with difficult preschoolers early on, before problems escalate.

CHAPTER 8

Follow-Up and Outcome Studies of Young Children

So far, I have considered the behavior and family context of children who are showing high levels of externalizing problems, that is, aggression, noncompliance, impulsivity, and overactivity in early childhood. But what happens to these children over the course of development? Which children were really showing early signs of serious problems that are likely to persist across the life span, and which children were showing only transient or less long-term adjustment difficulties? A growing body of research is beginning to suggest that specific risk factors are associated with persistent problems and that certain protective factors predict more positive outcomes. Overall, studies indicate that most children with early problems go on to show adequate adjustment despite early difficulties but that those children with more severe and pervasive early problems are more likely to have continuing difficulties in childhood and adolescence. In this chapter, I discuss the factors that predict which children with early problems will do well, which will have residual difficulties but function adequately, and which will show continuing problems. Not surprisingly, a range of child, family, and community factors appear to partially account for these different outcomes. Several longitudinal studies of community samples are reviewed, as are studies that have followed clinically diagnosed children with ADHD into adolescence and early adulthood. These studies were selected to throw light on questions of developmental course and predictors of outcome. In addition, data are presented from my own longitudinal study of hard-to-manage preschool children, tracking their development from kindergarten entry through middle childhood (Cohort 2) and early adolescence (Cohort 1). Finally, I return to the descriptions of individual children to illustrate the course of problems in early childhood.

LONGITUDINAL STUDIES OF TODDLERS AND PRESCHOOLERS INTO SCHOOL AGE AND BEYOND

Studies that have followed small samples of young children in the general population from infancy through school age indicate that problem behaviors are relatively common and that they often are associated with a particular developmental period. For example, difficulties with sleeping, eating, and crying are most common during infancy and early toddlerhood; concerns with bowel and bladder functions and with struggles for independence and autonomy become more salient at about age 2; by age 3, management and discipline problems predominate; fears and worries, as well as aggression with peers, may concern parents during the late preschool period or at kindergarten entry; and school difficulties emerge as more serious parental concerns by age 6 or 7. Early longitudinal data indicated that such difficulties are usually transient in nonclinical samples of children (MacFarlane, Allen, & Honzik, 1954). More recent, large-scale studies with much larger samples indicate that this is the case for *most*, but *not all*, young children with early difficulties. Findings are consistent in indicating that child characteristics and adverse family environments predict poor outcome (see Campbell, 1995; Campbell et al., 2000, for reviews).

In a classic large-scale epidemiological study, Werner and her colleagues (Werner, Bierman, & French, 1971; Werner & Smith, 1977) followed a cohort of children born in Hawaii in 1955. Birth records were obtained; maternal ratings of infant behavior were gathered at 1 year; children and families were assessed at 2, 10, and 18 years of age. Learning and behavior problems at age 10 were predicted by mild perinatal stress, particularly in the context of a high activity level at age 1, and by a poor mother–child relationship, family instability, and low maternal educational level, assessed during infancy or toddlerhood. Werner and Smith (1977) concluded that the interaction among biological impairment, difficult infant behavior, and environmental factors, including a low standard of living, predicted moderate mental health problems at age 10. Furthermore, once learning and behavior problems had stabilized at age 10, they tended to persist. These earlier and persistent learning and behavior problems were more likely to develop into antisocial behavior in adolescence among boys living in poorly functioning families; of the children who became delinquent in adolescence, most had been identified as having significant problems by age 10. Werner and Smith (1977) interpreted their data within a transactional model and emphasized the interacting contributions of biological vulnerability, environmental instability, and the quality of parent–child relationships in determining outcome.

The epidemiological study conducted by Richman, Stevenson, and Graham (1982) in London leads to similar conclusions in that problems persisted in a relatively high proportion of children who were identified as showing *clinically significant* problems at age 3, especially if they were overactive, inattentive, attention seeking, difficult to control, irritable, and negative in mood. However, only a small percentage of children (fewer than 10%) were initially identified as showing serious behavior problems at preschool age, and they showed a constellation of problems. At initial assessment, childhood problems were associated with a range of adverse family factors, including maternal depression, a poor marital relationship, punitive childrearing practices including frequent spankings, parental disagreements over childrearing, high parental criticism of the child, and lack of maternal warmth. A significant proportion of children in the problem group continued to have difficulties when followed up 1 year later. Problems persisted in 63% of this group at age 4 and in 62% at age 8. Furthermore, teacher ratings confirmed more problems at age 8 in the group rated by mothers as more difficult to handle at ages 3 and 4. Overactivity, concentration difficulties, discipline problems, unhappiness, and poor sibling relationships were still the primary concerns at the age 8 follow-up. Serious peer problems were also evidenced. Although early family adversity did not predict outcome, persistent difficulties were associated with *ongoing* family problems, including continued marital dysfunction, maternal illness and depression, and more external psychosocial stresses. Finally, persistent problems were related to the children's poorer cognitive and academic functioning, especially among boys. It is also important to note that some children developed problems over the course of the follow-up period and that family conflict and maternal depression were associated with the onset of new problems, as well as with the persistence of problems.

A cluster analysis of symptom ratings at age 3 indicated that most children fell into clusters defined primarily by bowel and bladder control and other transient and developmentally appropriate difficulties, such as feeding problems related to maturation and self-regulation. Of the two clinically significant clusters, one, describing 23% of the sample, was defined by feeding difficulties and a high activity level. Of most relevance is the *multiproblem* cluster, describing 10% of the sample: children high on restlessness and overactivity, tantrums, discipline problems, poor concentration, negative mood, and difficulties with siblings at age 3. Children in this cluster also had the most family problems and the worst outcomes. This cluster of symptoms was associated with low maternal warmth, high criticism of the child, and a poor marriage. At age 4, 89% of this group was still having difficulties; at age 8, 67% were still considered to have clinically significant problems. Taken together, these findings indicate that moderate to severe levels of overactivity, attentional problems, and management difficulties at age 3, especially in the context of family problems, are associated with poor outcome at school age. These findings were particularly strong for boys.

McGee and his colleagues reported on a large epidemiological study of a birth cohort of children in Dunedin, New Zealand (McGee & Silva, 1982; McGee, Silva, & Williams, 1984). Children were first recruited into the study at birth, and psychosocial data were first collected at age 3. Problems at various ages were defined by cutoff scores on parent and teacher rating scales. Children with behavior problems that persisted from age 5 to age 7 came from more discordant families characterized by higher rates of separation and single parenting, poorer family relationships, and more frequent school changes. In addition, their mothers were younger, of lower mental ability, and more likely to report symptoms of anxiety, depression, and minor physical complaints than mothers of children without problems. Thus it is likely that these children received poorer parenting than comparison children. Consistent with our own data and those of Richman et al. (1982), children with persistent problems were described by both parents and teachers as primarily hyperactive and aggressive rather than as sad, anxious, or withdrawn. In addition, stable behavior problems were associated with reading difficulties and poor school achievement. On the other hand, most indices of pregnancy and delivery complications, neonatal difficulties, neurological impairment, and developmental milestones did not differentiate children with stable behavior problems from those without. McGee et al. (1984) concluded that children with stable behavior problems have experienced a range of stresses in their lives that interact in complex fashion to produce and/or maintain disordered functioning.

In more recent follow-up data from the Dunedin sample, the researchers have emphasized early child characteristics, conceptualized as temperamental indicators of risk. An explosive personality style (Caspi, Henry, McGee, Moffitt, & Silva, 1995; Moffitt et al., 1996) was hypothesized to be a major predictor of continuing problems, especially antisocial behavior and difficulties with stable relationships. Children who were rated by testers at age 3 as showing a "lack of control," defined as poor impulse control, low persistence, and negative reactions to challenge, were seen as having more externalizing problems at ages 9, 11, 13, and 15 according to both parent and teacher reports. However, one may question whether this result reflects temperament or already emerging oppositional defiant disorder or ADHD. Boys whose early problems persisted into adolescence were more likely to come from families marked by chronic psychosocial adversity, including low education, occupational level, and income, single-parent status, and poor maternal mental health, than boys whose early problems did not persist. Thus, although Moffitt et al. (1996) emphasize child characteristics, they did not directly assess parenting behaviors, and their data are just as consistent with a transactional model in which early child characteristics interact with ongoing family adversity and poor parental support to predict chronic problems in the child through adolescence. This interpretation also is bolstered by recent data from the Minnesota High Risk Study (Aguilar, Sroufe, Egeland, & Carlson, 2000), which also indicated that early family risk predicted ongoing problems in adolescence in high-risk children followed from infancy.

Other recent longitudinal studies also have followed community samples of children from preschool or kindergarten to middle childhood and adolescence. These studies also have been consistent in demonstrating links between parenting and family characteristics and children's later adjustment. In general, negative, harsh, and inconsistent parental behavior has been repeatedly found to predict disruptive and aggressive behavior, even after controlling for initial levels of children's noncompliance (e.g., Campbell et al., 1996; McFadyen-Ketchum, Bates, Dodge, & Pettit, 1996; Pettit, Bates, & Dodge, 1993; Shaw et al., 1996).

In addition, studies have begun to try to examine subgroups of children following different developmental pathways in an attempt to identify precursors and correlates of increases and decreases in problem behavior (e.g., Keiley, Bates, Dodge, & Pettit, 2000; McFadyen-Ketchum et al., 1996; Nagin & Tremblay, 1999), as well as moderators of outcome.

One important and consistent finding is that only a small number of children show either stable or increasing problem behavior over time (Campbell et al., 2000; McFadyen-Ketchum et al., 1996; Nagin & Tremblay, 1999). Most children show a decrease in aggression and disruptive behavior whether assessed by parent, teacher, or peer report. For example, in the McFadyen-Ketchum et al. (1996) study, roughly 5% of boys and 6% of girls were identified as showing increasing aggression. Nagin and Tremblay (1999) likewise followed a large sample of boys from poor neighborhoods in Montreal from kindergarten through late adolescence and tracked the development of physical aggression and oppositionality, as well as hyperactivity, as assessed by teachers. In general most boys started out low to moderate in problem behavior and decreased over time. However, between 4% and 5% of boys showed high and stable levels of physical aggression, oppositionality, and/or hyperactivity, with only moderate overlap among these behavioral indicators. Self-reported serious delinquency and violence at ages 15, 16, and 17 were predicted by membership in the chronic-aggression and oppositional groups from early childhood on. Hyperactivity did not improve prediction and, by itself, it was not associated with later delinquency. Furthermore, even elevated levels of disruptive behaviors decreased over time in most boys, and no evidence was found for late-onset aggression.

Moffitt and colleagues (Moffitt, 1990, 1993; Moffitt et al., 1996) identified four groups of boys in the Dunedin data set who differed with respect to antisocial history and developmental course: an early-onset, persistent group; an adolescent-onset group; an early-onset group that was no longer aggressive in adolescence; and a comparison group of nonaggressive boys. Although the two early-onset groups received similar ratings on early "lack of control," the persistent group differed from the improved group in quality of family relationships and level of family dysfunction. About 7% of the sample had early and persistent problems, and, as already noted, these boys lived in more adverse family environments that reflected higher levels of sociodemographic and family risk than other boys in the sample. Boys whose early problems abated lived in more stable and harmonious families, suggesting that family context can also play a protective role. These data are consistent with other studies that have identified small groups of boys with early-onset and ongoing problems who lived in dysfunctional families (Patterson & Yoerger, 1997) and also indicate that not all aggressive boys are at risk for continuing problems that become serious in adolescence.

In a large sample of children from three communities who were screened prior to kindergarten entry and followed longitudinally, McFadyen-Ketchum et al. (1996) found that, in boys, increases in aggressive and disruptive behavior from kindergarten through Grade 3 were predicted by negative, coercive, and nonaffectionate maternal behavior observed at home prior to school entry. In contrast, girls living in families characterized by harsh parenting and low levels of affection showed high levels of aggression early but decreasing levels of aggression over the course of the study; surprisingly, maternal affection was unrelated to changes in levels of aggression in girls. These findings have important implications for understanding the different pathways that boys and girls may follow from early externalizing behavior to later externalizing and internalizing patterns. Using data from this same study, Pettit, Bates, and Dodge (1997) reported that supportive parenting—defined as positive involvement, inductive discipline, proactive teaching, and warmth—assessed prior to kindergarten entry predicted better academic performance and social adjustment at the end of sixth grade. In addition, supportive parenting interacted with SES and single-parent status to predict levels of externalizing problems. Higher levels of supportive parenting in the context of lower SES and single-parent status predicted lower levels of externalizing problems as reported by teachers. These studies, then, indicate that a small group of children are at risk for serious ongoing problems and that aspects of positive and negative parenting can serve to ameliorate or exacerbate risk, especially in the context of other indicators of family adversity.

Research on children's peer relations also indicates that by middle childhood the peer group can serve as a powerful influence, either positive or negative, on children's adjustment. Data from two large-scale studies suggest that early behavior problems, especially aggression, place children at high risk to become victims of bullying (Schwartz et al., 1999), which in turn is associated with more serious behavior problems later (Schwartz et al., 1998). Moreover, harsh parenting is associated with aggressive peer encounters (Strassberg et al., 1994), but reciprocal friendships can buffer children against the negative effects of harsh parenting and help them to avoid becoming victims of aggressive peers (Schwartz et al., 2000). This complex longitudinal process may reflect the fact that children who are capable of reciprocated friendships learn social skills and develop self-esteem that facilitates their further social development, despite the lack of supportive and appropriate role models at home. Other studies also suggest that friendships with prosocial peers can buffer children who may be at risk for the development of behavior problems. These findings have motivated several intervention trials that use peers to promote social competence and social skills in children at risk for disorder (Conduct Problems Prevention Research Group, 1992; Dumas, Prinz, Smith, & Laughlin, 1999; Vitaro et al., 1999).

At the same time, a wealth of data indicates that early peer difficulties and the association with deviant peers can encourage antisocial and delinquent behavior in children at risk (Coie & Dodge, 1998). Thus high levels of physical aggression, bullying, and proactive aggression are associated with significant negative outcomes (Vitaro, Gendreau, Tremblay, & Oligny, 1998; Schwartz et al., 1999). Peer rejection is also associated with aggressive behavior in the peer group, and it predicts ongoing behavior problems. For example, Keiley et al. (2000) followed children from the Pettit et al. (1997) sample from kindergarten through Grade 7, and found that peer rejection assessed in kindergarten was associated with mother-reported increases in internalizing problems, as well as relatively high and stable externalizing problems, across the elementary school years. However, SES and gender differences were also in evidence, with low-SES rejected boys having the highest initial and increasing levels of externalizing problems, followed by low-SES rejected girls. Low-SES rejected boys also had the highest levels of teacher-reported externalizing and internalizing behavior that showed slight increases across the follow-up period. Overall, the data suggest that a combination of early aggression and peer rejection is especially likely to be associated with a range of other behavior problems and also to predict longer term problems, especially when chronic peer problems and family adversity occur together (Coie & Dodge, 1998).

It has also been established that adolescents, especially adolescent boys, are more likely to engage in aggressive and antisocial activities with others in the peer group, and it has been well documented that aggressive boys are likely to seek out aggressive peers (e.g., Cairns,

Cairns, & Neckerman, 1989) and to engage in hostile exchanges that escalate (e.g., Dishion, Andrews, & Crosby, 1995). Patterson et al. (1989) suggest that aggressive boys, because they are rejected by more popular and prosocial peers, drift into relationships with other aggressive rejected boys and that they are likely to get into trouble together. To round out the picture, it also has been noted that family adversity and psychosocial risk predict which boys will associate with deviant peers at school age and adolescence (Fergusson & Horwood, 1999; Patterson et al., 1989).

Taken together, then, an accumulating body of evidence suggests that problems, particularly externalizing problems, persist in a small proportion of children who show early behavior management difficulties and aggression. Isolated symptoms or constellations of mild symptoms are usually indicative only of transient problems that are likely to disappear with development, but constellations of more serious problems appearing in early childhood may signify difficulties that can interact with ongoing family adversity and harsh or inconsistent parenting to place young children on a developmental pathway toward more long-term problems in social and academic functioning. As development proceeds, the peer group also becomes a fertile arena for problems to escalate, especially if problematic children are rejected by more prosocial classmates and are then surrounded by deviant peers who reinforce each other's antisocial behavior. However, it is important to emphasize that not all children with early and severe problems continue to have difficulties; furthermore, the nature of their problems may change or become less severe with development, depending on the environmental supports available to them in the family, peer group, school, and community. In particular, supportive parenting and reciprocated friendships with more prosocial peers may serve a buffering or protective role for children at risk.

As noted throughout this book, the combination of family adversity and persistent and worsening problems most likely reflects gene–environment correlations and gene–environment interactions. For example, children elicit certain patterns of parenting and certain responses from peers, and they also select and/or are selected into certain peer groups, partly as a function of their temperaments, personality characteristics, and social behaviors. Parents, by virtue of their own personalities and childrearing histories, also favor certain approaches to their difficult children over others (e.g., harsh punishment over reasoning). In addition, parents and children with similarly explosive or aggressive personality styles may escalate their negative and coercive interactions, whereas aggressive children with calmer parents who react less impulsively and angrily to their children's transgressions may help their children overcome, or at least control, some of their own tendencies to be aggressive, angry, or impulsive. Thus, although the data clearly implicate both child and family characteristics in the prediction of longer term problems, the ways in which genetic and environmental influences work together over time to lead to a particular outcome are just beginning to be explored (Collins et al., 2000; Lahey et al., 1999; Rutter et al., 1997).

FOLLOW-UP STUDIES OF CLINICALLY DIAGNOSED HYPERACTIVE/ADHD CHILDREN

There also is a growing body of research on children with diagnoses of hyperactivity or ADHD in childhood who have been followed into adolescence and young adulthood. Consistent with the findings from longitudinal studies of preschool and kindergarten children, problems are likely to persist, especially among children with ADHD with co-occurring oppositional and aggressive behavior who live in more conflict-ridden and dysfunctional families. For example, Biederman et al. (1996) provided data on a large clinically diagnosed sample of school-age boys with ADHD who were followed up 4 years after initial referral. Overall, 85% continued to meet diagnostic criteria for ADHD, and of these about 70% also met criteria for either ODD or conduct disorder (CD). Predictors of continuing ADHD included comorbid conduct problems, a family history of ADHD, and family conflict.

Barkley and colleagues have conducted a large follow-up study of children with ADHD (90% male) seen 8 years after initial diagnosis. Children were followed up in middle adolescence, at a mean age of 15 (Barkley, Fischer, Edelbrock, & Smallish, 1990). Consistent with the follow-up study of Biederman et al. (1996), 72% of the children with ADHD continued to meet DSM-III-R diagnostic criteria for ADHD; 67% also met criteria for either ODD or CD. In addition to continuing diagnoses, there were other indicators of poorer functioning in these children with ADHD at follow-up. Boys with ADHD, especially those who had co-occurring conduct problems, were more likely to have been expelled or suspended from school and to perform more poorly on measures of academic achievement, even after controlling for child IQ and maternal education (Fischer, Barkley, Edelbrock, & Smallish, 1990). Further, children with ADHD continued to perform more poorly on measures of sustained attention and impulsivity. Mothers of boys with both ADHD and co-occurring conduct problems also reported more family conflict, marital distress, stressful life events, and symptoms of depression and hostility. Observations of mother–adolescent interaction revealed more conflict and poorer communication in the comorbid group. Other follow-up studies have also indicated that children with ADHD often do not outgrow their symptoms and that cognitive and academic functioning remain impaired, especially when ADHD occurs together with aggression or conduct problems (Gittelman, Mannuzza, Shenker, & Bonagura, 1985; McGee, Partridge, Williams, & Silva, 1991). In the Gittelman et al. study, boys with ADHD were more likely to show symptoms of antisocial personality disorder and higher rates of substance abuse than comparison boys.

Although these studies all suggest that symptoms persist in children with ADHD, they also indicate that comorbidity plays an important role in predicting outcome, as does family stress and adversity. There is a growing consensus that especially poor outcome may be specific to children with ADHD who have co-occurring conduct problems (Hinshaw, 1994; Moffitt, 1990, 1993) and that children living in more dysfunctional families are more likely to have poor outcomes. The cause–effect relations among these factors have not been disentangled, but one possibility is that children with ADHD who live in more poorly functioning families are also at higher risk to develop conduct problems (Hinshaw, 1994; Hinshaw, Lahey, & Hart, 1993). Together, the more severe and pervasive symptoms and chronic family problems fuel one another, as well as a continuing disorder in the child. Among the processes implicated in this sequence are the modeling of negative and aggressive behavior of angry parents, and limited monitoring and supervision (e.g., Patterson et al., 1989), as well as peer influences. Aggressive and poorly achieving students are likely to be rejected by peers and to gravitate toward others like themselves (Coie & Dodge, 1998; Patterson et al., 1989). These complex determinants also appear to reflect biological vulnerability (Hinshaw, 1994), as indexed by parental psychopathology, cognitive deficits, and a family history of ADHD symptoms. These configurations of co-occurring problems within families also appear to illustrate patterns of gene–environment correlation and gene–environment interaction (Rutter et al., 1997).

The two major studies of adult outcome in children with ADHD are consistent with this formulation and suggest different outcomes for those with and without co-occurring conduct problems. Mannuzza and colleagues (Mannuzza, Klein, Bessler, Malloy, & Hynes, 1997; Mannuzza, Klein, Bessler, Malloy, & LaPadula, 1993) followed two cohorts of boys with ADHD and matched controls into early adulthood. Weiss and Hechtman (1993) also followed a sample of children diagnosed as hyperactive into young adulthood. Results of both these follow-up studies indicated that children with ADHD fared more poorly than controls in terms of educational and occupational attainment in adulthood. For example, Mannuzza et al. (1997) reported that the boys with ADHD averaged 2 fewer years of education than control-group boys and that about 25% did not finish high school, as compared with only 1% of controls—a difference that was not accounted for by antisocial personality characteristics or IQ differences. In the Weiss and Hechtman (1993) study, the hyperactive adults showed poorer job stability and employment satisfaction, as well as more interpersonal difficulties, including problems in forming stable intimate relationships.

In addition to adjustment problems, the adults with ADHD in both studies had higher rates of antisocial personality disorder, and in the Manuzza et al. (1993) sample, there were also higher rates of substance abuse and overall psychiatric diagnoses (33% met diagnostic criteria for a disorder vs. 16% of controls) at follow-up. Weiss and Hechtman (1993) also found that the hyperactive adults in their follow-up sample continued to report more restlessness, impulsivity, and/or difficulty paying attention and that these continuing symptoms interfered with their functioning at work and socially. In general, early indicators of aggression and family conflict were associated with poorer adult outcome in the Montreal sample. Thus, across numerous studies assessing children with ADHD at different ages, as well as studies assessing symptom ratings in the absence of a diagnosis, the combination of hyperactivity, aggression, and poor family relationships is associated with poorer adjustment at follow-up. Children whose ADHD symptoms are not associated with long-standing aggressive and oppositional behavior and who are not growing up in disturbed families appear to function better in adolescence and adulthood, even if they are not totally problem free.

FINDINGS FROM THE LONGITUDINAL STUDY OF HARD-TO-MANAGE PRESCHOOL CHILDREN

In our own studies, we have followed one cohort of parent-identified hard-to-manage preschool children and comparison children from age 3 to age 13; a second cohort of parent- and/or teacher-identified hard-to-manage preschool boys has been followed from age 4 to age 9, with periodic assessments of the children's functioning in a range of situations. Parent and teacher reports have been obtained, children have been observed in structured and unstructured laboratory situations, their classroom behavior has been observed, and family functioning has been assessed. As pointed out in Chapter 3, both cohorts of hard-to-manage children differed from comparison children without problems on a range of measures obtained at the time of entry into the study. These included parent and teacher reports of hyperactive–distractible behavior and aggressive–noncompliant behavior. Independent laboratory observations revealed that problem youngsters differed from controls on measures of activity level, inattention, and impulsivity obtained during both free play and experimenter-administered structured tasks (Campbell et al., 1982, 1994). Mothers of hard-to-manage children in Cohort 1 were more likely to provide direction and negative control during an unstructured play period, but problem children showed only a nonsignificant tendency to be more aggressive and noncompliant than controls in this setting (Campbell, Breaux, Ewing, Szumowski, & Pierce, 1986). Similarly, in Cohort 2, mothers of hard-to-manage boys were more likely to use negative control attempts to gain compliance during a toy cleanup procedure, although hard-to-manage boys were only marginally more noncompliant than control boys (Campbell, 1994). Observations in the preschool classrooms of study participants in both cohorts indicated that hard-to-manage children also were more disruptive and aggressive with peers than controls were; problem boys in both cohorts were less compliant with teacher requests than were other children. Problem children, however, did not differ from controls in their tendency to approach peers or to engage with them in cooperative play (Campbell & Cluss, 1982; Campbell et al., 1994). Finally, although the families of the problem children were, on average, from a lower social class and experiencing higher levels of psychosocial stress, there were wide individual differences on background measures.

Follow-Up to School Entry and Middle Childhood

In both cohorts, follow-up data were obtained 1 and 2 years after initial assessment. Results indicated that problems were relatively stable. In Cohort 1, children in the problem group were still rated as more hyperactive–distractible and aggressive–noncompliant by their mothers at age 4, and they differed on laboratory observations of activity, inattention, and impulsivity. Hard-to-manage boys in Cohort 2 were likewise rated by their mothers as more problematic at age 5 than were comparison boys (Campbell et al., 1984; Campbell et al., 1991). At age 6, hard-to-manage children in Cohort 1 continued to differ from controls on maternal and teacher ratings of externalizing, but not internalizing, symptoms. Both mothers and teachers rated the problem youngsters as significantly more hyperactive, inattentive, and aggressive than controls. In addition, mothers rated them as less competent with peers, and teachers rated them as showing less adaptive functioning in school. Classroom observations confirmed that children in the initial problem group tended to be more active and distractible, as well as more disruptive and aggressive, than comparison children. Laboratory observations of free play, of activity level during structured tasks, and of mother–child interaction during problem solving did not reveal group differences at age 6 (Campbell, Ewing, et al., 1986). Cohort 2 youngsters were observed in the laboratory on measures of attention and self-regulation, and maternal and teacher reports were obtained at age 6. Results indicated that, as a group, hard-to-manage boys made more impulsive errors and were more restless, fidgety, and distractible during structured tasks assessing vigilance and attention to detail (Campbell et al., 1994; Marakovitz & Campbell, 1998). They were also seen as more problematic and less socially competent than control boys by both parents and teachers (Campbell, 1994).

These findings indicate continued group differences at the time of entry into school in both cohorts of children. However, there also were wide individual differences in children's functioning at school entry. Some problem youngsters were doing fine at follow-up; some had mild problems; still others continued to have relatively severe problems. Thus we narrowed our focus to examine subgroups of children with clear evidence of continuing problems at follow-up and those whose initial problems appeared to have improved. We began by asking how many children in the initial-problem group met objective criteria for disorder at age 6; these youngsters ("persistent problems") were then compared with those who did not meet criteria ("improved group") and with controls on both follow-up and initial measures. Overall, findings from both cohorts indicated that children with persistent problems could be identified on the basis of higher initial symptom ratings and more family adversity, especially a negative mother–child interaction.

Children in Cohort 1 were identified as persistent problems if they met DSM-III criteria for attention deficit disorder at age 6, if they scored at or above the clinically significant cutoff score of 70 on the Aggression dimension of the CBCL (Achenbach, 1991), or if they were rated by their mothers as showing either moderate or severe problems on a follow-up interview. Exactly 50% of the original-problem group met one or more of these clinical criteria at age 6 and were considered to be showing persistent problems; the remainder were considered improved because they did not meet any of these criteria. When persistent-problem children, improved children, and controls were compared, only a few measures discriminated persistent and improved children initially (i.e., at age 3). However, consistent with findings reported earlier, mothers of children with persistent problems were observed to be more negative and controlling during play, and the children themselves received more severe initial ratings of both hyperactivity and aggression when compared with the improved group. Improved children also differed from controls at initial assessment. In contrast, most group differences at age 6 were accounted for by the children with persistent problems: Improved youngsters did not differ from controls on most measures, and they were rated as significantly less symptomatic than the persistent-problem group by teachers as well as parents. In addition, when the pattern of initial symptoms and symptom changes over time were examined, children with persistent problems were found to have both more numerous early signs of ODD or CD, to have higher overall symptom ratings, and to show less developmental change in symptoms from ages 3 to 4 and 4 to 6 than children who improved (Campbell, 1987).

At the age 9 follow-up assessment (Campbell & Ewing, 1990), mothers were administered a structured diagnostic interview, the Diagnostic Interview Schedule for Children—Parent Version (Edelbrock, Costello, Dulcan, Kalas, & Conover, 1985), which incorporated DSM-III criteria for major childhood disorders. Symptoms were scored on a 3-point scale, from 0—*absent* to 2—*definitely present*. The interviewers were both blind and independent; they knew nothing of the children's earlier behavior or group status. In addition, mothers and classroom teachers again completed questionnaires. Data were examined in terms of group status at age 6 (i.e., persistent problems, improved, control). Children in the persistent-problem group were more likely than children in the other two groups to meet diagnostic criteria for at least one externalizing disorder (attention deficit disorder, oppositional defiant disorder, or conduct disorder) at follow-up. In fact, 67% of the persistent group continued to meet diagnostic criteria at age 9, as compared with only 29% of the improved group and 16% of controls, a statistically significant difference. On the other hand, groups did not differ in the proportion that met criteria for an internalizing disorder (separation anxiety, overanxious disorder, dysthymia). However, several children in the persistent group who were reported at age 9 to show symptoms of an externalizing disorder were also described as depressed and/or anxious.

Maternal ratings on the CBCL were consistent with the diagnostic data. Children in the persistent-problem group received significantly higher ratings than their improved peers and than the comparison group on the dimensions Hyperactive, Aggressive, and Delinquent and significantly lower ratings on Social Competence (including behavior with peers, participation in organized activities, and behavior at home). They also were rated as more socially withdrawn than comparison children. However, by age 9, children seemed to be better controlled in school. Relatively few received elevated ratings from teachers on the Teacher Report Form (TRF), and group differences were significant only on the Nervous–Overactive and Externalizing scales, with persistent-problem youngsters differing from controls. It should be kept in mind that three children from the persistent-problem group were in special classes either full- or part-time by the age 9 follow-up; another four were receiving some form of school-based remedial help; two had repeated a grade. Five children were on stimulant medication for their hyperactivity. All of these factors may have influenced teacher ratings, because study children may not have stood out relative to classmates. Further, despite these teacher ratings, most children in the persistent-problem group had received some form of educational and/or psychological service by age 9, as detailed in Chapter 7.

We also examined several earlier predictors of maternal ratings of behavior problems at age 9 (Campbell & Ewing, 1990). Negative maternal control during play and the free-play composite score (derived from observations of the child's attention to toys), which were both observed in the laboratory playroom at age 3, continued to predict maternal ratings of hyperactivity at age 9, even when gender, IQ, and social class were controlled. Thus mothers who were more negative when observed with their preschoolers during semistructured play and whose children were more unfocused during independent free play at preschool age continued to rate their youngsters as more overactive and difficult to control 6 years later. In addition, both maternal and teacher ratings of externalizing problems at age 6 predicted maternal ratings of similar problems at age 9. These data indicate predictability over time and across informants, confirming that ratings of persistent problems reflect more than negative and biased assessments of children's behavior by their mothers.

Similar analyses were conducted on the data obtained from Cohort 2 at ages 6 and 9. Overall, 67% of the hard-to-manage boys were identified as showing disruptive behavior problems according to *either* a parent *or* a teacher at age 6 (i.e., elevated symptoms, T > 67, on the externalizing scale of the CBCL and/or elevated ratings of at least eight ADHD symptoms or five symptoms of ODD). However, classification into the persistent-problem group was made more stringent. At age 6, a boy had to be identified as showing elevated symptoms by at least *two* informants (both parents or parent and teacher; Campbell, 1994). Using this much stricter criterion, only 28% of the original hard-to-manage group was classified as showing clinically significant problems at age 6. When these boys were compared with those hard-to-manage boys who did not meet these cutoff scores, according to two informants, and with the comparison group, the three groups differed significantly from one another on both parent and teacher ratings of social competence. Persistent-problem boys also were rated by their mothers as higher in internalizing symptoms, and they rated themselves as less socially competent than boys in the other two groups did.

When groups were compared on initial family functioning and parenting, consistent with the findings from Cohort 1, continuing problems were associated with maternal reports of more stressful life events, less marital satisfaction, and more maternal depressive symptoms, as well as more use of negative control during the cleanup task observed in the laboratory at intake. Comparison boys and boys without significant problems did not differ on these initial maternal report measures, although mothers of hard-to-manage boys who did not have continuing problems were somewhat more negative than mothers of controls during toy cleanup. In addition, mothers of boys with continuing problems reported more depressive symptoms and less parenting competence at the age 6 follow-up. Thus continuing maternal depressive symptoms and higher levels of initial externalizing problems in children, as well as more observed negative maternal control, differentiated between hard-to-manage boys with continuing problems at age 6 and those whose problems became less severe over time.

At age 9, 59% of the hard-to-manage boys with persistent problems at age 6 met DSM-III-R diagnostic criteria for at least one disruptive behavior disorder (ADHD, ODD, or CD; Pierce, Ewing, & Campbell, 1999). Structured clinical interviews (Child Assessment Schedule—Parent Version [CAS-P]; Hodges, Kline, Stern, Cytryn, & McKnew, 1982) were conducted independently from earlier interviews, and they were scored by individuals blind to earlier information about children and families. Boys who met ADHD criteria at age 9 (including two controls) also were more active, inattentive, and impulsive on laboratory tasks (Marakovitz & Campbell, 1998); they had also been more active when observed in the laboratory at age 6, although they did not make more errors of either omission or commission on a standard vigilance task (the Continuous Performance Test, CPT). At age 4, these boys had a more difficult time resisting the prohibition not to touch an attractive toy than did hard-to-manage boys who did not meet ADHD criteria at age 9; however, the undiagnosed group, surprisingly, was more active and impulsive on other observational measures obtained in the laboratory at age 4. Overall, in fact, family measures (maternal stress and depression) and negative maternal control were more robust predictors of continuing problems at age 9 than were observational measures of child behavior (Campbell et al., 1996), and it is important to note that similar measures of family adversity and negative maternal control were both predictive of and correlated with the onset of problems in a small sample of control boys who developed symptoms by school age (Campbell, 1994; Campbell et al., 1996). Finally, negative maternal control assessed at ages 4 and 9 mediated associations between family stress and children's externalizing symptoms at each age, and earlier negative control predicted externalizing symptoms at age 9 after controlling for initial levels of symptoms and concurrent levels of control. This suggests a process whereby family stress undermines parenting, and a troubled mother–child interaction predicts continuing problems.

Follow-Up in Early Adolescence

The children in Cohort 1 were followed up in early adolescence at an average age of 13 years (Pierce et al., 1999). The hard-to-manage group continued to differ from controls on maternal reports of externalizing symptoms on the CBCL (aggression, delinquency, externalizing). The adolescents in the hard-to-manage group also acknowledged more problems on the Youth Self-Report (Achenbach & Edelbrock, 1987); they rated themselves as showing more aggression and delinquent behaviors and as lower in social competence than control adolescents. Over half the hard-to-manage group continued to meet DSM-III-R diagnostic criteria for ADHD on a structured and independently scored interview that was administered to mothers of study participants; 41% met criteria for ODD or CD; and 41% received more than one diagnosis. These rates were all much higher than in the control group, which ranged from 0 (comorbid, CD) to 8% (ADHD or ODD).

Diagnostic status at age 13 also was examined as a function of earlier course, focusing on children who were classified as showing persistent problems at both ages 6 and 9. Once children showed continuing problems through ages 6 and 9, they were almost certain to continue to receive an externalizing diagnosis at age 13. Indeed, 94% met criteria for a diagnosis at age 13, in contrast to only 12% of the hard-to-manage 3-year-olds, whose problems were no longer in evidence by age 6 or who showed an inconsistent pattern between ages 6 and 9 (i.e., they showed continuing problems at one age but not at both). Examination of symptom trajectories suggests a stably high group, a stably low group, and a moderately high but decreasing group. Indeed, within the hard-to-manage group, the initial ADHD symptom ratings of those with a continuing diagnosis at age 13 had been significantly higher at age 3 than the ratings of those without continuing problems. It is also interesting that the improved group was at the level of the controls by age 9 in terms of maternal reports of ADHD symptoms. In terms of ratings of externalizing problems on the CBCL, children with persistent problems received significantly higher ratings than improved children at age 6, and these groups continued to differ at ages 9 and 13. By age 9, the improved children no longer differed from controls. A similar pattern of symptom levels and changes was evident in Cohort 2. That is, boys whose problems persisted started out at a higher level of symptom severity as preschoolers than boys who improved; improved boys did not differ from controls at age 9. Unfortunately, we were not able to follow Cohort 2 beyond age 9.

Summary of Follow-Up Data

The follow-up data from these two cohorts of hard-to-manage preschool children provide converging findings on the developmental course of problems. Two subsets of hard-to-manage children could be pretty clearly identified by school entry. When problems were fairly severe initially and persisted to Grade 1, the likelihood increased that problems would also be evident and at a diagnosable level by age 9. Moreover, the data from Cohort 1 indicate that, when problems persisted through age 9, it was almost certain that problems would continue into early adolescence. Thus problem trajectories appeared to be well established by school entry and to stabilize by middle childhood. It also seems clear that family context is an important predictor of outcome. The family context includes both the quality and affective tone of mother–child interaction and other aspects of the family environment, including stressful events, marital status and satisfaction, and maternal mood and depressive symptoms. These findings are consistent with the arguments made throughout this book, as well as with the data from a number of longitudinal studies examining the developmental course of problems in young children. These general conclusions reflect data examined at the aggregate or group level.

At an idiographic and more clinical level, we were struck by the range of outcomes in the sample. Some children were doing fine at follow-up; others had learning problems that emerged in the early school years. In some cases, these problems were evident earlier in delayed language development or articulation and expression difficulties; in others, they were a surprise. Other children clearly met criteria for attention-deficit/hyperactivity disorder, and some were on medication or had been at some time between ages 6 and 9. As might be expected, learning problems and hyperactivity tended to co-occur in some children. Others appeared more oppositional than hyperactive at follow-up, although, again, the two also co-occurred in other youngsters. A few children met objective criteria for conduct problems, but in general these problems showed a low level of severity, partly reflecting overly lax criteria and the inclusion of some mildly antisocial behaviors that appear to reflect age-related activities that are not likely to presage serious antisocial behavior in late adolescence. Finally, despite early aggression and hyperactivity, a few children seemed to be more anxious and/or depressed at follow-up. Again, anxiety or high levels of dysphoric mood either coexisted with other difficulties (hyperactivity, noncompliance, or learning problems) or occurred alone in the context of family change. It is also worth noting that, whereas comparison children also showed signs of anxiety, these signs tended to be more isolated fears and worries rather than part of a symptom picture that included a range of difficulties with psychosocial functioning and academic achievement. Finally, some children whose problems appeared to continue were living in quite stable and well-functioning families, whereas in others, family problems were obvious. These issues are illustrated more specifically with a discussion of the four children described in previous chapters.

ILLUSTRATIONS BASED ON PROTOTYPIC CHILDREN

The four children discussed throughout this book are considered in terms of their continuing development and their outcomes at age 13. Recall that in each instance parents complained of problems from infancy onward and that these youngsters all showed some difficulties with self-regulation when seen at age 3. However, the four prototypic children differed widely in terms of the pattern and severity of initial problems, the quality of the mother–child relationship, the nature of the family environment, and their development at age 4.

Jamie L.

Jamie was among the more aggressive and difficult children in our sample, despite a stable and supportive family. Although he had made some gains by age 4, difficulties were still apparent, and he continued to have many more problems with compliance, restlessness, impulse control, overactivity, and peer relations than the average 4-year-old in our sample.

Jamie was followed up again just after his sixth birthday. He was reportedly much better able to focus his attention and control his activity. However, Mrs. L. stated that her current concerns about Jamie included his tendency to test limits, his difficulty confronting new situations, and his attention-seeking behavior in school. She noted, when questioned about specific behaviors, that he tended not to listen in school, that he still had difficulty controlling his temper, that he needed constant structure and discipline, and that he continued to get into fights at school, especially at recess. Mrs. L. continued to use time-out, reasoning, and the withdrawal of privileges as preferred disciplinary strategies, although Jamie's father was inclined to get angrier and to be less patient. According to both interview and questionnaire measures, Jamie was no longer seen as particularly hyperactive or distractible; he did not meet DSM-III criteria for ADD at age 6. However, on the CBCL his mother rated him in the clinical range on scales assessing aggression and disobedience. During the laboratory observation of free play at age 6, Jamie did not appear disorganized or unfocused. However, he was quite restless, fidgety, and impulsive on structured tasks, and he left his seat frequently.

Jamie was on a behavioral program at school and was also receiving professional help in an attempt to deal with his anger and poor self-control. At school, he tended to get into fights with other children, to talk out in class inappropriately, and to interrupt the ongoing activities of the teacher and other children. However, Jamie's experienced classroom teacher reported that his behavior was under control, and she did not rate him in the clinical range on any scales on the TRF. Furthermore, despite his social and discipline problems, Jamie continued to function at a superior level intellectually, and he was doing excellent school work; he also participated in extracurricular activities. Thus, at age 6, although problems were still in evidence, it was difficult to predict how he would fare over the course of the next few years. Protective factors included his good intelligence and academic achievement, as well as his strong family support, despite his continued problems with self-control.

At age 9, Jamie was still having significant problems at home and at school. He met DSM-III criteria for conduct disorder, socialized, because he continued to get into fairly frequent, sometimes intense, fights with other children and had begun to steal small amounts of money from his parents. However, he would not have met the more stringent DSM-IV criteria for conduct disorder. Jamie was still a discipline problem as well. Although Jamie also was described as impulsive and fairly active, he did not meet criteria for ADD because he was not having difficulty paying attention. He would, however, have been likely to meet DSM-IV criteria for ADHD, hyperactive–impulsive subtype, had these been available. His mother also described him as a youngster who was chronically unhappy, had low self-esteem, and was socially immature. On the CBCL, Jamie was rated in the clinical range on the Social Withdrawal, Aggressive, and Delinquent scales, consistent with the clinical picture at age 6. Although his mother reported that Jamie wanted to play with other children, his immature social behavior and aggressiveness tended to alienate peers. At age 9, he was reported to have no close friends. His fourth-grade teacher noted his excellent intellectual ability, high achievement test scores, and presence in a program for gifted youngsters. However, she also saw him as having significant problems with peers, with classroom discipline, and with self-control; on the TRF, he was rated just below the clinical range on the Aggression scale. Jamie and his family were being seen by a psychologist.

Jamie was followed up again at age 13, and problems continued to be in evidence, including difficulties with compliance and self-regulation in the classroom and at home. School achievement was adequate but likely not up to his high level of ability. Classroom discipline continued to be a problem, and Jamie's parents were somewhat concerned about his unwillingness to accept responsibility, his lack of respect for adults, and his moodiness. Although peer problems had continued through middle childhood, Jamie had a large circle of friends by early adolescence and was described as very sociable and well liked by peers. He also had a range of interests. Many of the conflicts described by both Jamie and his mother sounded age appropriate and normative (the degree and nature of parental monitoring and limit setting, privacy issues, moodiness), but these have assumed more importance given his earlier history of noncompliance, poor impulse control, and aggression. According to the Child Assessment Schedule—Parent Version (Hodges et al., 1982), Jamie met DSM-III-R diagnostic criteria for ADHD, ODD, and CD, consistent with earlier concerns. It is likely that he would have met DSM-IV criteria for ADHD, hyperactive–impulsive subtype, and for ODD. However, as at age 9, he would not have met the more stringent DSM-IV criteria for conduct disorder, given the relatively minor nature of his transgressions. Complaints revolved around frequent lying to his parents and aggression toward siblings. On the CBCL, Jamie's mother rated him high on delinquency, aggression, and externalizing problems, with above-average scores on internalizing as well. Jamie also rated himself relatively high on the Externalizing scale of the Youth Self-Report, although he did not acknowledge internalizing or peer problems. Further, Jamie indicated pride in his academic success and intellectual abilities and his large group of friends.

It is instructive to examine the developmental course of Jamie's difficulties. Problems with attention have abated since the preschool years, and he no longer appears particularly distractible. He is able to sit still and attend to things that interest him; he is performing adequately in school and succeeding in extracurricular activities that require concentration and practice. The peer problems that persisted through middle childhood have also abated, and he apparently is popular with peers. Thus, his superior intelligence, curiosity, and the considerable environmental support provided by his family and school appear to have paid off. However, he continues to demonstrate poor impulse control and signs of antisocial behavior, which may be especially evident when he is with peers with whom he shares similar rebellious qualities. This problem also leads to conflict with his parents. Paired with his moodiness, these problems may or may not presage persistent social and interpersonal difficulties as Jamie reaches late adolescence. Although Jamie met DSM-III-R criteria for disruptive behavior problems, he does not appear to be a seriously impaired adolescent, given his school achievement and success in the peer group. Family conflict appears to be primary, which may reflect appropriate parental involvement and monitoring, typical peer-focused antisocial behavior, and normative parent–adolescent conflict. On the other hand, although it is unlikely that Jamie will grow up to be violent or seriously antisocial, his chronic difficulties with self-control and moodiness may well continue in the form of more subtle relationship difficulties as he gets older, with implications for both professional and interpersonal functioning.

In terms of predictive factors, Jamie's initially high levels of both hyperactivity and aggression, as well as the intensity of his aggressive encounters with peers, seemed significant initially. His early problems with self-regulation and undercontrol are still reflected in his family relationships and the concerns voiced by his parents at the adolescent follow-up. At the same time, family support and involvement are likely to account for the fact that he is doing reasonably well with the developmental tasks of early adolescence, and he is not evidencing serious problems with antisocial behavior or school functioning.

Annie J.

Annie was a youngster whose difficulties seemed to derive, at least in part, from a poor mother–child relationship reflected in low warmth and high criticism, as well as inconsistent and inappropriate parental expectations. Annie was involved in an intense struggle with her mother over who was in control; her parents had difficulties providing her the needed environmental supports for developmental change, so that each developmental hurdle became a source of conflict. Despite this, Annie made a smooth transition to preschool, where she got along well with both teachers and peers. When followed up at age 6, the marked discrepancy between Annie's behavior with her mother and with others was still apparent, and her mother's perceptions of Annie's behavior appeared to be somewhat distorted. In the intervening 2 years, Mrs. J. had given birth to a daughter who was developing normally, although the younger daughter was also being overwhelmed by an intrusive and sometimes demanding mother. However, Mrs. J. reported that she was having an easier time with her second child, whom she perceived as easier to care for, more cuddly, and less irritable and defiant than Annie had been.

Annie eagerly greeted the home visitors, and there were certainly no longer any signs of separation anxiety. She was friendly and cooperative, ready to begin each new task, and almost never fidgety, bored, or off task. She performed at the superior level on the Wechsler Preschool and Primary Scale of Intelligence and was disappointed when testing was over. She took the examiner to her room to show off her favorite toys. Overall, she was a cooperative and sociable, but sadly needy, youngster who appeared hungry for attention, affection, and positive feedback. During the laboratory assessment, Annie likewise became engaged with the tasks easily; her play was focused and directed to a few salient toys; she was not at all impulsive or inattentive. In school she was also performing well, and her first-grade teacher saw her as showing no problems except a tendency "to talk too much to her neighbors." On the TRF, she was rated as a socially competent youngster with no behavior problems. Observations in the classroom confirmed the teacher's report that she was behaving appropriately in school.

Unfortunately, Mrs. J. painted a very different picture. She reported that Annie had had a difficult time adjusting to kindergarten and that there had been several instances of school refusal. She complained of continued difficulties with discipline, inattention, overactivity, and poor impulse control. Indeed, Annie met DSM-III criteria for ADHD, according to a maternal interview. On the CBCL, her mother rated her above the clinical range on Depression, Social Withdrawal, Somatic Complaints, and Aggression. Furthermore, she reported problems with bedwetting, nightmares, anxiety, fearfulness, and loneliness, providing a picture of an anxious, unhappy, and possibly angry youngster rather than a child with primarily externalizing problems. This report is in stark contrast to that of her teacher, who did not endorse any problems.

The marked discrepancy between maternal and teacher reports was still apparent at the age 9 follow-up. Annie's third-grade teacher reported that she was functioning at grade level and above in all academic areas and that she was getting along well socially. The third-grade teacher, like the first-grade teacher, did not endorse any problems on the TRF. Mrs. J. did acknowledge that Annie was doing well in school and reported that Annie had friends and was involved in a number of outside activities. In particular, Mrs. J. noted that Annie was taking ballet lessons and that she excelled at dancing. Although Mrs. J. was able, then, to recognize some of Annie's strengths, she also continued to report numerous problems at home. She complained of a number of externalizing and internalizing symptoms that she saw as relatively specific to her own relationship with Annie. Annie was still described by her mother as impulsive, overactive, inattentive, defiant, angry, immature, and aggressive. In addition, Mrs. J. was concerned about Annie's anxiety, sadness, moodiness, and tendency to worry about things. She described Annie as an overly sensitive child who tended to become easily upset by events around her, such as the death of a neighbor's dog and the move of a close friend. Mrs. J. rated Annie above the clinical range on five scales of the CBCL: Depression, Social Withdrawal, Somatic Complaints, Hyperactivity, and Aggression. According to the structured diagnostic interview with Mrs. J., administered by an interviewer who knew nothing of Annie's earlier history, she met DSM-III criteria for ADHD, for overanxious disorder, and for chronic dysphoric mood. This picture of relatively severe and pervasive psychopathology is certainly inconsistent with Annie's behavior at school and with peers. Mrs. J. also noted that her younger daughter had recently started preschool and had experienced very severe separation anxiety, suggesting that a pattern of mother–daughter problems with separation and individuation was about to be repeated.

At age 13, Annie was still having significant problems. Her mother endorsed symptoms on the CAS-P that qualified Annie for a diagnosis of overanxious disorder, separation anxiety, and ADHD, according to DSM-III-R criteria. Her symptom pattern, examined according to DSM-IV criteria, suggested that she might meet criteria for ADHD, inattentive subtype, and she would likely meet criteria for separation anxiety and generalized anxiety disorder. On the CBCL, she was rated especially high on internalizing symptoms, particularly anxiety, although she was also rated high on the depression and aggression scales. Despite these concerns, Annie was reportedly doing well in school, had many friends, and was active in sports and other extracurricular activities. Annie, however, did acknowledge concerns about being away from home overnight, and she reported some physical symptoms of distress, as well as worry about school and about meeting new people and confronting new situations. It is noteworthy that a potentially serious family illness was diagnosed during this time, which appeared to exacerbate Annie's separation anxiety and her worries about the family remaining intact. Like Jamie's, Annie's early problems appear to be evidenced in a somewhat different form as she makes the transition to adolescence, despite her good school achievement and success in the peer group.

Annie's early problems appeared to reflect a troubled relationship with her parents; her parents seemed somewhat insensitive, and at times they had difficulties responding to and meeting her emotional needs. They also did not always seem to recognize and appreciate her many strengths. Her mother also appeared intrusive and overconcerned, primarily about what she saw as Annie's problems, and she seemed to lack genuine warmth, acceptance, and affection. At age 6, Annie appeared to be a highly anxious youngster with low self-esteem and an overwhelming need to please. At age 9, despite her many accomplishments, Annie was still apparently highly anxious and possibly depressed. As noted earlier, it is possible, even likely, that Annie was indeed a more difficult than average infant and that her early behavior contributed to an escalating pattern of mother–daughter conflict, although this is impossible to assess. In any case, it seems clear that relatively low levels of positive maternal engagement paired with her mother's overintrusiveness and poor understanding of the developmental and psychological needs of young children played a significant role in the persistence of Annie's problems at home.

Annie's continued difficulties at age 9 with her mother also appeared to reflect desperate efforts for acceptance and recognition in the face of continuing criticism and conflict, which may have served to exacerbate her anxiety, sadness, concerns about separation, and anger even further. In addition, Mrs. J. seemed to have difficulty empathizing with Annie or helping her cope with major developmental transitions (such as entry into kindergarten) or other stresses that are understandably upsetting to young children (such as her friend's move). At age 6, Annie's dependent behavior with other adults and her neediness were seen as partly reflecting an earlier insecure and anxious attachment relationship (see Sroufe, 1983). On the other hand, her ability to relate to other adults and to function relatively adequately in the peer group since early childhood suggest that Annie has adapted reasonably well to her family situation and that she has learned alternative ways of having some of her emotional needs met, at least superficially. At the age 9 follow-up, we concluded that Annie was not really likely to be showing ADD but that she may well be at risk for continued problems with anxiety, dysphoria, and low self-esteem, which all appear to be quite realistic reactions to her history of mother–child conflict. This still seems to be the case at age 13. Although Annie met DSM-III-R diagnostic criteria for ADHD and her mother reported primarily problems with inattention, these symptoms may well be reflections of her ongoing anxiety rather than true inattention; it is hard to determine this, but her above-average school performance and her acknowledged worry and anxiety make this a likely interpretation. Moreover, she would not be likely to meet DSM-IV criteria for ADHD, because her problems seem situation specific and do not spill over to affect her school performance. Annie's separation anxiety and overall concerns with performance and acceptance appear linked to her earlier difficulties in the family. Furthermore, if one accepts Bowlby's (1969) hypothesis that the relationship with the primary caregiver is the prototype for all later attachments, it is logical to predict that Annie may well have difficulty establishing trusting relationships with significant others in early adulthood. On the other hand, she may be resilient enough to develop into an intellectually and socially competent young woman, despite these early setbacks, possibly buffered by her ability to establish supportive friendships with peers.

Robbie S.

Robbie initially presented as a fairly active and impulsive youngster with poor self-control. Although he was relatively noncompliant at home, he got along well with peers in preschool and was not described as aggressive. However, as his family situation deteriorated and his parents ultimately separated, his behavior problems worsened. He was showing a variety of symptoms at age 5, some consistent with his initial difficulties with attentional control and compliance, others characteristic of young children coping with separation. At the age 6 follow-up, things had not improved. The conflict between Robbie's parents had resulted in an unstable family situation. He continued to be sad and anxious and to have sleep problems. He was also active, inattentive, noncompliant, and angry much of the time, both at home and at school. He met DSM-III criteria for ADD and received high ratings on both the internalizing and externalizing portions of the CBCL. Laboratory observations were consistent with maternal reports of problem behavior. Robbie was aggressive in his play and somewhat out of control. He was also quite restless, impulsive, and inattentive on structured tasks, and he tended to test the limits with the examiner.

Teacher reports also indicated problems with attention, compliance with classroom rules, and task completion. In addition, Robbie was getting into some relatively serious fights with other children. Finally, he was making very limited academic progress, despite better than average intellectual abilities. Classroom observations indicated that he was disruptive and irritating with other children, uncooperative with the teacher, and frequently out of his seat and that he often did not listen to the ongoing lesson. By the end of first grade, Robbie had not learned to read. Ultimately, he was enrolled in a special class for children with learning and behavior problems, where he began to make some progress.

At age 9, problems were still in evidence, although Robbie also had made some progress academically. His family situation had stabilized over the intervening years, but there was still conflict between his parents over visitation, and his father did not always follow through on planned visits and outings, leaving Robbie upset and angry. At school, Robbie remained in a special class for children with behavior problems, although he was mainstreamed for most academic subjects. He was functioning at grade level in reading and arithmetic, despite his earlier problems. Robbie's special class teacher was particularly concerned about his inattention and poor self-control and his consequent need for constant direction and structure, although she felt that he had made considerable gains, both socially and academically, and that he was well motivated. She saw Robbie as very responsive to feedback and praise.

However, Robbie also had been getting into fights during recess and at lunch with two boys who tended to tease and harass him, and he had been spending a portion of each day sitting in the principal's office. Mrs. S. painted a similar picture. She was primarily concerned about Robbie's attentional and discipline problems. According to the structured diagnostic interview administered to Mrs. S., Robbie met DSM-III criteria for ADHD. On the CBCL, his mother endorsed items leading to elevated scores on the dimensions of Social Withdrawal and Aggression, reflecting his recent fights with peers and some discipline problems at home.

At the age 13 follow-up, Robbie was on stimulant medication for his attentional problems and in a special program for children with learning problems. He also has received speech therapy. According to a maternal interview, Robbie clearly met DSM-III-R criteria for both ADHD and ODD; he would also meet DSM-IV criteria for ADHD, combined type, as well as for ODD. The combination of medication and a strictly controlled classroom, however, have made it easier for Robbie to cope at school, and he has made relatively good academic progress. He also gets along socially with other children, consistent with his sociability in preschool. Robbie continues to have an excellent relationship with his mother. He also now has regular contacts with his biological father.

It appears that Robbie is a youngster whose initial difficulties reflected a combination of temperamental difficultness, a possible genetic vulnerability to psychopathology, and family tensions. His earlier problems appear to have been exacerbated by the instability in his life. Indeed, although we may characterize him as consistently active, inattentive, and noncompliant since early childhood, his aggression, anxiety, and cognitive problems appear to wax and wane in tandem with environmental stressors. In addition, Robbie's somewhat delayed language development probably contributed to his early reading problems. It is possible to speculate that he was a youngster at biological risk for problems and that, given the severity and chronicity of early family problems, his difficulties worsened and became more stable at age 9. However, it is also important to note that Robbie is not engaged in serious delinquency and that he seems to have adjusted fairly well to school, the peer group, and his family situation. In terms of predictive factors, the combined contribution of high initial symptoms and ongoing family disruption appear to account for Robbie's relatively poor outcome at age 9, consistent with research findings from other follow-up studies. However, his strong relationship with his mother, ongoing treatment, an appropriate school placement, and a stable family situation appear to have helped him to function adequately. Overall, considering the severity of his initial problems and the unstable family situation he experienced in early childhood, Robbie is doing fairly well. Despite continuing academic and other difficulties, he is functioning much better than one might have predicted after the age 9 follow-up. However, it is difficult to determine how well he will do in later adolescence and early adulthood, given his ongoing, albeit relatively low, level of chronic problems.

Teddy M.

Teddy was the least problematic of the four children described when seen initially. It was our impression that his parents' interpretations of his early behavior and their expectations for quiet and compliance were somewhat unrealistic and that Teddy's behavior was pretty much age appropriate. Although his play was somewhat unfocused when observed in the lab at age 4, he seemed to be doing well in general, and there were few signs of any real problems.

At the time of the age 6 follow-up, the M. family was still living in the same house, and the family situation remained unchanged. Mrs. M. no longer saw Teddy as overactive or distractible. She described him as "happy" and "pretty easy going," although he was somewhat fearful of the dark and of thunderstorms. Mrs. M. also reported that Teddy was somewhat shy with other children, waiting for them to initiate contacts, and that he was reluctant to visit them, preferring to remain at home with her. Despite his apparent shyness, he had several friends with whom he played regularly, and he was also involved in structured activities that brought him into contact with other children. His mother no longer saw him as showing significant problems, as indicated by her responses both to the interview and to structured questionnaires. She also reported that Teddy was doing well in school, something that was confirmed by his teacher, who described him as a "delightful child" who was "well liked by his classmates" and "enjoys learning." Teddy's teacher rated him well below the clinical range on all scales of the TRF. Observational measures confirmed parent and teacher reports of no significant problems. Teddy was cooperative and engaged during the laboratory assessment of free play; he performed willingly and well on structured tasks, with no signs of impulsivity, inattention, or fidgetiness.

When observed in the classroom, he was also involved in appropriate classroom activities, attentive to teacher directives, and cooperative with peers.

At the age 9 follow-up, we were surprised to discover that Teddy had repeated second grade because his parents had been concerned about his shyness and social immaturity. The school had not seen the need for him to remain behind, but because he was one of the younger children in his class, they acceded to his parents' wishes. Mrs. M. still expressed some concerns about Teddy's shyness and failure to initiate peer contacts. She also noted that his schoolwork was often disorganized and messy. On the other hand, he was apparently functioning at grade level and above in all academic areas. Both maternal and teacher reports indicated no significant behavior problems. At the age 13 follow-up, Teddy continued to function well socially, and he was not a discipline problem. No significant problems were noted on either interview or questionnaire measures of adjustment. Teddy did have some minor learning problems for which he was receiving extra help at school, but overall his academic progress was above average. He apparently had many friends and was engaged in extracurricular activities.

Teddy is a good example of a child whose development, although slightly uneven, was well within the normal range. During the preschool years, Teddy's parents tended to misinterpret his age-appropriate activity level, relatively short bouts of sustained play, and limited ability to share toys as problems. Mr. and Mrs. M.'s high expectations for good behavior and their earlier pressures for maturity may well have placed Teddy under some stress, and this may have been apparent in his anxiety and fearfulness at age 6. Or these may have been age-related fears and timidities that resulted from starting school. Teddy's difficulties appear to be minimal, well within the normal range for children his age; his shyness and mild fearfulness did not appear to affect his social and academic functioning negatively. Certainly, relative to most of the children in the study who had been seen by their parents as having significant difficulties in late toddlerhood and the early preschool period, Teddy has adjusted very well, and there is little reason to be seriously concerned about persistent problems as he enters adolescence. Teddy's outcome is consistent with findings from the few other longitudinal studies reported in this chapter. Low levels of initial symptoms, a stable family environment, and a positive parent–child relationship would be expected to predict a good outcome in elementary school and beyond.

SUMMARY

In this chapter, longitudinal studies of toddlers and preschoolers who were followed up to elementary school were discussed, as were follow-up studies of clinically diagnosed hyperactive children followed to adolescence and early adulthood. Although epidemiological studies of large population samples indicate that only a small proportion of children will show serious and ongoing problems from early childhood to adolescence, the studies of hard-to-manage children suggest that problems are more stable at the extremes. Roughly half to one-third of the children with severe externalizing problems in early childhood continued to show some degree of disturbance at school age; although gender differences were addressed only superficially and boys have been studied more systematically, it appears that boys were doing more poorly than girls at follow-up. Similarly, clinically referred school-age children, especially boys, who present with symptoms of both hyperactivity and oppositional or conduct disorders have a 50–50 chance of showing some form of continuing difficulty in adolescence or young adulthood. Further, it should be pointed out that some children do not come to clinical attention until they enter school; this may reflect parental tolerance or reluctance to seek help in some cases in which problems had their onset in the preschool period but, for one reason or another, they went unrecognized. However, problems in some children clearly have their onset with the stress of school entry or as a function of newly emerging difficulties in the family.

In addition, studies have examined predictors of good and poor outcome at various ages. Most studies suggest that family discord or disruption, negative and conflict-ridden parent–child relations, and maternal depression or anxiety are associated with both the onset and the persistence of problems. Some studies identify predictive relationships, whereas others suggest that ongoing family difficulties are associated with ongoing problems in the child. In addition, all follow-up studies are consistent in showing that high levels of initial symptoms in the child, especially in boys, are associated with continuing difficulties. In particular, high levels of aggression and disobedience in the context of a high activity level, as well as poor peer relations, are associated with persistent problems, both from preschool to elementary school and from elementary school to adolescence. Furthermore, children with lower IQs are more likely to have persistent difficulties that may also be reflected in specific learning disabilities or more general deficits in cognitive functioning and school achievement. These risk factors, however, must all be considered as part of a complex developmental process that sets particular children along a risk trajectory that is more or less likely to change depending on ongoing stresses and supports in the family, school, and peer group.

Whereas it is now fairly evident that earlier disorder predicts later difficulties in adjustment, it also appears that children with early symptoms can show a range of outcomes. Furthermore, it is likely that a variety of factors contribute to outcome and that the relevant factors and their complex interactions may be different for different children living in different family and social environments. That is, children with the same symptom picture at one point in time may have different outcomes, and these outcomes are likely to be mediated or moderated by different factors. This complexity was illustrated both by general findings from our own longitudinal study of parent-identified hard-to-manage preschoolers followed up at ages 6, 9, and 13 and by illustrations based on prototypic children from this study. Thus, in one instance, a child with high levels of initial hyperactivity and aggression had a mixed outcome, with residual difficulties in evidence, despite low levels of ongoing stressors or other risk factors for disorder. He continued to be somewhat aggressive, difficult to discipline, and rebellious at follow-up, although school achievement and peer relations were not problems. In a second example, a boy with relatively severe initial symptoms of hyperactivity and noncompliance (but not aggression), complicated by a family history of psychopathology and ongoing family turmoil, continued to show serious behavior problems at age 9; by age 13, although problems continued, treatment and a more stable family situation seemed to be associated with some lessening of problems and improvement in school achievement, despite a diagnosis of ADHD. These improvements were also apparent against a backdrop of a long-standing positive mother–child relationship, which is likely to have been a protective factor against worsening antisocial behavior at adolescence. In a third instance, a negative mother–child relationship was associated with sadness and anxiety in a girl who was functioning well outside the home. This youngster had made a reasonably good adjustment to family conflict, which may also reflect ongoing marital distress and maternal depression. However, her long-term prognosis remains unclear. Finally, one boy with relatively mild initial symptoms and no clearly identifiable risk factors or family problems was doing well at follow-up, despite initial parental concerns about high activity and inattention and later worries about immaturity and shyness. Taken together, these data and case illustrations underline the complexities inherent in identifying causal mechanisms in the development of disorders in children, in predicting future adjustment, and in delineating the specific factors contributing to outcome, both generally and in the individual case.

CHAPTER 9

Conclusions and Social Policy Implications

This book has discussed the major developmental transitions facing preschoolers. Early indicators of behavior problems were described, albeit with many caveats about the clinical implications of difficult behavior in early childhood. I have argued that child characteristics interact with family factors and features of the wider social environment to determine whether children will function well or poorly in early childhood and that complex transactions among these factors also will determine how well adjusted children are at school age and beyond. A warm and supportive parent–child relationship, paired with firm, reasonable, consistent, and flexible childrearing practices, and a generally positive emotional climate in the home are seen as particularly important factors that facilitate optimal child development, especially when young children are irritable and demanding. Conversely, a conflicted parent–child relationship, arbitrary, punitive, and/or uninvolved parenting, and high levels of family discord are associated with the development of problems in toddlerhood, particularly when children were already negative in mood or difficult to calm as infants. Problems that emerge early are more likely to persist and worsen over time if the family climate, including childrearing practices, also remains negative and parents are harsh and/or disengaged. These complex child, parent, and family interaction factors reflect a combination of genetic and environmental influences on child development and family climate.

Relationships with siblings and peers are also seen as having an important influence on young children's social development. Experiences with age-mates and with siblings help young children learn to negotiate the tasks required to become cooperative members of a social group, as they develop the skills needed to compromise, negotiate, inhibit aggression, share, and understand the other's point of view. Further parent–child relationships, sibling relationships, and peer relationships all appear to influence one another in systemic fashion. Thus problems at home can have ramifications in the peer group and vice versa; for example, children living in stressful family circumstances may become aggressive at school or children who are rejected by other children may become noncompliant and moody at home. Other factors in the preschool or day care environment, such as too little or too much structure or caregivers who are insensitive, harsh, and/or disengaged, may precipitate problems at home. Similarly, external stresses on the parents, such as problems at work or with extended family, may have an impact on parental availability or patience and thereby precipitate or exacerbate problems between parents and children. Children's problems may appear as transient situational disturbances or as reactions to stress that disappear as external stressors lessen. However, in the context of particular child characteristics, such as negative mood and poor self-regulatory abilities, especially when there are multiple and ongoing family stresses, problems may become more severe and persistent with development.

A transactional model is based on the assumption that development is neither linear nor necessarily predictable. Young children are often able to overcome early difficulties, given a relationship with a supportive and responsive caregiver. However, some proportion of children with early and relatively serious behavior problems will continue to have difficulties throughout the early childhood years, sometimes despite positive environmental influences. The data also suggest that problems may persist despite access to currently available treatments. Further, the combination of provocative and aggressive child behavior, inconsistent and rejecting parenting strategies, and continuing family adversity, reflecting multiple risks, is most clearly associated with chronic problems. It is also evident that individual children develop problems for different reasons and that there are likely to be a variety of routes to disorder, as well as different factors that influence problem persistence and severity. Thus different combinations of factors may lead to problem onset in the individual case; even when similar etiological factors appear to be present, their relative importance may vary from one individual to the next. Finally, one factor may be causal in one case and a consequence of problems in another. For example, rejection by peers may lead to provocative and attention-seeking behavior in one child, whereas in another, aggressive behavior may lead to peer rejection. As has been evident throughout this book, it is almost impossible to know where and how to draw causal inferences. Some of these issues were illustrated by case vignettes.

Despite the complexity inherent in this field of study and the difficulty establishing clear-cut causal links among particular genetic and environmental factors and the child's behavior, a number of conclusions have been drawn in preceding chapters that link aspects of family functioning and social context to the onset and/or persistence, as well as the amelioration, of children's problems. At a practical level, research findings regarding child and family development and later outcome have major social policy implications, and many current debates about social policy have important ramifications on young children and their families (e.g., White, 1996). Among the more heated debates are those revolving around policies concerning child care (Belsky, 2001; Scarr, 1998; Shonkoff & Phillips, 2000; Zigler & Gilman, 1996), early intervention (Ramey & Ramey, 1998; Shonkoff & Phillips, 2000; Thompson & Nelson, 2001), welfare reform (Duncan & Brooks-Gunn, 2000; Knitzer, Yoshikawa, Cauthen, & Aber, 2000; Zaslow, Tout, Smith, & Moore, 1998), and parental leave (e.g., Frank & Zigler, 1996; Kamerman, 2000). Educational programs for parents (Cowan, Powell, & Cowan, 1998) and for health professionals also need to be addressed. The lack of availability of comprehensive treatment programs for preschoolers with behavior problems needs to be given serious attention by the mental health and pediatric communities, especially in view of the growing awareness of the prevalence of problems in young children (Lavigne et al., 1998a) and the problems of access presented by managed care (American Academy of Pediatrics, 2000). Children and families like those described in this book have been widely neglected by the mental health community, which has targeted children of school age and adolescence for intervention efforts or has paid most attention to preschool children with more serious cognitive and emotional disorders such as autism. Other programs, such as Head Start, are appropriately available for children living in chronic poverty. Young children with less obvious problems tend to fall through the cracks because they are frequently ineligible and/or inappropriate for those programs that are available. Moreover, many insurance companies are loath to reimburse families for mental health services for young children.

Despite the increased attention to social policies that affect young children (Jacobs & Davies, 1991; Zigler & Styfco, 1996), the resources for comprehensive and sustained programs, especially for high-risk infants and preschool children, are still grossly inadequate (Kamerman, 1996; Shonkoff & Phillips, 2000). This situation reflects a combination of conflicting political priorities and agendas, differing political philosophies about the role of government in supporting children and families, and misinterpretations and oversimplifications of research findings (Hall, Kagan, & Zigler, 1996; Jacobs & Davies, 1991; Kamerman, 1996; Thompson & Nelson, 2001; White, 1996). It is noteworthy that the United States has a less coherent, focused, consistent, and universal family policy than most other Western democracies (Kamerman, 1996).

When translating developmental findings into social policies that affect infants and preschoolers, the need for transactional, ecological, and systems models seems obvious (Shonkoff & Phillips, 2000; Woodhead, 1988). In 1988, Woodhead cautioned against the overly simplistic interpretation of research findings that can lead cost-conscious legislators to favor one-shot and quick solutions to complex problems. This problem is still with us in 2002, and the likelihood is that it will worsen with the increasing move toward local control, devolution of power to the states, and huge tax cuts. Although there have been significant increases in funding for Head Start and other early childhood programs since the first edition of this book in 1990 (Raikes, 1998), there are still major gaps in services for needy children. For example, only half of the Head Start-eligible children in Pennsylvania could be accommodated in 1998 (Bergsten & Steketee, 1999), and this appears to be the case nationwide (Shonkoff & Phillips, 2000). There are also marked discrepancies in program availability and quality from one community to another. This is partly a function of the reliance on block grants to the states, ensuring disparities, for example, in the availability of basic health care for young children, as well as the regulation of child care and preschool programs (e.g., Raikes, 1998; Ripple, Gilliam, Chanana, & Zigler, 1999; Shonkoff & Phillips, 2000; Zigler & Styfco, 1996). Despite the increase in government spending on infancy and early childhood programs over the past 10 years, the number of children living in poverty has not diminished substantially, and serious social, behavioral, and cognitive problems are the continuing legacy of poverty and deprivation (Duncan & Brooks-Gunn, 2000; McLoyd, 1998; Ramey & Ramey, 1998; Shonkoff & Phillips, 2000; Zigler & Styfeo, 1996).

Funding for programs such as Head Start has increased, but the debate on its effectiveness has not subsided. This is, in part, a direct result of the failure (or lack of well-documented success) of various prevention and treatment programs to effect *sweeping* social changes or to have long-lasting effects on outcome. Zigler and Styfco (1996) discuss Head Start and other early-intervention programs for impoverished preschoolers, which have waxed and waned in popularity and consequently in funding levels over the past 35 years. Funding for such programs at any point in time appears to depend on the findings from specific studies, the nature of public expectations, the types of outcome measures employed, and the general political climate (e.g., whether the zeitgeist is toward activist government or not, the continuing tension between federal and state initiatives, and the ongoing debate about fiscal restraint).

Recent studies indicate that early-intervention programs for disadvantaged children are effective, even in the long term, when they are structured, have a reasonable staff-to-child ratio, and involve parents, although the nature of the change process is poorly understood (Ramey & Ramey, 1998; Shonkoff & Phillips, 2000; Zigler & Styfco, 1993). Early-intervention programs were initially based on the expectation that cognitive enrichment would lead to permanent gains in cognitive functioning (Hunt, 1961). Naive optimism about the effectiveness of early intervention led not only to expectations of significant and permanent gains in IQ but also to suggestions that enrichment programs for disadvantaged preschoolers would break the cycle of poverty. Woodhead (1988), Zigler (1987), and, more recently, Thompson and Nelson (2001), among others, have pointed out the negative social policy implications of overblown expectations. When expectations are unrealized because they are unrealistic, funding suffers, and funding cuts rarely take into account the relative merits of different programs. A more realistic appraisal of early intervention programs, one that is more consistent with the accumulated evidence, suggests that all programs, whether prevention programs for disadvantaged children or treatment programs for children with difficulties, must be targeted to the right group of children, must be comprehensive, intense, and appropriately timed, and must consider the child within a family context (Cummings et al., 2000; Ramey & Ramey, 1998; Shonkoff & Phillips, 2000). Similar caveats can be applied to a number of other social policy issues that have an effect on the lives of a large number of young children and their families.

EDUCATION FOR PARENTING

Although childbirth education classes of various sorts are widely available to pregnant women and their husbands, such programs tend to help couples prepare for and deal with the delivery. They do not prepare parents for the profound psychological impact of becoming a parent or for the multiple changes that occur in the marital relationship and the family system (e.g., Belsky, Rovine, & Fish, 1989; Cowan & Cowan, 1992). New parents do not routinely receive sufficient guidance about what to expect from a newborn or about how best to manage typical caretaking tasks that may seem overwhelming at first. The multitude of disparate programs that are available to teach parents more generally about children's early development or developmental needs have not been systematically evaluated (Cowan et al., 1998), so it is unclear what does and does not work. It also is often assumed that most parents just "know" what to do or that they discover the best methods of coping with a particular problem or developmental phase by learning from their social network, from their own parents, or, at worst, by trial and error. Although parenting groups often are available for parents who are "at risk," many educated, sensitive, and child-centered parents, as well as those with fewer resources, might benefit from educational programs that provide both support (especially to first-time parents) and information about the development of infants and toddlers.

For instance, it may be helpful to new parents to understand something about their infant's developing perceptual and sensory systems, as well as the fact that face-to-face social interaction and close bodily contact are important for early social-emotional development. Understanding that infants vary widely in temperament or personality and that they may have different needs depending on, for example, their self-soothing abilities, activity levels, and alertness, may also be helpful. As infants begin to explore the world of objects and show fear of strangers, understanding the developmental underpinnings of these major advances may help parents to cope with them more effectively, for example, by more appropriately childproofing the house to permit exploration and by being sensitive to their young child's response to the approach of strangers or to separations. The importance of parental responsiveness to distress is also something about which parents may need guidance. All too frequently parents worry about "spoiling" a 2-month-old by picking him up when he cries. Understanding that a 2-month-old and a 12-month-old differ greatly in their levels of cognitive and social development, their abilities to meet their own needs and communicate about them, and their understanding of cause–effect relations would appear to make parenting an easier task. Certainly, when children reach toddlerhood, many parents need help setting consistent and appropriate limits. In some instances, parents may require support to help them ride out the tantrums that may accompany this sometimes stormy and difficult developmental period. Often parents have a hard time providing a supportive environment that will facilitate exploration and the development of autonomy but not elicit conflict-ridden defiance. With this in mind, the Office of Child Development at the University of Pittsburgh has put together a series of parenting guides that are available online (*www.pitt.edu/~ocdweb/guides.htm*), based on the research literature and reviewed by a panel of experts.

Unfortunately, although numerous books and various programs for parents are available, it is difficult to sort out those that work from those that do not or those that are based on scientific findings from those based on popular misconceptions or ideologies about child-rearing. Tested programs that teach parents about the rudiments of development are rarely available. All too often parents enter "parenting" programs when things have gotten out of hand and it is clear that a 6-week or a 12-week parent training program by itself will do little as a therapeutic intervention over the long term (see Chapter 7). Furthermore, such programs often tend to be based on naive behaviorism, with little concern for the differing needs of children at different developmental levels. In addition, annoying behaviors are sometimes identified as the problem that requires modification, and parents are not encouraged to think about underlying causes or other ways of conceptualizing what the real problem might be. Rather, simple solutions, such as star charts and time-out, are prescribed for most if not all presenting complaints. Normal perturbations in development are rarely addressed, nor is a link made between stressful events in the family and a child's aggressive, defiant, or clingy behavior. It is indeed surprising how educated and sensitive parents sometimes think that their preschooler is buffered from ongoing stressful family events. Thus it would seem that many minor problems that can escalate and become more serious, even though they may remain transient, could be prevented or ameliorated by some relatively straightforward pointers for parents. Such programs could be made available through a range of pediatric, developmental, and educational facilities for a small fee. Parents of children like Annie and Teddy might benefit from more information on normal development when their children are infants and toddlers; increased awareness of what to expect during infancy and toddlerhood may make it easier to cope with early irritability or demandingness and normal developmental transitions. A parent education (i.e., normal developmental) component should also be incorporated into more comprehensive programs for families considered at risk. Finally, evaluation of the efficacy of these programs is essential if funds are to be spent wisely and healthy family development is to be facilitated.

EDUCATION FOR HEALTH PROFESSIONALS

When Robbie's mother contacted her pediatrician about her difficulties handling his behavior in infancy, she was told that he would outgrow the problem and not to worry about it. This was a common experience of parents in our project. Now, 10 years later, there is more emphasis on the problems of young children (Shonkoff & Phillips, 2000), but it is also true that mental and pediatric health professionals still do not routinely receive in-depth systematic training in developmental issues. This is especially the case for those in frontline positions who are often called on to make decisions about referral to specialists. Unfortunately, general training programs for pediatricians, family physicians, nurses, or other primary care providers rarely include comprehensive courses on *normal* social and cognitive development. Developmental issues are more likely to be covered in specialty programs such as developmental pediatrics or pediatric nursing, although individuals with such specialized training are more often found in teaching hospitals or specialty clinics, not in primary care. This is true despite the fact that parents bring their questions about common developmental problems and their concerns about behavior management to their pediatrician or family physician first. This situation prompted Routh, Schroeder, and Koocher

(1983) to propose that clinical psychologists (presumably those with developmental backgrounds) join forces with pediatricians working in group practices, health maintenance organizations, and other frontline facilities. I strongly agree with this recommendation; it should also be pointed out, however, that many psychiatrists, psychologists, and social workers receive little basic grounding in developmental issues; mental health training programs tend to focus on pathology and its ramifications. However, in-depth knowledge of normal child and family development would seem to be a crucial prerequisite for work with young children and their families, whether one is providing primary services or services to children on a referral basis. I would argue that work with young children and their families requires special training, training that helps the pediatric or mental health worker to understand parental concerns within a developmental framework, while not minimizing them as insignificant.

When the first edition of this book was written, managed care was just emerging. Its dominance of the health care system also has implications for the funding of pediatric care and overall access to mental health facilities for families with young children with special needs. Even with the emergence of the State Children's Health Insurance Program, a federally funded, state-run initiative meant to provide health insurance to children not covered by either Medicaid or their parents' health insurance, many children are lost to the system. Moreover, managed care means that many children have difficulty accessing specialty treatments for mental health services or for chronic conditions with developmental sequelae because of cost constraints, lack of coverage for long-term intervention, and guidelines that favor healthy children over those with chronic illnesses or disabilities. The American Academy of Pediatrics has taken the lead in issuing several policy statements aimed at rectifying some of these problems (AAP, 1998, 2000). Although the focus of these statements is on care across the age range from infancy to adolescence, they underscore the need for coordinated, comprehensive, and developmentally informed care for young children with special physical and mental health needs, for more access to appropriately trained developmental specialists in pediatrics and other professions, and the need for the various systems that impinge on children (education, child care, child welfare, social service agencies) to work together to provide needed services for children.

CHILD CARE

Reframing the Child-Care Debate

According to recent statistics from the 1999 National Household Education Survey (as cited in Shonkoff & Phillips, 2000, p. 298), nearly half of all infants under 1 year of age and over half of all 1- and 2-year-olds are enrolled in some type of nonparental care for part of each week. By age 3, over 70% of children in the United States are in child care. These data are consistent with those from the NICHD Study of Early Child Care, which found that half of all infants enrolled in the study were in nonparental care for at least 10 hours a week by the age of 6 months (NICHD Early Child Care Research Network, 1997). By age 3, this number rose to 66%. Thus, despite early debates on whether child care was good or bad for infants and toddlers (Belsky, 1988; Clarke-Stewart, 1989), the reality of family life in the United States at the beginning of the 21st century is that in most two-parent families, both parents work, and in single-parent families, work is a necessity for the primary caregiver. Thus child care in some form is a necessary aspect of family life, making debates about whether it is good or bad for children moot and inappropriate. The issue now must be reframed to focus on questions about age of entry and about type, amount, stability, and quality of child care (NICHD Early Child Care Research Network, 1997, 1999b, 2000a, 2000b, 2001b, 2002b). Under what conditions do children of different ages and from different family backgrounds do well or poorly in child care? Does age of entry make a difference? What type of care is better for children of different ages? How does one define and measure quality?

Parameters of Child Care

Obviously, child care is not a monolithic construct; young children of working parents may be cared for at home by a relative, a paid babysitter, or a nanny; at a neighbor's house; in a regulated family day care home; in a day care center; or in some combination of in-home and out-of-home care. In each type of care, the quality of care and the nature of the child–caregiver relationship will vary widely. In both family day care homes and child-care centers, adult–child ratio and group size will also vary considerably, and caregivers will differ in their levels of training, experience, and knowledge of child development (NICHD Early Child Care Research Network, 1997a, 1999b, in 2002b). Furthermore, family day care homes also differ in whether they are relatively informal arrangements that are unregulated or more formal settings that must meet state regulations (Kontos et al., 1995). Not surprisingly, given the documented range in quality and type of care, the accumulating evidence indicates clearly that child care per se is neither good nor bad (Kontos et al., 1995; NICHD Early Child Care Research Network, 1997b, 1998, 2002b). However, findings also indicate that both the quality of care and the quality of the family environment are important predictors of children's outcomes (e.g., Howes & Olenick, 1986; NICHD Early Child Care Research Network, 1997a, 1997b, 1998, 2000a, 2000b, 2002a, 2002b). Some studies indicate that features of child care (quality, stability, amount) interact with family factors to determine the impact of child care on children's development (e.g., Howes & Olenick, 1986; NICHD Early Child Care Research Network, 1997b). Thus, for example, the combination of poor quality child care and a less sensitive mother predicted insecure attachment at 15 months in the NICHD study. There is also some evidence to suggest that too many hours in care may be associated with less optimal development, as reflected in slightly higher levels of problem behavior, at least during the transition to school (NICHD Early Child Care Research Network, 2001b).

From a transactional and ecological perspective, one must consider the convergent factors in the child, family, and child-care facility that are associated with good versus poor adaptation to nonparental care (Hungerford, Brownell, & Campbell, 2000; Lamb, 1998). The anecdotes presented in Chapter 4 suggest that there may be negative effects of care when children spend too much time away from home, especially when the quality of care is poor, providing children with inadequate attention, affection, and emotional support from familiar and caring adults. When there are major tensions in the home that interfere with adequate parenting, children who spend many hours in substandard or rejecting care may be especially at risk to develop problems. Several of the children described earlier were reacting to a subtle, but insidious, form of emotional neglect. Dealing with only one facet of this complex interplay of factors will probably not be adequate to ameliorate children's problems. However, rigorously enforced and stringent standards for child-care facilities would make a small dent in one aspect of the problem by underscoring the need for adequate numbers of properly trained and/or experienced caregivers, presumably those who might be more sensitive to the needs of young children, and by promoting health and safety standards.

Structural and Process Definitions of Child-Care Quality

The quality of care, defined grossly in terms of the ratio of children to caregivers and staff training in child development, becomes crucial if the goal is optimizing children's development rather than simply providing custodial care (Scarr, 1998). To this end, staff-to-child ratios of 3:1 for infants and 4:1 for toddlers have been proposed by several professional associations (National Association for the Education of Young Children, 1984; American Public Health Association and American Academy of Pediatrics Collaborative Project, 1992), based on an analysis of the needs of young children for individual care, attention, and social interaction with adults (see Phillips, 1988; Whitebook, Sakai, & Howes, 1997). Evidence from a number of studies indicates that staff-to-child ratio, group size, staff training and experience, stable familiar caregivers, and emphasis on developmentally appropriate programming rather than on custodial care are associated with expected gains in children's cognitive functioning and social competence (Kontos et al., 1995; NICHD Early Child Care Research Network, 1999b, 2000b, 2002b; Whitebook et al., 1990).

Despite these findings, variability in standards and quality is the rule. For example, the NICHD Study of Early Child Care has followed children living in nine states across the country representing the northeast, midwest, south, and west, as well as rural, suburban, and urban centers (NICHD Early Child Care Research Network, 1999b). Of the 97 centers that were observed when study children were 6 months of age, only one in three met the standard of a 3:1 ratio of caregivers to babies. The upper range observed was 1:15; the mean was 4.24. Some caregivers had less than a high school education, although 65% had the recommended level of at least some college courses. Overall, however, only 10% of the settings in which 6-month-old study children were being cared for met all four guidelines for ratio, group size, caregiver education, and caregiver training, and 20% met none of them. By the time study children were 36 months of age, a higher proportion were in settings in which quality standards were met. Of the 250 observed centers, more than half met guidelines for the ratio of caregivers to children

(1:7), and 80% met the educational guidelines of some college course work. Overall, 34% met all four standards at 36 months. It is noteworthy that these were licensed centers, so presumably they all met the minimum state standards needed to achieve licensure. These data underscore the variability across settings and the need for standards that are more than just voluntary guidelines. Children in settings that met higher standards had better language development, higher scores on measures of early school readiness, and fewer behavior problems at 36 months, even with family income and maternal sensitivity controlled.

In addition to these structural features of quality that are subject to regulation (staff-to-child ratio, group size, and caregiver education and training), in the NICHD Study quality was also defined in process terms, conceptualized as the observed responsiveness, sensitivity, and appropriately timed stimulation provided by caregivers to the study children. This index of caregiving quality was found to be an important predictor of children's outcomes, even after controlling for demographic variables, aspects of family functioning, and other parameters of child care (NICHD Early Child Care Research Network, 1997b, 1998, 2000b, 2002b). Children with more responsive and stimulating caregivers were more cooperative and had fewer behavior problems, according to both maternal and caregiver reports at 24 and 36 months. They also had better language skills, concept development, and school readiness. Similar results were obtained at 54-month follow-up (NICHD Early Child Care Research Network, 2002b). Taken together, data from the NICHD Study of Early Child Care, the most comprehensive follow-up of children in infant and toddler care, indicates that both structural and process aspects of child-care quality are significant predictors of children's functioning at preschool age across social and cognitive domains. Moreover, structural features of quality exert some of their effects through the quality of the caregiver–child interaction, presumably because caregivers with fewer children to care for and with more training in child development are more responsive and stimulating. This aspect of quality, in turn, predicts better outcomes. It is also important to note, however, that in every instance family factors, especially maternal sensitivity, explained a larger share of the variance in outcomes than any child-care parameter did, including quality of care.

Although quality of child care can make a difference (Ramey & Ramey, 1998), it also is well known that children with the most needs are often those who are left in the least adequate facilities (Kontos et al.,1995; Phillips, Voran, Kisker, Howes, & Whitebook, 1994). For example, Phillips et al. (1994) found that even when centers meet structural standards of care, caregivers working with the poorest children are often more harsh and less responsive. Moreover, children living in poverty may be either in excellent subsidized care or in poor-quality relative or family day care (Kontos et al., 1995; Lamb, 1998; NICHD Early Child Care Research Network, 1997a), and some studies find a curvilinear relationship between quality of center care and income, with children of lower and middle-income working families receiving poorer quality care than families at the bottom and top of the income distribution (NICHD Early Child Care Research Network, 1997a).

Regardless of family circumstances, providers of care to young children should be trained to understand children and their development. The fact that caregivers are often untrained and unskilled, working for low wages in facilities with high turnover, should be a cause for concern among parents, child development specialists, and politicians alike. Staff-to-child ratios in some facilities are often inadequate to meet either necessary safety standards or the psychological needs of young children. One adult cannot possibly meet the needs of five or six infants or toddlers for basic caregiving, as well as social and cognitive stimulation, although a number of states permit such ratios (Young & Zigler, 1986). Poor pay and low status lead to rapid staff turnover, even though there is substantial evidence that consistent care from familiar people is important to young children's sense of security and well-being.

Federal Child-Care Standards and Child Care in the Era of Welfare Reform

The history of federal standards for day care centers and family day care homes provides a sobering picture of the interplay between political concerns and children's welfare (see Phillips, 1986; Zigler & Gilman, 1996). Although standards were drawn up and published as the HEW Federal Interagency Day Care Requirements (1980), they were withdrawn because of cost constraints; furthermore, these are *minimum* standards, "a standard below which the child's development could be impaired" (Young & Zigler, 1986). These standards are adequate in some areas (e.g., staff-to-child ratio and group size), but specifications for staff training and programming are more ambiguous. In 1985, Congress passed the Model Child Care Standards Act in response to highly publicized allegations of sexual abuse in day care and preschool facilities (see Phillips, 1986, for a detailed discussion of this legislation and its weaknesses). This legislation, consistent with government policies on deregulation and limited federal involvement in state-run programs, is seen as advisory rather than mandatory. Its main thrust is the requirement that states institute background checks on new staff, supposedly as a way of decreasing incidents of child abuse by caregivers. Certainly, every effort should be made to monitor and minimize such crimes against children, but this legislation fails to deal, except in vague and nonspecific terms, with general issues of quality of care. Thus it does not delineate specific requirements for staff training or supervision, staff-to-child ratios, or programming, although staff-to-child ratios and staff training and qualifications have been clearly related to outcomes. Despite this, the development of regulations is left to the discretion of the states. Clearly, this bill, which was reactive to a specific and highly publicized aspect of the child-care crisis rather than proactive, falls far short even of the minimum standards promulgated in 1980.

Given the inexorable move toward more state control and less federal regulation, as well as the move toward block grants for child-care initiatives (Raikes, 1998), how well are the states protecting children? Young and Zigler (1986) examined state licensing requirements for child-care facilities and compared them with the 1980 federal standards. As might be expected, there is wide variability. Although all 50 states have some form of regulation and licensing requirement for day care centers and most states also regulate family day care homes, standards range widely, and only a few states actually adhere to the federal guidelines for child-care quality (Zigler & Gilman, 1996). For example, many states do not require the director of a day care facility to have specialized training in child care or child development. Few states have program requirements that go much beyond custodial care (i.e., basic health and safety regulations), and in those that do, the requirements are vague, nonspecific, and often not enforced. This situation underscores the need for enforceable federal standards to establish uniformly adequate facilities for the growing number of young children in child care. Of course, problematic issues of funding and affordability are thereby raised and need to be addressed. However, the failure to make decisions about what constitutes minimum adequate care for young children may well have serious economic and human consequences, both immediately and in the long term, given the potential impact of inadequate facilities on the safety, health, cognitive, and social development of young children (Shonkoff & Phillips, 2000; Zigler & Gilman, 1996).

In view of the fact that women with children under 3 are returning to work in increasing numbers, federal standards that mandate quality care, that is, care that facilitates children's emotional, social, and cognitive development, should be among our society's highest priorities, as it is in several European countries, including France, Italy, and Sweden. There certainly are excellent facilities with caring staff, but places in these facilities are hard to come by. It is not uncommon for working women to place their names on the waiting lists of high-quality child-care centers as soon as they learn that they are pregnant. Needless to say, such centers are extremely expensive, and children living in less than comfortable circumstances rarely, if ever, have access to them. The increase in franchised, for-profit day care facilities is also a cause for concern. These facilities are often physically attractive, but issues of ratio, staff training, and programming may be ignored in the interests of profitability; it is unclear how the owners of such facilities balance children's and families' needs against their desire for profit. Lamb (1998) cites evidence suggesting that such for-profit centers may provide lower quality care. Finally, many family day care settings are unlicensed and, therefore, may not even meet their state's minimum requirements for adequacy.

It seems obvious that professionals concerned with young children must join forces with parents to put pressure on politicians to establish and enforce adequate federal standards. Organizations such as the Children's Defense Fund and the National Association for the Education of Young Children have been vocal on this issue. The recent report issued by the National Academy of Sciences (Shonkoff & Phillips, 2000) also highlights child care as a major national concern. Other educational, developmental, and mental health groups need to make this a top priority issue as well.

The Clinton administration was vocal in its support of child-care initiatives, and it earmarked a large increase in federal funds in fiscal year 1999 for child-care block grants, tax credits for working families using child care, and tax credits for businesses providing child-care facilities or resources to workers, among other initiatives meant to help working families with young children have access to quality child care (Raikes, 1998). However, these programs are in some ways diffuse, and the fact that the bulk of these funds went directly to the states in the form of block grants means that variable quality will be the rule rather than the exception. Moreover, the fate of some of these programs is now very much in question.

Furthermore, the 1996 legislation that ended Aid to Families with Dependent Children and substituted the Personal Responsibility and Work Opportunity Reconciliation Act of 1996 (PRWORA), paid through Temporary Assistance to Needy Families, has led to a marked increase in the need for child care, as women on welfare are expected to seek employment (Raikes, 1998; Zaslow, et al., 1998), in many states when infants are as young as 3 months old (Kamerman, 2000). As a result, many young women with infants and toddlers are using unregulated, and even illegal, child care that is paid for by the federal government via block grants to the states. However, the states often do not have the resources or the will to monitor the quality of care received by the infants and toddlers of poor women needing subsidized services (Raikes, 1998). Because the goal of welfare reform was to return poor single women to the labor force, the more comprehensive goal of family support and well-being has been overlooked in many states. Although some families living below the poverty level actually receive high-quality care because of government subsidies (e.g., NICHD Early Child Care Research Network, 1996), it is also true that many poor children are in substandard and even dangerous care (Kontos et al., 1995; Phillips et al., 1994; Raikes, 1998). Thus, despite the unprecedented increase in government funding for child care during the Clinton years, the devolution of power to the states and the lack of enforceable federal standards for child-care quality mean that the child-care system has numerous problems. These problems are unlikely to be addressed by the current administration, especially so given new fiscal constraints. Indeed, it appears that even maintaining the status quo will be a victory.

FAMILY/MATERNITY LEAVE AND FLEXIBLE WORK SCHEDULES FOR PARENTS

Related to debates about child care are those focused on parental-leave policies and flexible work schedules for parents with young children, another important aspect of family policy (Frank & Zigler, 1996; Kamerman, 2000). Policies on family leave and work schedules may permit some families with two working parents or single parents in the work force to rely less or not at all on infant child care. However, parental-leave policies have also been the subject of fierce debate in Congress, and the major bill dealing with this issue, the Family and Medical Leave Act (FMLA) of 1993, includes only weak provisions, and these only apply to a segment of society. The history of this bill is also a window into the complicated and difficult road to passage of family-friendly legislation that supports women in the work force but that is opposed by business groups as too costly.

Kamerman (2000) notes that the United States is one of only a handful of developed countries that does not have a national policy providing paid maternity leave for mothers after the birth of a baby or the adoption of a child. The FMLA, first introduced in Congress in 1985 and passed several times with bipartisan support, was vetoed twice by the first President Bush. Earlier versions had somewhat more generous provisions, but after much compromise and a 7-year struggle, the current bill was signed into law by President Clinton in 1993. It provides for up to 12 weeks of *unpaid* leave, with job security and the continuation of health insurance. However, eligibility requirements related to tenure, hours, job responsibilities, and size of business mean that only about half the workers in the country are covered under this law (Kamerman, 2000). This situation is in stark contrast to most European countries that provide from 14 weeks (Ireland, Germany) to a year (Norway, Sweden) of parental leave with from 70% to 100% pay. For example, Italy not only has a network of excellent state-supported child-care centers but also mandates that women be allowed 5 months of maternity leave with 80% pay and an additional 6 months at 30% pay, if desired. France permits both parents to take a leave for up to 16 weeks at full pay, with a number of other provisions for multiple births, sick infants, adoptions, and so on (Kamerman, 2000). Of the developed nations, only New Zealand and Australia, like the United States, have no paid leave provisions, although parents can take up to 1 year without fear of losing their jobs or benefits.

The need for a more generous family leave policy seems obvious. The FMLA of 1993 is a *small* step in the right direction. Importantly, some states have taken up the slack by instituting more family-friendly policies, often as a way of attracting business at a time of economic growth and low unemployment. However, as is the case with child-care regulation, states vary widely in guidelines and mandates on this issue.

A consistent national policy of paid family leave for mothers of young infants would help to deal with some of the problems of finding quality affordable infant care. Many parents who are forced to return to work because of fear of job loss would at least have the option of staying home with their newborn for the first few months, a time when early parent–infant relationships are being established. Certainly, it appears reasonable to grant paid or partially paid leave at least through the postpartum period (i.e., 3 months), although 6 months seems preferable. In a society that places so much emphasis on "family values," it seems logical that women not be required to return to work when they are still exhausted from the physical and psychological demands of childbirth and that young infants need not be placed in substitute care if one of their parents would prefer to remain at home.

Indeed, one recent study examined whether the length of maternity leave was related to the quality of mother–infant interaction in a large sample of new mothers. Clark, Hyde, Essex, and Klein (1997) studied 198 mothers and their infants at 4 months postpartum. Mothers who had to return to work at 6 weeks postpartum were less positive when observed with their infants during feeding and play at 4 months, and this was especially true for women who also reported depressive postpartum symptoms. Women who perceived their infants as fussy and irritable were also less positive when they returned to work after only 6 weeks; presumably, these mothers and infants had not had adequate time to adapt to one another or to establish a rhythm of mutual positive interaction (Stern, 1985). The implications of this study for family-leave policies seem obvious, in that longer leaves were associated with more harmonious interactions, even in the context of other stressors.

Although the need for a parental-leave policy is clear, there are also other changes in policy that seem important for families with young children. Because company-run, on-site day care centers are rare, there is a need for more flexible work hours for families with young children. This issue is addressed by Winett (1998), who suggests that part-time work arrangements that include flexible work hours and more opportunities to work at home can provide some relief for parents trying to juggle two careers and the care of young children. For example, Winett suggests that more part-time job opportunities that allow parents to work 75% time without jeopardizing promotions would permit one parent to return home in the late afternoon to spend time with preschool-age or younger children, making it unnecessary for the young child to spend 40 or more hours a week in a day care center. More flexible work hours also would permit parents to share childrearing, allowing one parent to be at home during part of the time the other worked, cutting down the expenses of child care, as well as the number of hours each week that children are in nonparental care. Although some parents have managed to work out such schedules, such as those who do shift work or work in certain types of positions, flexible work hours are rarely considered as an option that may assist young families who are dealing with child-care problems. However, there is some empirical evidence to suggest that flexible work hours ease the pressures on families with young children and increase the time parents spend with children without decreasing worker productivity (Winett, 1998). Certainly more thought needs to be given to various flexible work schedules in both the public and private sectors.

MENTAL HEALTH PROGRAMS FOR PRESCHOOL CHILDREN

As noted throughout this book, there is a serious lack of appropriate mental health programs for preschool children and their families. Although funds have been allocated for various mental health screening programs for infants and young children, adequate programs are rarely available to deal with problems once they are identified. This is particularly the case for preschool-age children with behavior and adjustment problems that are not accompanied by mental retardation, severe emotional withdrawal (e.g., autism), or marked poverty and psychosocial disadvantage. Thus the working-class or middle-class family whose 3- or 4-year-old has a significant behavior problem really has few places to turn. Few workers in mental health centers are knowledgeable about the special issues that confront preschoolers and their parents. As already noted, parents are often told that the problems will be outgrown, or they are coached in the use of behavior management procedures. Comprehensive treatment programs are almost nonexistent. (See also Saxe, Cross, & Silverman, 1988, for a more general discussion of this issue and of the fact that most treatment programs are not based on our current knowledge of development or of what works.) Thus children who are too difficult to manage in a regular preschool program, who require more specialized programs, but who are not appropriate for programs for retarded or severely disturbed youngsters tend to be overlooked. There are few programs available for such children, and those that do exist often have long waiting lists. Children such as Jamie and Robbie require small classes with structured programs that help children develop prosocial behaviors such as sharing, compromising, and playing cooperatively and that also help them to control their aggressive and angry impulses. Obviously, preschool programs that cater to such children must have a small teacher-to-child ratio, and the staff must be knowledgeable about young children's development and also be trained to deal with impulsive and defiant behavior, as well as social withdrawal. However, it is unknown whether aggressive and defiant preschoolers do better when mainstreamed into programs with children who are developing normally or whether they require a highly specialized program geared only to children with problems.

In addition, a therapeutic preschool program must meet the needs of the child's family as a whole to be effective as a mental health intervention. Thus parent groups that provide both support and help with childrearing are needed. As was made clear throughout this book, often children's behavior problems occur in the context of other family problems. Therefore, a comprehensive program would need to provide individual or marital therapy when it appeared to be indicated, as well as referrals for help with other problems confronting the child or family. The literature reviewed in Chapter 7 suggested some of the ingredients that may go into a successful comprehensive program for preschoolers and their families, but no treatment-outcome studies have evaluated the effectiveness of a truly comprehensive therapeutic program for preschoolers with behavior problems. In general, programs deal with only one or two facets of a complex problem; often they are not sufficiently intense to permit an assessment of whether the approach is viable or not. Because it is well documented that relatively severe behavior problems in preschool children can have long-term developmental consequences for some children and their families, the need for early-intervention programs seems obvious. Although comprehensive treatment programs for preschoolers may seem costly in the current economic climate, the successful amelioration of problems in young children should ultimately decrease the need for mental health and educational services later on.

SUMMARY

Research and theory on young children's development and on early indicators of behavior problems were reviewed and integrated. The discussion in this chapter focused on several social policy implications of both the research and clinical findings. In particular, educational programs for parents and health care providers were discussed. The quality and availability of child care also was discussed, and the need for uniform federal day care standards and for adequate funding was emphasized as among the major problems confronting families with young children. Parental leave and flexible work schedules were also addressed as ways of helping parents with young children juggle the multiple demands of career and family, while also providing their children some needed time at home with at least one parent. Finally, the lack of comprehensive treatment programs for preschool children with significant behavior problems was noted.

Although there are a myriad of programs that serve infants and preschoolers (Shonkoff & Phillips, 2000), programs that run the gamut from nutritional supplements to educational screening and intervention, there has also been a notable lack of planning, direction, integration, or assessment of priorities and outcomes. One particular gap is in the availability of comprehensive treatment programs for preschoolers with behavior problems. Findings from several studies now converge to indicate that preschoolers with severe externalizing problems, especially those living in more dysfunctional or disrupted family environments, are at risk for persistent problems that may last into elementary school and beyond. Therefore, the need for early-intervention programs appears obvious. Programs that include educational and therapeutic work with the parents, as well as intensive, structured work with troubled children in a preschool setting, remain an ideal goal. Furthermore, a parental-leave policy and the availability of adequate child care might help to alleviate the stresses on dysfunctional families or families with difficult children and make parents more available to meet their children's needs. In other instances, stable and nurturant caregivers might buffer some young children from the impact of parental unavailability, insensitivity, or rejection. It seems obvious that the ultimate cost to society that stems from not treating such problems early far outweighs the cost of instituting appropriately targeted intervention programs when children are young.

References

Abramovitch, R., Corter, C., & Pepler, D. (1980). Observations of mixed-sex sibling dyads. *Child Development, 51,* 1268–1271.

Achenbach, T. M. (1991). *Manual for the Child Behavior Checklist/4–18 and 1991 Profile.* Burlington, VT: University of Vermont, Department of Psychiatry.

Achenbach, T. M. (1992). *Manual for the Child Behavior Checklist/2–3 and 1992 Profile.* Burlington, VT: University of Vermont, Department of Psychiatry.

Achenbach, T. M., & Edelbrock, C. (1978). The classification of child psychopathology: A review and analysis of empirical efforts. *Psychological Bulletin, 85,* 1275–1301.

Achenbach, T. M., & Edelbrock, C. (1987). *Manual for the Youth Self-Report and Profile.* Burlington, VT: University of Vermont, Department of Psychiatry.

Achenbach, T. M., McConaughy, S. H., & Howell, C. T. (1987). Child/adolescent behavioral and emotional problems: Implications of cross-informant correlations for situational specificity. *Psychological Bulletin, 101,* 213–232.

Aguilar, B., Sroufe, L. A., Egeland, B., & Carlson, E. (2000). Distinguishing the early-onset/persistent and adolescent-onset/antisocial behavior types: From birth to 16 years. *Development and Psychopathology, 12,* 109–132.

Ainsworth, M. D. S., Blehar, M., Waters, E., & Wall, S. (1978). *Patterns of attachment.* Hillsdale, NJ: Erlbaum.

Alexander, J. F., & Malouf, R. E. (1983). Intervention with children experiencing problems in personality and social development. In P. H. Mussen (Series Ed.) & E. M. Hetherington (Vol. Ed.), *Handbook of child psychology: Vol. 4. Socialization, personality, and social development* (4th ed., pp. 913–980). New York: Wiley.

American Academy of Pediatrics. (1996). *The classification of child and adolescent mental diagnoses in primary care (DSM-PC).* Elk Grove, IL: Author.

American Academy of Pediatrics. (1998). Managed care and children with special health care needs: A subject review. *Pediatrics, 102,* 657–660.

American Academy of Pediatrics. (2000). Guiding principles for managed care arrangements for the health care of newborns, infants, children, adolescents, and young adults. *Pediatrics, 105,* 132–135.

American Psychiatric Association. (1980). *Diagnostic and statistical manual of mental disorders* (3rd ed.). Washington, DC: Author.

American Psychiatric Association. (1987). *Diagnostic and statistical manual of mental disorders* (3rd ed., rev.). Washington, DC: Author.

American Psychiatric Association. (1994). *Diagnostic and statistical manual of mental disorders* (4th ed.). Washington, DC: Author.

American Public Health Association and American Academy of Pediatrics Collaborative Project. (1992). *Caring for our children—National health and safety performance standards: Guidelines for out-of-home child care programs.* Washington, DC: American Public Health Association.

Andrews, S. R., Blumenthal, J. B., Johnson, D. L., Kahn, A. J., Ferguson, C. J., Lasater, T. M., Malone, P. E., & Wallace, D. B. (1982). The skills of mothering: A study of Parent Child Development Centers. *Monographs of the Society for Research in Child Development, 47*(Serial No. 198).

Asher, S. (1983). Social competence and peer status: Recent advances and future directions. *Child Development, 54,* 1427–1434.

Axline, V. (1969). *Play therapy.* New York: Ballantine.

Barkley, R. A. (1997). *Defiant children: A clinician's manual for assessment and parent training* (2nd ed.). New York: Guilford Press.

Barkley, R. A., Fischer, M., Edelbrock, C. S., & Smallish, L. (1990). Adolescent outcome of hyperactive children diagnosed by research criteria: I. An 8-year prospective follow-up study. *Journal of the American Academy of Child and Adolescent Psychiatry, 29,* 546–557.

Barkley, R. A., Shelton, T. L., Crosswaite, C., Moorehouse, M., Fletcher, K., Barrett, S., Jenkins, L., & Metavia, L. (2000). Multi-method psycho-educational intervention for preschool children with disruptive behavior: Preliminary results at post-treatment. *Journal of Child Psychology and Psychiatry, 41,* 319–332.

Bates, J. E. (1987). Temperament in infancy. In J. Osofsky (Ed.), *Handbook of infant development* (2nd ed., pp. 1101–1149). New York: Wiley.

Bates, J. E., & Bayles, K. (1988). Attachment and the development of behavior problems. In J. Belsky & T. Nezworski (Eds.), *Clinical implications of attachment* (pp. 253–299). Hillsdale, NJ: Erlbaum.

Bates, J. E., & MacFadyen-Ketchum, S. (2000). Temperament and parent–child relations as interacting factors in children's behavioral adjustment. In V. J. Molfese & D. L. Molfese (Eds.), *Temperament and personality development across the life span* (pp. 141–176). Mahwah, NJ: Erlbaum.

Bates, J. E., Maslin, C. A., & Frankel, K. A. (1985). Attachment security, mother–child interaction, and temperament as predictors of behavior problem ratings at age three years. In I. Bretherton & E. Waters (Eds.), Growing points in attachment theory and research. *Monographs of the Society for Research in Child Development, 50*(Serial No. 209), 167–193.

Bates, J. E., Pettit, G. S., Dodge, K. A., & Ridge, B. (1998). Interaction of temperamental resistance to control and restrictive parenting in the development of externalizing behavior. *Developmental Psychology, 34,* 982–995.

Bates, J. E., Viken, R. J., Alexander, D. B., Beyers, J., & Stockton, L. (2002). Sleep and adjustment in preschool children: Sleep diary reports by mothers relate to behavior reports by teachers. *Child Development, 73,* 62–74.

Baumrind, D. (1967). Child care practices anteceding three patterns of preschool behavior. *Genetic Psychology Monographs, 75,* 43–88.

Bayley, N., & Schaefer, E. S. (1964). Correlations of maternal and child behaviors with the development of mental abilities: Data from the Berkeley Growth Study. *Monographs of the Society for Research in Child Development, 29*(Serial No. 97).

Bell, R. Q. (1968). A reinterpretation of the direction of effects in studies of socialization. *Psychological Review, 75,* 81–95.

Belsky, J. (1984). The determinants of parenting: A process model. *Child Development,* 55, 83–96.

Belsky, J. (1988). The "effects" of infant day care reconsidered. *Early Childhood Research Quarterly,* 3, 235–272.

Belsky, J. (2001). Developmental risks (still) associated with early child care. *Journal of Child Psychology and Psychiatry,* 42, 845–859.

Belsky, J., Campbell, S., Cohn, J. F., & Moore, G. (1996). Instability of infant–parent attachment security. *Developmental Psychology,* 32, 921–924.

Belsky, J., Hsieh, K., & Crnic, K. (1998). Mothering, fathering, and infant negativity as antecedents of boys' externalizing problems and inhibition at age 3 years: Differential susceptibility to rearing experience? *Development and Psychopathology,* 10, 301–319.

Belsky, J., & Rovine, M. (1988). Nonmaternal care in the first year of life and security of infant–parent attachment. *Child Development,* 59, 157–168.

Belsky, J., Rovine, M., & Fish, M. (1989). The developing family system. In M. Gunnar & E. Thelen (Eds.), *Minnesota Symposium on Child Psychology* (Vol. 22, pp. 119–166). Hillsdale, NJ: Erlbaum.

Belsky, J., Rovine, M., & Taylor, D. G. (1984). The Pennsylvania Infant and Family Development Project III: The origins of individual differences in infant–mother attachment: Maternal and infant contributions. *Child Development,* 55, 718–728.

Belsky, J., Woodworth, S., & Crnic, K. (1996). Trouble in the second year: Three questions about family interaction. *Child Development,* 67, 556–568.

Bennett, K. J., Lipman, E. L., Racine, Y. C., & Offord, D. R. (1998). Do measures of externalizing behavior in normal populations predict later outcome?: Implications for targeted interventions to prevent conduct disorder. *Journal of Child Psychology and Psychiatry,* 39, 1059–1070.

Bergsten, M. C., & Steketee, M. W. (1999). *The state of the child in Pennsylvania: A 1999 guide to child well-being in Pennsylvania.* Harrisburg, PA: Pennsylvania Kids Count Partnership.

Biederman, J., Faraone, S., Milberger, S., Curtis, S., Chen, L., Marrs, A., Ouelette, C., Moore, P., & Spencer, T. (1996). Predictors of persistence and remission of ADHD into adolescence: Results from a four-year prospective follow-up. *Journal of the American Academy of Child and Adolescent Psychiatry,* 35, 343–351.

Bjorklund, D. F. (2000). *Children's thinking: Developmental function and individual differences.* Belmont, CA: Wadsworth.

Block, J. H., & Block, J. (1980). The role of ego control and ego resiliency in the organization of behavior. In W. A. Collins (Ed.), *Minnesota Symposium on Child Psychology: Development of cognition, affect, and social relations* (Vol. 13, pp. 39–102). Hillsdale, NJ: Erlbaum.

Block, J. H., Block, J., & Morrison, A. (1981). Parental agreement–disagreement on childrearing orientations and gender-related personality correlates in children. *Child Development,* 52, 965–974.

Booth, C. L., Rose-Krasnor, L., & Rubin, K. H. (1991). Relating preschoolers' social competence and their mothers' parenting behaviors to early attachment security and high risk status. *Journal of Personal and Social Relationships,* 8, 363–382.

Bornstein, M. H., & Sigman, M. D. (1986). Continuity in mental development from infancy. *Child Development,* 57, 251–274.

Bowlby, J. S. (1969). *Attachment and loss: Vol. I. Attachment.* New York: Basic Books.

Bowlby, J. S. (1973). *Attachment and loss: Vol. II. Separation.* New York: Basic Books.

Brendgen, M., Vitaro, F., Bukowski, W. M., Doyle, A. B., & Markiewicz, D. (2001). Developmental profiles of peer social preference over the course of elementary school: Associations with trajectories of internalizing behavior. *Developmental Psychology,* 37, 308–320.

Brestan, E. V., & Eyberg, S. M. (1998). Effective psychosocial treatments of conduct-disordered children and adolescents: 29 years, 82 studies, and 5,272 kids. *Journal of Clinical Child Psychology,* 27, 180–189.

Bretherton, I. (1985). Attachment theory: Retrospect and prospect. In I. Bretherton & E. Waters (Eds.), Growing points in attachment theory and research. *Monographs of the Society for Research in Child Development,* 50(Serial No. 209), 3–35.

Brim, O., & Kagan, J. (1980). *Constancy and change in human development.* Cambridge, MA: Harvard University Press.

Brody, G. H., & Forehand, R. (1985). The efficacy of parent training with maritally distressed and nondistressed mothers: A multimethod assessment. *Behaviour Research and Therapy,* 23, 291–296.

Brody, G. H., Stoneman, Z., & Burke, M. (1987a). Child temperaments, maternal differential behavior, and sibling relationships. *Developmental Psychology,* 23, 354–362.

Brody, G. H., Stoneman, Z., & Burke, M. (1987b). Family system and individual child correlates of sibling behavior. *American Journal of Orthopsychiatry,* 57, 561–569.

Bronfenbrenner, U. (1986). Ecology of the family as a context for human development: Research perspectives. *Developmental Psychology,* 22 ,723–741.

Brown, A. L., Bransford, J. D., Ferrara, R. A., & Campione, J. C. (1983). Learning, remembering, and understanding. In P. H. Mussen (Series Ed.) & J. H. Flavell & E. M. Markman (Vol. Eds.), *Handbook of child psychology: Vol. 3. Cognitive development* (4th ed., pp. 77–166). New York: Wiley.

Brown, G. W., & Harris, T. (1980). *Social origins of depression.* London: Tavistock.

Brownell, C. A. (1986). Convergent developments: Cognitive-developmental correlates of growth in infant-toddler peer skills. *Child Development,* 57, 275–286.

Brownell, C. A. (1988). Combinatorial skills: Converging developments over the second year. *Child Development,* 59, 675–685.

Buss, A., & Plomin, R. (1975). *A temperament theory of personality development.* New York: Wiley.

Buss, D. M., Block, J. H., & Block, J. (1980). Preschool activity level: Personality correlates and developmental implications. *Child Development,* 51, 401–408.

Cairns, R. B., Cairns, B. D., & Neckerman, H. J. (1989). Early school dropout: Configurations and determinants. *Child Development,* 60, 1437–1452.

Calkins, S. (1994). Origins and outcomes of individual differences in emotion regulation. In N. A. Fox (Ed.), The development of emotion regulation. *Monographs of the Society for Research in Child Development,* 59(2–3, Serial No. 240), 53–72.

Campbell, F. A., Pungello, E. P., Miller-Johnson, S., Burchinal, M., & Ramey, C.T. (2001). The development of cognitive and academic abilities: Growth curves from an early childhood educational experiment. *Developmental Psychology,* 37, 231–242.

Campbell, F. A., & Ramey, C. T. (1994). Effects of early intervention on intellectual and academic achievement: A follow-up study of children from low-income families. *Child Development,* 51, 684–698.

Campbell, S. B. (1985). Hyperactivity in preschoolers: Correlates and prognostic implications. *Clinical Psychology Review,* 5, 502–524.

Campbell, S. B. (1986). Developmental issues. In R. Gittelman (Ed.), *Anxiety disorders of childhood* (pp. 24–57). New York: Guilford Press.

Campbell, S. B. (1987). Changes in symptoms over time in young children seen as hard-to-manage preschoolers. *Journal of Child Psychology and Psychiatry,* 28, 835–845.

Campbell, S. B. (1990). Socialization and social development of hyperactive (ADD) children. In M. Lewis & S. Miller (Eds.), *Handbook of developmental psychopathology* (pp. 77–92). New York: Plenum Press.

Campbell, S. B. (1991). Longitudinal studies of active and aggressive preschoolers: Individual differences in early behavior and in outcome. In D. Cicchetti & S. Toth (Eds.), *The Rochester Symposium on Developmental Psychopathology: Vol. 2. Internalizing and externalizing expressions of dysfunction* (pp. 57–90). Hillsdale, NJ: Erlbaum.

Campbell, S. B. (1994). Hard-to-manage preschool boys: Externalizing behavior, social competence, and family context at two-year follow-up. *Journal of Abnormal Child Psychology, 22,* 147–166.

Campbell, S. B. (1995). Behavior problems in preschool children: A review of recent research. *Journal of Child Psychology and Psychiatry, 36,* 113–149.

Campbell, S. B. (1997). Behavior problems in preschool children: Developmental and family issues. In T. Ollendick & R. Prinz (Eds.), *Advances in clinical child psychology* (Vol. 19, pp. 1–26). New York: Plenum Press.

Campbell, S. B., & Breaux, A. M. (1983). Maternal ratings of activity level and symptomatic behavior in a nonclinical sample of young children. *Journal of Pediatric Psychology, 8,* 73–82.

Campbell, S. B., Breaux, A. M., Ewing, L. J., & Szumowski, E. K. (1984). A one-year follow-up of parent-identified behavior problem toddlers. *Journal of the American Academy of Child Psychiatry, 23,* 243–249.

Campbell, S. B., Breaux, A. M., Ewing, L. J., & Szumowski, E. K. (1986). Correlates and predictors of hyperactivity and aggression: A longitudinal study of parent-referred problem preschoolers. *Journal of Abnormal Child Psychology, 14,* 217–234.

Campbell, S. B., Breaux, A. M., Ewing, L. J., Szumowski, E. K., & Pierce, E. W. (1986). Parent-referred problem preschoolers: Mother–child interaction during play at intake and one-year follow-up. *Journal of Abnormal Child Psychology, 14,* 425–440.

Campbell, S. B., Brownell, C. A., Hungerford, A., Spieker, S., Mohan, R., & Blessing, J. S. (2001). *The course of maternal depressive symptoms and maternal sensitivity as predictors of preschool attachment security at 36 months.* Manuscript submitted for publication.

Campbell, S. B., & Cluss, P. (1982). Peer relations in young children with behavior problems. In H. Ross & K. Rubin (Eds.), *Peer relationships and social skills in childhood* (pp. 323–352). New York: Springer-Verlag.

Campbell, S. B., & Cohn, J. F. (1997). The timing and chronicity of postpartum depression. In L. Murray & P. J. Cooper (Eds.), *Postpartum depression and child development* (pp. 165–197). New York: Guilford Press.

Campbell, S. B., Cohn, J. F., & Meyers, T. (1995). Depression in first-time mothers: Mother–infant interaction and depression chronicity. *Developmental Psychology, 31,* 349–357.

Campbell, S. B., Ewing, L. J., Breaux, A. M., & Szumowski, E. K. (1986). Behavior problem toddlers: Follow-up status at school entry. *Journal of Child Psychology and Psychiatry, 27,* 237–241.

Campbell, S. B., March, C., Pierce, E., & Ewing, L. J. (1991). Hard-to-manage preschool boys: Family context and stability of externalizing behavior. *Journal of Abnormal Child Psychology, 19,* 301–318.

Campbell, S. B., Pierce, E. W., March, C. L., Ewing, L. J., & Szumowski, E. K. (1994). Hard-to-manage preschool boys: Symptomatic behavior across contexts and time. *Child Development, 65,* 836–851.

Campbell, S. B., Pierce, E. W., Moore, G., Marakovitz, S., & Newby, K. (1996). Boys' externalizing problems at elementary school: Pathways from early behavior problems, maternal control, and family stress. *Development and Psychopathology, 8*, 701–720.

Campbell, S. B., Shaw, D. S. , & Gilliom, M. (2000). Early externalizing behavior problems: Toddlers and preschoolers at risk for later maladjustment. *Development and Psychopathology, 12*, 467–488.

Campbell, S. B., Szumowski, E. K., Ewing, L. J., Gluck, D. S., & Breaux, A. M. (1982). A multidimensional assessment of parent-identified behavior problem toddlers. *Journal of Abnormal Child Psychology, 10*, 569–591.

Campos, J. J., Barrett, K. C., Lamb, M. E., Goldsmith, H. H., & Stenberg, C. (1983). Socioemotional development. In P. H. Mussen (Series Ed.) & H. H. Haith & J. J. Campos (Eds.), *Handbook of child psychology: Vol. 2. Infancy and developmental psychobiology* (4th ed., pp. 783–916). New York: Wiley.

Cantwell, D., Baker, L., & Mattison, R. (1979). The prevalence of psychiatric disorder in children with speech and language disorders: An epidemiological study. *Journal of the American Academy of Child Psychiatry, 18*, 450–461.

Carlson, E., & Sroufe, L. A. (1995). Contribution of attachment theory to developmental psychopathology. In D. Cicchetti & D. Cohen (Eds.), *Developmental psychopathology: Vol. 1. Theory and methods* (pp. 581–617). New York: Wiley.

Caspi, A., Henry, B., McGee, R., Moffit, T., & Silva, P. (1995). Temperamental origins of child and adolescent behavior problems: From ages three to fifteen. *Child Development, 66*, 887–895.

Cassidy, J. (1986). The ability to negotiate the environment: An aspect of infant competence as related to quality of attachment. *Child Development, 57*, 331–337.

Cicchetti, D., & Cohen, D. J. (1995). Perspectives on developmental psychopathology. In D. Cicchetti & D. J. Cohen (Eds.), *Developmental psychopathology: Vol. 1. Theory and methods* (pp. 3–20). New York: Wiley.

Cicchetti, D., Cummings, E. M., Greenberg, M. T., & Marvin, R. S. (1990). An organizational perspective on attachment beyond infancy: Implications for theory, research, and measurement. In M. T. Greenberg, D. Cicchetti, & E. M. Cummings (Eds.), *Attachment in the preschool years: Theory, research, and intervention* (pp. 3–50). Chicago: University of Chicago Press.

Cicchetti, D., & Rogosch, F. (1996). Equifinality and multifinality in developmental psychopathology. *Development and Psychopathology, 8*, 597–600.

Cicchetti, D., Rogosch, F. A., & Toth, S. L. (1998). Maternal depressive disorder and contextual risk: Contributions to the development of attachment insecurity and behavior problems in toddlerhood. *Development and Psychopathology, 10*, 283–300.

Cicchetti, D., Rogosch, F. A., & Toth, S. L. (2000). The efficacy of toddler–parent psychotherapy for fostering cognitive development in offspring of depressed mothers. *Journal of Abnormal Child Psychology, 28*, 135–148.

Clark, E. (1983). Meanings and concepts. In P. H. Mussen (Series Ed.) & J. H. Flavell & E. M. Markman (Vol. Eds.), *Handbook of child psychology: Vol. 3. Cognitive development* (4th ed., pp. 787–840). New York: Wiley.

Clark, R., Hyde, J. S., Essex, M. J., & Klein, M. H. (1997). Length of maternity leave and quality of mother–infant interactions. *Child Development, 68*, 364–383.

Clarke-Stewart, K. A. (1989). Infant day care: Maligned or malignant? *American Psychologist, 44*, 266–273.

Cochran, M., & Brassard, J. (1979). Child development and personal social networks. *Child Development, 50*, 601–616.

Cohen, N. J., Davine, M., & Meloche-Kelly, M. (1989). The prevalence of unsuspected language disorders in a child psychiatric population. *Journal of the American Academy of Child and Adolescent Psychiatry, 28,* 107–111.

Cohen, N. J., Lojkasek, M., Muir, E., Muir, R., & Parker, C. (2002). Six-month follow-up of two mother–infant psychotherapies: Convergence of therapeutic outcomes. *Infant Mental Health Journal, 23.*

Cohen, N. J., Muir, E., Lojkasek, M., Muir, R., Parker, C., Barwick, M., & Brown, M. (1999). Watch, Wait, and Wonder: Testing the effectiveness of a new approach to mother–infant psychotherapy. *Infant Mental Health Journal, 20,* 429–451.

Cohen, N. J., Sullivan, J., Minde, K., Novak, C., & Helwig, C. (1981). The relative effectiveness of methlyphenidate and cognitive behavior modification in the treatment of kindergarten-aged hyperactive children. *Journal of Abnormal Child Psychology, 9,* 43–54.

Coie, J. D., & Dodge, K. A. (1998). Aggression and antisocial behavior. In W. Damon (Series Ed.) & N. Eisenberg (Vol. Ed.), *Handbook of child psychology: Vol. 3. Social, emotional, and personality development* (5th ed., pp. 779–862). New York: Wiley.

Coie, J. D., Watt, N. F., West, S. G., Hawkins, J. D., Asarnow, J. R., Markman, H. J., Ramey, S. L., Shure, M. B., & Long, B. (1993). The science of prevention: A conceptual framework and some directions for a national research program. *American Psychologist, 48,* 1013–1022.

Coleman, J., Wolkind, S., & Ashley, L. (1977). Symptoms of behavior disturbance and adjustment to school. *Journal of Child Psychology and Psychiatry, 18,* 201–210.

Collins, W. A., Maccoby, E., Steinberg, L., Hetherington, E. M., & Bornstein, M. (2000). Contemporary research on parenting: The case for nature and nurture. *American Psychologist, 55,* 218–232.

Conduct Problems Prevention Research Group. (1992). A developmental and clinical model for the prevention of conduct disorder: The Fast Track Program. *Development and Psychopathology, 4,* 509–527.

Conduct Problems Prevention Research Group. (1999). Initial impact of the Fast Track Prevention Trial for conduct problems: I. The high risk sample. *Journal of Consulting and Clinical Psychology, 67,* 631–647.

Conduct Problems Prevention Research Group. (2002). The implementation of the Fast Track Program: An example of a large-scale prevention science efficacy trial. *Journal of Abnormal Child Psychology, 30,* 1–18.

Cooper, P. J., & Murray, L. (1997). The impact of psychological treatments of postpartum depression on maternal mood and infant development. In L. Murray & P. J. Cooper (Eds.), *Postpartum depression and child development* (pp. 201–220). New York: Guilford Press.

Corsaro, W. A. (1981). Friendship in the nursery school: Social organization in a peer environment. In J. Gottman & S. Asher (Eds.), *The development of children's friendships* (pp. 207–241). New York: Cambridge University Press.

Corter, C., Abramovitch, R., & Pepler, D. (1983). The role of the mother in sibling interaction. *Child Development, 54,* 1599–1605.

Cowan, P. A. (1997). Beyond meta-analysis: A plea for a family systems view of attachment. *Child Development, 68,* 600–603.

Cowan, P. A., & Cowan, C. P. (1992). *When partners become parents.* New York: Basic Books.

Cowan, P. A., Powell, D., & Cowan, C. P. (1998). Parenting interventions: A family systems perspective. In W. Damon (Series Ed.) & I. Sigel & A. K. Renninger (Vol.

Eds.), *Handbook of child psychology: Vol. 4. Child psychology in practice* (5th ed., pp. 3–72). New York: Wiley.

Coyle, J. T. (2000). Psychotropic drug use in very young children. *Journal of the American Medical Association, 283,* 1021–1023.

Crick, N. R., & Grotpeter, J. (1995). Relational aggression, aggression, and social psychological adjustment. *Child Development, 66,* 313–322.

Crockenberg, S. B. (1981). Infant irritability, mother responsiveness, and social support influences on the security of infant–mother attachment. *Child Development, 52,* 857–865.

Crockenberg, S. B., & Litman, C. (1990). Autonomy as competence in 2-year-olds: Maternal correlates of child defiance, compliance and self-assertion. *Developmental Psychology, 26,* 961–971.

Crowther, J. K., Bond, L. A., & Rolf, J. E. (1981). The incidence, prevalence, and severity of behavior disorders among preschool-aged children in day care. *Journal of Abnormal Child Psychology, 9,* 23–42.

Crnic, K. A., Greenberg, M. T., Ragozin, A. S., Robinson, N. M., & Basham, R. B. (1983). Effects of stress and social support on mothers and preterm and full-term infants. *Child Development, 54,* 209–217.

Cummings, E. M., & Davies, P. T. (1999). Depressed parents and family functioning: Interpersonal effects and children's functioning and development. In T. Joiner & J. C. Coyne (Eds.), *The interactional nature of depression: Advances in interpersonal approaches* (pp. 299–327). Washington, DC: American Psychological Association.

Cummings, E. M., Davies, P. T., & Campbell, S. B. (2000). *Developmental psychopathology and family process.* New York: Guilford Press.

Cummings, E. M., Zahn-Waxler, C., & Radke-Yarrow, M. (1981). Young children's responses to expressions of anger and affection by others in the family. *Child Development, 52,* 1274–1282.

Cummings, E. M., Zahn-Waxler, C., & Radke-Yarrow, M. (1984). Developmental changes in children's reactions to anger in the home. *Journal of Child Psychology and Psychiatry, 25,* 63–74.

Cunningham, C. E., Bremner, R., & Boyle, M. (1995). Large group community-based parenting programs for families of preschoolers at risk for disruptive behaviour disorders: Utilization, cost effectiveness, and outcome. *Journal of Child Psychology and Psychiatry, 36,* 1141–1160.

Dadds, M. R., Schwartz, S., & Sanders, M. R. (1987). Marital discord and treatment outcome in behavioral treatment of child behavior problems. *Journal of Consulting and Clinical Psychology, 55,* 396–403.

Daehler, M. W., & Greco, C. (1985). Memory in very young children. In M. Pressley & C. J. Brainerd (Eds.), *Cognitive learning and memory in children* (pp. 49–80). New York: Springer-Verlag.

Damon, W. (1977). *The social world of the child.* San Francisco: Jossey-Bass.

Davies, P. T., & Cummings, E. M. (1994). Marital conflict and child adjustment: An emotional security hypothesis. *Psychological Bulletin, 116,* 387–411.

Davies, P. T., & Cummings, E. M. (1998). Exploring children's emotional security as a mediator of the link between marital relations and child adjustment. *Child Development, 69,* 124–139.

Deater-Deckard, K., Dodge, K. A., Bates, J. E., & Pettit, G. S. (1996). Physical discipline among African American and European American mothers: Links to children's externalizing behavior. *Developmental Psychology, 32,* 1065–1072.

DeKlyen, M., Speltz, M. L., & Greenberg, M. T. (1998). Fathering and early onset conduct problems: Positive and negative parenting, father–son attachment, and marital conflict. *Clinical Child and Family Psychology Review, 1,* 3–22.

DeLoache, J. S., Cassidy, D. J., & Brown, A. L. (1985). Precursors of mnemonic strategies in very young children. *Child Development, 56,* 125–137.

DeMulder, E. K., & Radke-Yarrow, M. (1991). Attachment with affectively ill and well mothers: Concurrent behavioral correlates. *Development and Psychopathology, 3,* 227–242.

Denham, S., & Auerbach, S. (1995). *Mother–child dialogue about emotions and preschoolers' emotional competence.* Paper presented at the biennial meeting of the Society for Research in Child Development, Indianapolis, IN.

De Wolff, M., & Van IJzendoorn, M. H. (1997). Sensitivity and attachment: A meta-analysis of parental antecedents of infant attachment. *Child Development, 68,* 571–591.

Dishion, T. J., Andrews, D. W., & Crosby, L. (1995). Antisocial boys and their friends in early adolescence: Relationship characteristics, quality, and interactional process. *Child Development, 66,* 139–151.

Dodge, K. A. (1983). Behavioral antecedents of peer social status. *Child Development, 54,* 1386–1399.

Dodge, K. A., Pettit, G. S., & Bates, J. E. (1994). Effects of physical maltreatment on the development of peer relations. *Development and Psychopathology, 6,* 43–55.

Dumas, J. E., Prinz, R. J., Smith, E. P., & Laughlin, J. (1999). The EARLY ALLIANCE prevention trial: An integrated set of interventions to promote competence and reduce risk for conduct disorder, substance abuse, and school failure. *Clinical Child and Family Psychology Review, 2,* 37–53.

Dumas J. E., & Wahler, R. G. (1985). Indiscriminate mothering as a contextual factor in aggressive-oppositional child behavior: "Damned if you do and damned if you don't." *Journal of Abnormal Child Psychology, 13,* 1–18.

Duncan, G., & Brooks-Gunn, J. (2000). Family poverty, welfare reform, and child development. *Child Development, 71,* 188–196.

Dunn, J. (1983). Sibling relationships in early childhood. *Child Development, 54,* 787–811.

Dunn, J. (1985). *Siblings.* Cambridge, MA: Harvard University Press.

Dunn, J., Bretherton, I., & Munn, P. (1987). Conversations about feeling states between mothers and their young children. *Developmental Psychology, 23,* 132–139.

Dunn, J., Brown, J., & Beardsall, L. (1991). Family talk about emotions, and children's later understanding of other's emotions. *Developmental Psychology, 27,* 448–455.

Dunn, J., Brown, J., & Maguire, M. (1995). The development of children's moral sensibility: Individual differences and emotion understanding. *Developmental Psychology, 31,* 649–659.

Dunn, J., & Kendrick, C. (1981). Social behavior of young siblings in the family context: Differences between same-sex and different-sex dyads. *Child Development, 52,* 1265–1273.

Dunn, J., & Kendrick, C. (1982). *Siblings: Love, envy, and understanding.* Cambridge, MA: Harvard University Press.

Dunn, J., & Munn, P. (1985). Becoming a family member: Family conflict and the development of social understanding in the second year. *Child Development, 56,* 480–492.

Dunn, J., & Munn, P. (1986). Sibling quarrels and maternal intervention: Individual differences in understanding and aggression. *Journal of Child Psychology and Psychiatry, 27,* 583–595.

Dunn, J., Plomin, R., & Nettles, M. (1985). Consistency of mothers' behavior toward infant siblings. *Developmental Psychology, 21,* 1188–1195.

Earls, F. (1980). The prevalence of behavior problems in 3-year-old children. *Archives of General Psychiatry, 37,* 1153–1159.

Edelbrock, C. S., Costello, A. J., Dulcan, M. K., Kalas, N. C., & Conover, N. C. (1985). Age differences in the reliability of the psychiatric interview of the child. *Child Development, 56,* 265–275.

Eisenberg, N., & Fabes, R. (1998). Prosocial development. In W. Damon (Series Ed.) & N. Eisenberg (Vol. Ed.), *Handbook of child psychology: Vol. 3. Social, emotional, and personality development* (5th ed., pp. 701–778). New York: Wiley.

Emery, R.E. (1999). *Marriage, divorce, and children's adjustment* (2nd ed.). Thousand Oaks, CA: Sage.

Erikson, E. (1963). *Childhood and society.* New York: Norton.

Eron, L. D., & Huesmann, L. R. (1990). The stability of aggressive behavior—even unto the third generation. In M. Lewis & S. Miller (Eds.), *Handbook of developmental psychopathology* (pp. 147–156). New York: Plenum Press.

Eyberg, S. M. (1987, August). *Assessing therapy outcomes with preschool children: Progress and problems.* Presidential address to the Section on Clinical Child Psychology of the American Psychological Association, New York.

Eyberg, S. M., Boggs, S., & Algina, J. (1995). Parent–child interaction therapy: A psychosocial model for the treatment of young children with conduct problem behavior and their families. *Psychopharmacology Bulletin, 31,* 83–91.

Eyberg, S. M., Schuhmann, E., & Rey, J. (1998). Psychosocial treatment research with children and adolescents: Developmental issues. *Journal of Abnormal Child Psychology, 26,* 71–81.

Fabes, R. A., Eisenberg, N., Jones, S., Smith, M., Guthrie, I., Poulin, R., Shepard, S., & Friedman, J. (1999). Regulation, emotionality, and preschoolers' socially competent peer interactions. *Child Development, 55,* 432–442.

Feldman, R., Greenbaum, C. W., & Yirimiya, N. (1999). Mother–infant affect synchrony as an antecedent of the emergence of self-control. *Developmental Psychology, 35,* 223–231.

Fergusson, D. M., & Horwood, L. J. (1999). Prospective childhood predictors of deviant peer affiliations in adolescence. *Journal of Child Psychology and Psychiatry, 40,* 581–593.

Field, T. M. (1992). Infants of depressed mothers. *Development and Psychopathology, 4,* 49–66.

Field, T. M., & Reite, M. (1984). Children's responses to separation from mother during the birth of another child. *Child Development, 55,* 1308–1316.

Fincham, F., & Osborn, L. N. (1993). Marital conflict and children: Retrospect and prospect. *Clinical Psychology Review, 13,* 75–88.

Fischer, M. E., Barkley, R. A., Edelbrock, C. S., & Smallish, L. (1990). Adolescent outcome of hyperactive children diagnosed by research criteria: II. Academic, attentional, and neuropsychological status. *Journal of Consulting and Clinical Psychology, 58,* 580–588.

Fischer, M. E., Rolf, J. E., Hasazi, J. E., & Cummings, L. (1984). Follow-up of a preschool epidemiological sample: Cross-age continuities and predictions of later adjustment with internalizing and externalizing dimensions of behavior. *Child Development, 55,* 137–150.

Flavell, J. (1963). *The developmental psychology of Jean Piaget.* Princeton, NJ: Van Nostrand.

Fraiberg, S. (Ed.). (1980). *Clinical studies in infant mental health*. New York: Basic Books.

Framo, J. (1975). Personal reflections of a therapist. *Journal of Marriage and Family Counseling, 1*, 15–28.

Frank, M., & Zigler, E. F. (1996). Family leave: A developmental perspective. In E. F. Zigler, S. L. Kagan, & N. W. Hall (Eds), *Children, families, and government: Preparing for the twenty-first century* (pp. 117–131). New York: Cambridge University Press.

Frankel, K. A., & Harmon, R. J. (1996). Depressed mothers: They don't always look as bad as they feel. *Journal of the American Academy of Child and Adolescent Psychiatry, 35*, 289–298.

Frodi, A., Bridges, L., & Grolnick, W. (1985). Correlates of mastery related behavior: A short-term longitudinal study of infants in their second year. *Child Development, 56*, 1291–1298.

Garcia, M. M., Shaw, D. S., Winslow, E. B., & Yaggi, K. (2000). Destructive sibling conflict and the development of conduct problems in young boys. *Developmental Psychology, 36*, 44–53.

Gardner, F. E. (1987). Positive interaction between mothers and conduct-problem children: Is there training for harmony as well as fighting? *Journal of Abnormal Child Psychology, 15*, 283–293.

Gardner, F. E. (1989). Inconsistent parenting: Is there evidence for a link with children's conduct problems? *Journal of Abnormal Child Psychology, 17*, 223–233.

Gardner, F. E., Sonuga-Barke, E., & Sayal, K. (1999). Parents anticipating misbehavior: An observational study of strategies parents use to prevent conflict with behavior problem children. *Journal of Child Psychology and Psychiatry, 40*, 1185–1196.

Garvey, C. (1977). *Play*. Cambridge, MA: Harvard University Press.

Garvey, C. (1990) *Play* (2nd ed.). Cambridge, MA: Harvard University Press.

Gelfand, D., Teti, D. M., Seiner, S. A., & Jameson, P. B. (1996). Helping mothers fight depression: Evaluation of a home-based intervention program for depressed mothers and their infants. *Journal of Clinical Child Psychology, 25*, 406–422.

Gittelman, R., Mannuzza, S., Shenker, R., & Bonagura, N. (1985). Hyperactive boys almost grown up: Psychiatric status. *Archives of General Psychiatry, 42*, 937–947.

Goldsmith, H. H., & Campos, J. J. (1982). Toward a theory of infant temperament. In R. N. Emde & R. J. Harmon (Eds.), *The development of attachment and affiliative systems* (pp. 161–193). New York: Plenum Press.

Goodman, S. H., & Brumley, H. L. (1990). Schizophrenic and depressed mothers: Relational deficits in parenting. *Developmental Psychology, 26*, 31–39.

Gopnik, A., & Meltzoff, A. (1988). The development of categorization in the second year and its relation to other cognitive and linguistic developments. *Child Development, 58*, 1523–1531.

Gottman, J. M., & Parkhurst, J. T. (1980). A developmental theory of friendship and acquaintanceship processes. In W. A. Collins (Ed.), *Minnesota Symposium on Child Psychology: Vol. 13. Development of cognition, affect, and social relations* (pp. 197–254). Hillsdale, NJ: Erlbaum.

Greenberg, M. T., Lengua, L. J., Coie, J. D., & Pinderhughes, E. E.(1999). Predicting developmental outcomes at school entry using a multiple risk model: Four American communities. *Developmental Psychology, 35*, 403–417.

Greenberg, M.T., Speltz, M. L., & DeKlyen, M. (1993). The role of attachment in the development of disruptive behavior problems. *Development and Psychopathology, 5*, 191–214.

Greenberg, M. T., Speltz, M. L., DeKlyen, M., & Jones, K. (2001). Correlates of clinic referral for early conduct problems: Variable and person-oriented approaches. *Development and Psychopathology, 13,* 255–276.

Haley, J. (1976). *Problem-solving therapy.* San Francisco: Jossey-Bass.

Hall, N. W., Kagan, S. L., & Zigler, E. F. (1996). The changing nature of child and family policy: An overview. In E. F. Zigler, S.L. Kagan, & N. W. Hall (Eds.), *Children, families, and government: Preparing for the twenty-first century* (pp. 3–9). New York: Cambridge University Press.

Harnish, J. D., Dodge, K. A., Valente, E., and the Conduct Problems Prevention Research Group. (1995). Mother–child interaction quality as a partial mediator of the roles of maternal depressive symptomatology and socioeconomic status in the development of child behavior problems. *Child Development, 66,* 739–753.

Harper, L. V., & Huie, K. S. (1985). The effects of prior group experience, age, and familiarity on the quality and organization of preschoolers' social relationships. *Child Development, 56,* 704–717.

Harris, J. R. (1998). *The nurture assumption.* New York: Free Press.

Hart, C. H., DeWolf, D. M., Wozniak, P., & Burts, D. C. (1992). Maternal and paternal disciplinary styles: Relations with preschoolers' playground behavioral observations and peer status. *Child Development, 63,* 879–892.

Harter, S. (1983). Cognitive-developmental considerations in the conduct of play therapy. In C. Schaeffer & K. J. O'Connor (Eds.), *Handbook of play therapy* (pp. 95–127). New York: Wiley.

Harter, S. (1998). The development of self-representations. In W. Damon (Series Ed.) & N. Eisenberg (Vol. Ed.), *Handbook of child psychology: Vol. 3. Social, emotional, and personality development* (5th ed., pp. 553–618). New York: Wiley.

Hartup, W. W. (1983). Peer relations. In P. H. Mussen (Series Ed.) & E. M. Hetherington (Ed.), *Handbook of child psychology: Vol. 4. Socialization, personality, and social development* (pp. 103–196). New York: Wiley.

Hartup, W. W., Laursen, B., Stewart, M. A., & Eastenson, A. (1988). Conflicts and friendship relations of young children. *Child Development, 59,* 1590–1600.

Health, Education, and Welfare Federal Intra-Agency Day Care Requirements (1980). Washington, DC: U.S. Government Printing Office.

Hetherington, E. M. (1989). Coping with family transitions: Winners, losers, and survivors. *Child Development, 60,* 1–14.

Hetherington, E. M., Bridges, M., & Insabella, G. (1998). What matters? What does not?: Five perspectives on the association between marital transitions and children's adjustment. *American Psychologist, 53,* 167–184.

Hinshaw, S. P. (1994). *Attention deficits and hyperactivity in children.* Thousand Oaks, CA: Sage.

Hinshaw, S. P., & Cicchetti, D. (2000). Stigma and mental disorder: Conceptions of illness, public attitudes, personal disclosure, and social policy. *Development and Psychopathology, 12,* 555–598.

Hinshaw, S. P., Lahey, B. B., & Hart, E. (1993). Issues of taxonomy and comorbidity in the development of conduct disorder. *Development and Psychopathology, 5,* 31–49.

Hodges, K., Kline, J., Stern, L., Cytryn, L., & McKnew, D. (1982). The development of a child assessment interview for research and clinical use. *Journal of Abnormal Child Psychology, 10,* 173–189.

Howes, C. (1988). Peer interaction of young children. *Monographs of the Society for Research in Child Development, 53*(Serial No. 217), 1–77.

Howes, C., & Olenick, M. (1986). Family and child care influences on toddler's compliance. *Child Development, 57,* 202–216.

Hungerford, A., Brownell, C. A., & Campbell, S. B. (2000). Child care in infancy: An ecological perspective. In C. Zeanah (Ed.), *Handbook of infant mental health* (2nd ed., pp. 519–532). New York: Guilford Press

Hunt, J. M. (1961). *Intelligence and experience.* New York: Ronald Press.

Jacobs, F., & Davies, M. (1991, Winter). Rhetoric or reality? Child and family policy in the United States. *SRCD Social Policy Report, 5.*

Jellinek, M. S. (1999). Changes in the practice of child and adolescent psychiatry: Are our patients better served? *Journal of the American Academy of Child and Adolescent Psychiatry, 38,* 115–117.

Jenkins, S., Bax, M., & Hart, H. (1980). Behaviour problems in preschool children. *Journal of Child Psychology and Psychiatry, 21,* 5–18.

Jensen, A. (1969). How much can we boost IQ and scholastic achievement? *Harvard Educational Review, 29,* 1–23.

Jouriles, E. N., Murphy, C. M., Farris, A. M., Smith, D. A., Richters, J. E., & Waters, E. (1991). Marital adjustment, parental disagreements about child rearing, and behavior problems in boys: Increasing the specificity of the marital assessment. *Child Development, 62,* 1424–1433.

Kagan, J. (1971). *Change and continuity in infancy.* New York: Wiley.

Kagan, J. (1981). *The second year: The emergence of self-awareness.* Cambridge, MA: Harvard University Press.

Kagan, J. (1984). *The nature of the child.* New York: Basic Books.

Kagan, J. (1997). Temperament and reactions to unfamiliarity. *Child Development, 68,* 139–143.

Kagan, J., Kearsley, R. B., & Zelazo, P. R. (1978). *Infancy: Its place in human development.* Cambridge, MA: Harvard University Press.

Kagan, J., & Moss, H. (1962). *Birth to maturity.* New York: Wiley.

Kamerman, S. B. (1996). Child and family policies: An international overview. In E. F. Zigler, S. L. Kagan, & N. W. Hall (Eds.), *Children, families, and government: Preparing for the twenty-first century* (pp. 31–47). New York: Cambridge University Press.

Kamerman, S. B. (2000). Parental leave policies: An essential ingredient in early childhood education and care policies. *SRCD Social Policy Report, 15*(2).

Kaslow, N. J., & Thompson, M. P. (1998). Applying the criteria for empirically supported treatments to studies of psychosocial interventions for child and adolescent depression. *Journal of Clinical Child Psychology, 27,* 146–155.

Kazdin, A. E. (1997). A model for developing effective treatments: Progression and interplay of theory, research, and practice. *Journal of Clinical Child Psychology, 26,* 114–129.

Keenan, K., Shaw, D. S., Walsh, B., Delliquadri, E., & Giovannelli, J. (1997). DSM-III-R disorders in preschool children from low income families. *Journal of the American Academy of Child and Adolescent Psychiatry, 36,* 620–627.

Keenan, K., & Wachschlag, L. S. (2000). More than the terrible twos: The nature and severity of behavior problems in clinic-referred preschool children. *Journal of Abnormal Child Psychology, 28,* 33–46.

Keiley, M. K., Bates, J. E., Dodge, K. A., & Pettit, G. A. (2000). A cross-domain growth analysis: Externalizing and internalizing behaviors during 8 years of childhood. *Journal of Abnormal Child Psychology, 28,* 161–179.

Klein, M. (1932). *The psycho-analysis of children.* New York: Norton.

Knitzer, J., Yoshikawa, H., Cauthen, N. K., & Aber, J. L. (2000). Welfare reform, family support, and child development: Perspectives from policy analysis and developmental psychopathology. *Development and Psychopathology, 12,* 619–632.

Kochanska, G. (1993). Toward a synthesis of parental socialization and child temperament in early development of conscience. *Child Development, 64,* 325–347.

Kochanska, G. (1995). Children's temperament, mothers' discipline, and security of attachment: Multiple pathways to emerging internalization. *Child Development, 66,* 597–615.

Kochanska, G. (1997). Mutually responsive orientation between mothers and their young children: Implications for early socialization. *Child Development, 68,* 94–112.

Kohn, M. (1977). *Social competence, symptoms, and underachievement in childhood: A longitudinal perspective.* Washington, DC: Winston.

Kontos, S., Howes, C., Shinn, M., & Galinsky, E. (1995). *Quality in family child care and in relative care.* New York: Columbia University, Teachers College Press.

Koot, H. M. (1993). *Problem behavior in Dutch preschoolers.* Rotterdam: Erasmus University.

Koot, H. M., Van Den Oord, E. J., Verhulst, F., & Boomsma, D. I. (1997). Behavioral and emotional problems in young preschoolers: Testing the validity of the Child Behavior Checklist/2–3. *Journal of Abnormal Child Psychology, 25,* 183–196.

Kopp, C. B. (1982). Antecedents of self-regulation: A developmental perspective. *Developmental Psychology, 18,* 199–214.

Kopp, C. B. (1989). Regulation of distress and negative emotions: A developmental view. *Developmental Psychology, 25,* 343–354.

Korner, A. F., Zeanah, C. H., Linden, J., Berkowitz, R. I., Kraemer, H. C., & Agras, W. S. (1985). The relation between neonatal and later activity and temperament. *Child Development, 56,* 38–42.

Kovacs, M., & Paulauskas, S. (1986). The traditional psychotherapies. In H. C. Quay & J. S. Werry (Eds.), *Psychopathological disorders of childhood* (3rd ed., pp. 496–522). New York: Wiley.

Kramer, L., Perozynski, L. A., & Chung, T. (1999). Parental responses to sibling conflict: The effects of development and gender. *Child Development, 70,* 1401–1414.

Kuczynski, L., Radke-Yarrow, M., Kochanska, G., & Girnius-Brown, O. (1987). A developmental interpretation of young children's noncompliance. *Developmental Psychology, 23,* 799–806.

Ladd, G. W., & Burgess, K. B. (1999). Charting the relationship trajectories of aggressive, withdrawn, and aggressive/withdrawn children during early grade school. *Child Development, 70,* 910–929.

Ladd, G. W., & Price, J. M. (1987). Predicting children's social and school adjustment following the transition from preschool to kindergarten. *Child Development, 58,* 1168–1189.

Lahey, B. B., Pelham, W. E., Stein, M. A., Loney, J., Trapani, C., Nugent, K., Kipp, H., Schmidt, E., Lee, S., Cales, M., Gold, E., Hartung, C. M., Willcutt, E., & Baumann, B. (1998). Validity of DSM-IV Attention Deficit/Hyperactivity Disorder for young children. *Journal of the American Academy of Child and Adolescent Psychiatry, 37,* 695–702.

Lahey, B. B., Waldman, I. D., & McBurnett, K. (1999). The development of antisocial behavior: An integrative causal model. *Journal of Child Psychology and Psychiatry, 39,* 669–682.

Lamb, M. E. (1987a). Predictive implications of individual differences in attachment. *Journal of Consulting and Clinical Psychology, 55,* 817–824.

Lamb, M. E. (1987b). *The father's role: Cross-cultural perspectives.* Hillsdale, NJ: Erlbaum.

Lamb, M. E. (1998). Nonparental child care: Context, quality, correlates, and consequences. In W. Damon (Series Ed.) & I. Sigel & A. K. Renninger (Vol. Eds.), *Handbook of child psychology: Vol. 4. Child psychology in practice* (5th ed., pp. 73–133). New York: Wiley.

Lavigne, J. V., Arend, R., Rosenbaum, D., Binns, H., Christoffel, K. K., & Gibbons, R.D. (1998a). Psychiatric disorders with onset in the preschool years: I. Stability of diagnoses. *Journal of the American Academy of Child and Adolescent Psychiatry, 37,* 1246–1254.

Lavigne, J. V., Arend, R., Rosenbaum, D., Binns, H., Christoffel, K. K., & Gibbons, R. D. (1998b). Psychiatric disorders with onset in the preschool years: II. Correlates and predictors of stable case status. *Journal of the American Academy of Child and Adolescent Psychiatry, 37,* 1255–1261.

Lavigne, J. V., Arend, R., Rosenbaum, D., Smith, A., Weissbluth, M., Binns, H. J., & Christoffel, K. K. (1999). Sleep and behavior problems among preschoolers. *Journal of Developmental and Behavioral Pediatrics, 20,* 164–169.

Lavigne, J. V., Gibbons, R. D., Christoffel, K. K., Arend, R., Rosenbaum, D., Binns, H., Dawson, N., Sobel, H., & Isaacs, C. (1996). Prevalence rates and correlates of psychiatric disorders among preschool children. *Journal of the American Academy of Child and Adolescent Psychiatry, 35,* 204–214.

Lazar, I., & Darlington, R. (1982). Lasting effects of early education: A report from the consortium for longitudinal studies. *Monographs of the Society for Research in Child Development, 47*(Serial No. 1195).

Leach, G. M. (1972). A comparison of the social behaviour of some normal and problem children. In N. Blurton Jones (Ed.), *Ethological studies of child behaviour* (pp. 244–284). London: Cambridge University Press.

Lee, C. L., & Bates, J. E. (1985). Mother–child interaction at age two years and perceived difficult temperament. *Child Development, 56,* 1314–1323.

Lee, V. E., Brooks-Gunn, J., & Schnur, E. (1988). Does Head Start work? A 1-year follow-up comparison of disadvantaged children attending Head Start, no preschool, and other preschool programs. *Developmental Psychology, 24,* 210–222.

Lewis, M. (2000). Toward a development of psychopathology: Models, definition, and prediction. In A. J. Sameroff, M. Lewis, & S. Miller (Eds.), *Handbook of developmental psychopathology* (2nd ed., pp. 3–22). New York: Plenum Press.

Lewis, M., Alessandri, S., & Sullivan, M. W. (1992). Differences in shame and pride as a function of children's gender and task difficulty. *Child Development, 63,* 630–638.

Lewis, M., & Brooks-Gunn, J. (1979). Toward a theory of social cognition: The development of the self. In I. Uzgiris (Ed.), *New directions in child development: Social interaction and communication during infancy* (pp. 54–83). San Francisco: Jossey-Bass.

Lewis, M., Feiring, C., McGuffog, C., & Jaskir, J. (1984). Predicting psychopathology in six-year-olds from early social relations. *Child Development, 55,* 123–136.

Lewis, M., Feiring, C., & Rosenthal, S. (2000). Attachment over time. *Child Development, 71,* 707–720.

Lieberman, A. F., Silverman, R., & Pawl, J. H. (2000). Infant–parent psychotherapy: Core concepts and current approaches. In C. Zeanah (Ed.), *Handbook of infant mental health* (2nd ed., pp. 472–484). New York: Guilford Press.

Lonigan, C. J., Elbert, J. C., & Johnson, S. B. (1998). Empirically supported psychosocial interventions for children: An overview. *Journal of Clinical Child Psychology, 27,* 138–145.

Lyons-Ruth, K. (1996). Attachment relationships among children with aggressive behavior problems: The role of disorganized early attachment patterns. *Journal of Consulting and Clinical Psychology, 64,* 64–73.

Lytton, H. (1980). *Parent–child interaction: The socialization process observed in twin and singleton families.* New York: Plenum Press.

Maccoby, E. E. (1988). Gender as a social category. *Developmental Psychology, 24,* 755–765.

Maccoby, E. E. (1990). Gender and relationships: A developmental account. *American Psychologist, 45,* 513–520.

Maccoby, E. E., & Martin, J. A. (1983). Socialization in the context of the family: Parent–child interaction. In P. H. Mussen (Series Ed.) & E. M. Hetherington (Vol. Ed.), *Handbook of child psychology: Vol. 4. Socialization, personality, and social development* (4th ed., pp.1–101). New York: Wiley.

MacFarlane, J. W., Allen, L., & Honzik, M. P. (1954). *A developmental study of the behavior problems of normal children between twenty-one months and fourteen years.* Berkeley: University of California Press.

Mahler, M. S. (1968). *On human symbiosis and the vicissitudes of individuation: Vol. 1. Infantile psychosis.* New York: International Universities Press.

Main, M., & Solomon, J. (1990). Procedures for identifying infants as disorganized–disoriented during the Ainsworth Strange Situation. In M. T. Greenberg, D. Cicchetti, & E. M. Cummings (Eds.), *Attachment in the preschool years: Theory, research, and intervention* (pp. 121–160). Chicago: University of Chicago Press.

Mannuzza, S., Klein, R. G., Bessler, A., Malloy, P., & Hynes, M. E. (1997). Educational and occupational outcome of hyperactive boys grown up. *Journal of the American Academy of Child and Adolescent Psychiatry, 36,* 1122–1127.

Mannuzza, S., Klein, R. G., Bessler, A., Malloy, P., & LaPadula, M. (1993). Adult outcome of hyperactive boys: Educational achievement, occupational rank, and psychiatric status. *Archives of General Psychiatry, 50,* 565–576.

Marakovitz, S., & Campbell, S. B. (1998). Inattention, impulsivity, and hyperactivity from preschool to school age: Performance of hard-to-manage boys on laboratory measures. *Journal of Child Psychology and Psychiatry, 39,* 841–851.

Marshall, E. (2000) Planned Ritalin trial for tots heads into uncharted waters. *Science, 290,* 1280–1282.

Martin, C. L., & Fabes, R. A. (2001). The stability and consequences of young children's same-sex peer interactions. *Developmental Psychology, 37,* 431–446.

Mash, E. J., & Johnston, C. (1982). Comparison of the mother–child interactions of younger and older hyperactive and normal children. *Child Development, 53,* 1371–1381.

Mash, E. J., & Johnston, C. (1983). Sibling interactions of hyperactive and normal children and their relationship to reports of maternal stress and self-esteem. *Journal of Clinical Child Psychology, 12,* 91–99.

Masten, A., & Coatsworth, J. D. (1998). The development of competence in favorable and unfavorable environments: Lessons from research on successful children. *American Psychologist, 53,* 205–220.

Matas, L., Arend, R. A., & Sroufe, L. A. (1978). Continuity of adaptation in the second year: The relationship between quality of attachment and later competence. *Child Development, 49,* 547–556.

McCall, R. B. (1977). Challenges to a science of developmental psychology. *Child Development, 48,* 333–344.

McCall, R. B. (1981). Nature–nurture and the two realms of development: A proposed integration. *Child Development, 52,* 1–12.

McDonough, S. C. (2000). Interaction guidance: An approach for difficult to engage families. In C. Zeanah (Ed.), *Handbook of infant mental health* (2nd ed., pp. 485–493). New York: Guilford Press.

McFadyen-Ketchum, S. A., Bates, J. E., Dodge, K. A., & Pettit, G. S. (1996). Patterns of change in early childhood aggressive disruptive behavior: Gender differences in predictions from early coercive and affectionate mother–child interactions. *Child Development, 67,* 2417–2433.

McGee, R., Partridge, F., Williams, S., & Silva, P. A. (1991). A twelve-year follow-up of preschool hyperactive children. *Journal of the American Academy of Child and Adolescent Psychiatry, 30,* 224–232.

McGee, R., & Silva, P. A. (1982). *A thousand New Zealand children: Their health and development from birth to seven* (Special Report, Series No. 8). Aukland, NZ: Medical Council of New Zealand.

McGee, R., Silva, P. A., & Williams, S. (1984). Perinatal, neurological, environmental, and developmental characteristics of seven-year-old children with stable behaviour problems. *Journal of Child Psychology and Psychiatry, 25,* 573–586.

McHale, J. P., & Rasmussen, J. L.(1998). Co-parental and family group level dynamics during infancy: Early family precursors of child and family functioning during preschool. *Development and Psychopathology, 10,* 39–59.

McLoyd, V. C. (1990). The impact of economic hardship on Black families and children: Psychological distress, parenting, and socio-emotional development. *Child Development, 61,* 311–346.

McLoyd, V. C. (1998). Socieconomic disadvantage and child development. *American Psychologist, 53,* 185–204.

Milich, P., Landau, S., Kilby, G., & Whitten, P. (1982). Preschool peer perceptions of the behavior of hyperactive and aggressive children. *Journal of Abnormal Child Psychology, 10,* 497–510.

Minton, C., Kagan, J., & Levine, J. A. (1971). Maternal control and obedience in the two-year-old. *Child Development, 42,* 1873–1894.

Moffitt, T. E. (1990). Juvenile delinquency and attention deficit disorders: Boys' developmental trajectories from age 3 to age 15. *Child Development, 61,* 893–910.

Moffitt, T. E. (1993). Adolescence-limited and life-course-persistent antisocial behavior: A developmental taxonomy. *Psychological Review, 100,* 674–701.

Moffitt, T. E., Caspi, A., Dickson, N., Silva, P. A., & Stanton, W. (1996). Childhood onset versus adolescent onset antisocial conduct in males: Natural history from age 3 to 18. *Development and Psychopathology, 8,* 399–424.

Moore, G., Cohn, J., & Campbell, S. B. (1997). Mothers' affective behavior with infant siblings: Stability and change. *Developmental Psychology, 33,* 856–860.

Musten, L. M., Firestone, P., Pisterman, S., Bennett, S., & Mercer, J. (1997). Effects of methlyphenidate on preschool children with ADHD: Cognitive and behavioral functions. *Journal of the American Academy of Child and Adolescent Psychiatry, 36,* 1407–1415.

Myers, N. A., & Perlmutter, M. (1978). Memory in the years from two to five. In P. A. Ornstein (Ed.), *Memory development in children* (pp. 191–218). Hillsdale, NJ: Erlbaum.

Nagin, D., & Tremblay, R. (1999). Trajectories of physical aggression, opposition, and hyperactivity on the path to physically violent and non-violent juvenile delinquency. *Child Development, 70,* 1181–1196.

National Association for the Education of Young Children. (1984). *Accreditation criteria* and procedures of the National Academy of Early Childhood Programs. Washington, DC: Author.

National Center for Clinical Infant Programs. (1994). 0–3: Diagnostic classification of mental health and developmental disorders of infancy and early childhood. Arlington, VA: Author.

Nelson, K. (1996). Language in cognitive development: The emergence of the mediated mind. New York: Cambridge University Press.

NICHD Early Child Care Research Network. (1996). Poverty and patterns of child care. In J. Brooks-Gunn & G. J. Duncan (Eds.), Consequences of growing up poor (pp. 100–131). New York: Russell Sage Foundation.

NICHD Early Child Care Research Network. (1997a). Child care experiences during the first year of life. Merrill–Palmer Quarterly, 43, 340–360.

NICHD Early Child Care Research Network. (1997b). The effects of infant child care on infant-mother attachment security: Results of the NICHD Study of Early Child Care. Child Development, 68, 860–879.

NICHD Early Child Care Research Network. (1998). Early child care and cooperation, compliance, defiance, and problem behavior at 24 and 36 months of age. Child Development, 69, 1145–1170.

NICHD Early Child Care Research Network. (1999a). Chronicity of maternal depressive symptoms, maternal sensitivity, and child functioning at 36 months. Developmental Psychology, 35, 1399–1413.

NICHD Early Child Care Research Network. (1999b). Child outcomes when child-care center classes meet recommended standards for quality. American Journal of Public Health, 89, 1072–1077.

NICHD Early Child Care Research Network. (2000a). Characteristics and quality of child care for toddlers and preschoolers. Applied Developmental Science, 4, 116–135.

NICHD Early Child Care Research Network. (2000b). The relation of child care to cognitive and language development. Child Development, 71, 960–980.

NICHD Early Child Care Research Network. (2001a). Child care and family predictors of MacArthur preschool attachment and stability from infancy. Developmental Psychology, 37, 847–862.

NICHD Early Child Care Research Network. (2001b). Does amount of time spent in child care predict socioemotional adjustment during the transition to kindergarten? Manuscript submitted for publication.

NICHD Early Child Care Research Network. (2002a). The NICHD Study of Early Child Care: Contexts of development and developmental outcomes over the first seven years of life. In J. Brooks-Gunn & L. J. Berlin (Eds.), Young children's education, health, and development: Profile and synthesis project report. Washington, DC: Department of Education.

NICHD Early Child Care Research Network. (2002b). Child care structure → process → outcome: Direct and indirect effects of caregiving quality on young children's development. Psychological Science, 13, 199–206.

Offord, D. R., Boyle, M. H., Fleming, J., Munroe-Blum, H., & Rae-Grant, N. (1989). Ontario Child Health Study: Summary of selected results. Canadian Journal of Psychiatry, 34, 483–491.

Offord, D. R., Kraemer, H. C., Kazdin, A. E., Jensen, P. S., & Harrington, R. (1998). Lowering the burden of suffering from child psychiatric disorder: Trade-offs among clinical, targeted, and universal interventions. Journal of the American Academy of Child and Adolescent Psychiatry, 37, 686–694.

Ollendick, T. H., & King, N. J. (1998). Empirically supported treatments for children with phobic and anxiety disorders. *Journal of Clinical Child Psychology, 27*, 156–167.

Olson, G., & Sherman, T. (1983). Attention, learning, and memory in infants. In P. H. Mussen (Series Ed.) & M. M. Haith & J. J. Campos (Vol. Eds.), *Handbook of child psychology: Vol. II. Infancy and developmental psychobiology* (pp. 1001–1080). New York: Wiley.

Olweus, D. (1979). Stability of aggressive reaction patterns in males: A review. *Psychological Bulletin, 86*, 852–875.

Ornstein, P. A. (1978). The study of children's memory. In P. A. Ornstein (Ed.), *Memory development in children* (pp. 1–20). Hillsdale, NJ: Erlbaum.

Overton, W. F., & Reese, H. W. (1981). Conceptual prerequisites for an understanding of stability-change and continuity-discontinuity. *International Journal of Behavioral Development, 4*, 99–123.

Parke, R., & Buriel, R. (1998). Socialization in the family: Ethnic and ecological perspectives. In W. Damon (Series Ed.) & N. Eisenberg (Vol. Ed.), *Handbook of child psychology: Vol. 3. Social, emotional, and personality development* (5th ed., pp. 463–552). New York: Wiley.

Parke, R., & Slaby, R. G. (1983). The development of aggression. In P. H. Mussen (Series Ed.) & E. M. Hetherington (Vol. Ed.), *Handbook of child psychology: Vol. 4. Socialization, personality, and social development* (pp. 547–661). New York: Wiley.

Parker, J. G., & Asher, S. R. (1987). Peer relations and later personal adjustment: Are low-accepted children at risk? *Psychological Bulletin, 102*, 357–389.

Patterson, G. R. (1980). Mothers: The unacknowledged victims. *Monographs of the Society for Research in Child Development, 45*(Serial No. 186).

Patterson, G. R. (1984). Siblings: Fellow travelers in coercive family processes. In R. J. Blanchard (Ed.), *Advances in the study of aggression* (pp. 235–261). New York: Academic Press.

Patterson, G. R., DeBaryshe, B., & Ramsey, E. (1989). A developmental perspective on antisocial behavior. *American Psychologist, 44*, 329–335.

Patterson, G. R., & Yoerger, K. (1997). A developmental model for late-onset delinquency. *Nebraska Symposium on Motivation, 44*, 119–177.

Pavuluri, M. N., Luk, S., & McGee, R. (1996) Help-seeking for behavior problems by parents of preschool children: A community study. *Journal of the American Academy of Child and Adolescent Psychiatry, 35*, 215–222.

Peery, J. C. (1979). Popular, amiable, isolated, rejected: A reconceptualization of sociometric status in preschool children. *Child Development, 50*, 1231–1234.

Pelham, W., & Bender, M. E. (1982). Peer relations in hyperactive children: Description and treatment. In K. Gadow & I. Bialer (Eds.), *Advances in learning and behavioral disabilities* (Vol. 1, pp. 364–436). Greenwich, CT: JAI Press.

Pelham, W., Wheeler, T., & Chronis, A. (1998). Empirically supported treatments for Attention Deficit Hyperactivity Disorder. *Journal of Clinical Child Psychology, 27*, 190–205.

Pepler, D., Corter, C., & Abramovitch, R. (1982). Social relations among children: Comparison of sibling and peer interaction. In K. H. Rubin & H. S. Ross (Eds.), *Peer relationships and social skills in childhood* (pp. 209–228). New York: Springer-Verlag.

Perlman, M., & Ross, H. S. (1997). The benefits of parent intervention in children's disputes: An examination of concurrent changes in fighting. *Child Development, 68*, 690–700.

Pettit, G. S., Bates, J. E., & Dodge, K. A. (1993). Family interaction patterns and children's conduct problems at home and at school: A longitudinal perspective. *School Psychology Review, 22,* 401–418.

Pettit, G. S., Bates, J., & Dodge, K. (1997). Supportive parenting, ecological context, and children's adjustment: A seven-year longitudinal study. *Child Development, 68,* 908–923.

Phillips, D. (1986). The Federal Model Child Care Standards of 1985: Step in the right direction or hollow gesture? *American Journal of Orthopsychiatry, 56,* 56–64.

Phillips, D. (1988). *Quality in child care: What does research tell us?* Washington, DC: National Association for the Education of Young Children.

Phillips, D. A., Voran, M., Kisker, E., Howes, C., & Whitebook, M. (1994). Child care for children in poverty: Opportunity or inequity? *Child Development, 65,* 472–492

Piaget, J. (1926). *The language and thought of the child.* London: Routledge & Kegan Paul.

Piaget, J. (1928). *Judgment and reasoning in the child.* London: Routledge & Kegan Paul

Piaget, J. (1932). *The moral judgment of the child.* New York: Free Press.

Pierce, E. W., Ewing, L. J., & Campbell, S. B. (1999). Diagnostic status and symptomatic behavior of hard-to-manage preschool children in middle childhood and early adolescence. *Journal of Clinical Child Psychology, 28,* 44–57.

Pliszka, S. R., McCracken, J.T., & Maas, J.W. (1996). Catecholamines in attention-deficit hyperactivity disorder: Current perspectives. *Journal of the American Academy of Child and Adolescent Psychiatry, 35,* 264–272.

Raikes, H. (1998). Investigating the child care subsidy: What are we buying? *SRCD Social Policy Report, 12*(2).

Ramey, C. T., & Ramey, S. L. (1998). Early intervention and early experience. *American Psychologist, 58,* 109–120.

Reynolds, A. J., Temple, J. A., Robertson, D. L., & Mann, E. A. (2001). Long-term effects of an early childhood intervention on educational achievement and juvenile arrest. *Journal of the American Medical Association, 285,* 2339–2346.

Richman, N., Stevenson, J., & Graham, P. J. (1982). *Preschool to school: A behavioural study.* London: Academic Press.

Ripple, C. H., Gilliam, W., Chanana, N., & Zigler, E. (1999). Will fifty cooks spoil the broth? The debate over entrusting Head Start to the states. *American Psychologist, 54,* 327–343.

Rogers, S. (1998). Empirically supported comprehensive treatments for young children with autism. *Journal of Clinical Child Psychology, 27,* 168–179.

Rothbart, M. K., & Bates, J. E. (1998). Temperament. In W. Damon (Series Ed.) & N. Eisenberg (Vol. Ed.), *Handbook of child psychology: Vol. 3. Social, emotional, and personality development* (5th ed., pp. 105–176). New York: Wiley.

Rothbart, M. K., Posner, M., & Hershey, K. (1995). Temperament, attention, and developmental psychopathology. In D. Cicchetti & D. Cohen (Eds.), *Developmental psychopathology: Vol. 1. Theory and methods* (pp. 315–340). New York: Wiley.

Routh, D., Schroeder, C. S., & Koocher, G. (1983). Psychology and primary health care for children. *American Psychologist, 38,* 95–98.

Rubin, K. H. (1982). Social and social-cognitive developmental characteristics of young isolate, normal, and sociable children. In K. H. Rubin & H. S. Ross (Eds.), *Peer relationships and social skills in childhood* (pp. 353–374). New York: Springer-Verlag.

Rubin, K. H., Bukowski, W., & Parker, J. G. (1998). Peer interactions, relationships, and groups. In W. Damon (Series Ed.) & N. Eisenberg (Vol. Ed.), *Handbook of child psychology: Vol. 3. Social, emotional, and personality development* (5th ed., pp. 619–700). New York: Wiley.

Rubin, K. H., Fein, G. G., & Vandenberg, B. (1983). Play. In P. H. Mussen (Series Ed.) &

E. M. Hetherington (Vol. Ed.), *Handbook of child psychology: Vol. 4. Socialization, personality, and social development* (pp. 693–774). New York: Wiley.

Ruffman, T., Perner, J., Naito, M., Parkin, L., & Clements, W. A. (1998). Older (but not younger) siblings facilitate false belief understanding. *Developmental Psychology, 34,* 161–174.

Russ, S. W. (1995). Play psychotherapy research. In T. H. Ollendick & R. J. Prinz (Eds.), *Advances in clinical child psychology* (Vol. 17, pp. 365–391). New York: Plenum Press.

Rutter, M. (1981). Stress, coping, and development: Some issues and some questions. *Journal of Child Psychology and Psychiatry, 22,* 323–356.

Rutter, M. (1994). Beyond longitudinal data: Causes, consequences, changes, and continuity. *Journal of Consulting and Clinical Psychology, 62,* 928–940.

Rutter, M. (2000). Genetic studies of autism: From the 1970s into the millennium. *Journal of Abnormal Child Psychology, 28,* 3–14.

Rutter, M., Dunn, J., Plomin, R., Simonoff, E., Pickles, A., Maughan, B., Ormel, J., Meyer, J., & Eaves, L. (1997). Integrating nature and nurture: Implications of person–environment correlations and interactions for developmental psychopathology. *Development and Psychopathology, 9,* 335–364.

Rutter, M., & the English and Romanian Adoptees Study Team. (1998). Developmental catch-up and deficit following adoption after severe early global privation. *Journal of Child Psychology and Psychiatry, 39,* 465–476.

Rutter, M., Silberg, J. L., O'Connor, T. G., & Simonoff, E. (1999). Genetics and child psychiatry: I. Advances in quantitative and molecular genetics. *Journal of Child Psychology and Psychiatry, 40,* 19–55.

Rutter, M., & Sroufe, L. A. (2000). Developmental psychopathology: Concepts and challenges. *Development and Psychopathology, 12,* 265–296.

Saarni, C., Mumme, D., & Campos, J. (1998). Emotional development: Action, communication, and understanding. In W. Damon (Series Ed.) & N. Eisenberg (Vol. Ed.), *Handbook of child psychology: Vol. 3. Social, emotional, and personality development* (5th ed., pp. 237–309). New York: Wiley.

Sameroff, A. J. (1975). Early influences on development: Fact or fancy? *Merrill–Palmer Quarterly, 21,* 265–294.

Sameroff, A. J. (1995). General systems theories and developmental psychopathology. In D. Cicchetti & D. Cohen (Eds.), *Developmental psychopathology: Vol. 1. Theory and methods* (pp. 659–695). New York: Wiley

Sameroff, A. J. (2000). Dialectical processes in developmental psychopathology. In A. J. Sameroff, M. Lewis, & S. Miller (Eds.), *Handbook of developmental psychopathology* (2nd ed., pp. 23–40). New York: Plenum Press.

Sameroff, A. J., & Chandler, M. (1975). Reproductive risk and the continuum of caretaking casualty. In F. Horowitz (Ed.), *Review of child development research* (Vol. 4, pp. 187–244). Chicago: University of Chicago Press.

Sameroff, A. J., Seifer, R., Baldwin, A., & Baldwin, C. P. (1993). Stability of intelligence from preschool to adolescence: The influence of social and family risk factors. *Child Development, 64,* 88–97.

Sameroff, A. J., Seifer, R., & Zax, M. (1982). Early development of children at risk for emotional disorder. *Monographs of the Society for Research in Child Development, 47*(Serial No. 199).

Sanders, M. R., & Christensen, A. P. (1985). A comparison of the effects of child management and planned activities training in five parenting environments. *Journal of Abnormal Child Psychology, 13,* 101–117.

Saxe, L., Cross, T., & Silverman, N. (1988). Children's mental health: The gap between what we know and what we do. *American Psychologist, 43,* 800–807.

Scarr, S. (1998). American child care today. *American Psychologist, 53,* 95–108.

Scarr, S., & McCartney, K. (1983). How people make their own environments: A theory of genotype–environment effects. *Child Development, 54,* 424–435.

Schwartz, D., Dodge, K. A., & Coie, J. D. (1993). The emergence of chronic peer victimization in boys' play groups. *Child Development, 64,* 1755–1772.

Schwartz, D., Dodge, K. A., Pettit, G. S., & Bates, J. E. (1997). The early socialization of aggressive victims of bullying. *Child Development, 68,* 571–591.

Schwartz, D., Dodge, K. A., Pettit, G. S., Bates, J. E., & the Conduct Problems Prevention Research Group. (2000). Friendship as a moderating factor in the pathway between early harsh home environment and later victimization in the peer group. *Developmental Psychology, 36,* 646–662.

Schwartz, D., McFadyen-Ketchum, S. A., Dodge, K. A., Pettit, G. S., & Bates, J. E. (1998). Peer victimization as a predictor of behavior problems at home and in school. *Development and Psychopathology, 10,* 87–100.

Schwartz, D., McFadyen-Ketchum, S. A., Dodge, K. A., Pettit, G. S., & Bates, J. E. (1999). Early behavior problems as a predictor of later peer group victimization: Moderators and mediators in the pathways of social risk. *Journal of Abnormal Child Psychology, 27,* 191–201.

Selman, R. (1980). *The growth of interpersonal understanding.* New York: Academic Press.

Selman, R. (1981). The child as friendship philosopher. In J. Gottman & S. Asher (Eds.), *The development of children's friendships* (pp. 242–272). New York: Cambridge University Press.

Shantz, C. U. (1987). Conflicts between children. *Child Development, 58,* 282–305.

Shatz, M. (1983). Communication. In P. H. Mussen (Series Ed.) & J. H. Flavell & E. M. Markman (Vol. Eds.), *Handbook of child psychology: Vol. 3. Cognitive development* (4th ed., pp. 841–889). New York: Wiley.

Shatz, M., & Gelman, R. (1973). The development of communication skills: Modifications in the speech of young children as a function of the listener. *Monographs of the Society for Research in Child Development, 38*(Serial No. 152).

Shaw, D. S., Bell, R. Q., & Gilliom, M. (2000). A truly early starter model of antisocial behavior. *Clinical Child and Family Psychology Review, 3,* 155–172.

Shaw, D. S., Keenan, K., & Vondra, J. I. (1994). Developmental precursors of externalizing behavior: Ages 1 to 3. *Developmental Psychology, 30,* 355–364.

Shaw, D. S., Owens, E. B., Vondra, J. I., Keenan, K., & Winslow, E. B. (1996). Early risk factors and pathways in the development of early disruptive behavior problems. *Developmental Psychopathology, 8,* 679–699.

Shaw, D. S., & Vondra, J. I. (1993). Chronic family adversity and infant attachment security. *Journal of Child Psychology and Psychiatry, 34,* 1205–1215.

Shaw, D. S., Winslow, E. B., Owens, E. B., Vondra, J. I., Cohn, J. F., & Bell, R.Q. (1998). The development of early externalizing problems among children from low-income families: A transformational perspective. *Journal of Abnormal Child Psychology, 26,* 95–108.

Shelton, T. L., Barkley, R. A., Crosswaite, C., Moorehouse, M., Fletcher, K., Barrett, S., Jenkins, L., & Metavia, L. (2000). Multi-method psycho-educational intervention for preschool children with disruptive behavior: Two-year post-treatment follow-up. *Journal of Abnormal Child Psychology, 28,* 253–266.

Shepherd, M., Oppenheim, B., & Mitchell, S. (1971). *Childhood behaviour and mental health.* New York: Grune & Stratton.

Shonkoff, J., & Phillips, D. (2000). *From neurons to neighborhoods*. Washington, DC: National Academy Press.

Shonkoff, J. P., Lippitt, J., & Cavanaugh, D. (2000). Early childhood policy: Implications for infant mental health. In C. Zeanah (Ed.), *Handbook of infant mental health* (2nd ed., pp. 503–518). New York: Guilford Press.

Slaughter, D. T. (1983). Early intervention and its effects on maternal behavior and child development. *Monographs of the Society for Research in Child Development, 48*(Serial No. 202).

Snow, C. E. (1972). Mothers' speech to children learning language. *Child Development, 43,* 549–565.

Sonuga-Barke, E. J. S., Daley, D., Thompson, M., Laver-Bradbury, C., & Weeks, A. (2001). Parent-based therapies for preschool attention deficit/hyperactivity disorder: A randomized controlled trial with a community sample. *Journal of the American Academy of Child and Adolescent Psychiatry, 40,* 402–408.

Speltz, M. L., DeKlyen, M., & Greenberg, M.T. (1999). Attachment in boys with early onset conduct problems. *Development and Psychopathology, 11,* 269–286.

Speltz, M. L., DeKlyen, M., Greenberg, M. T., & Dryden, M. (1995). Clinical referral for oppositional defiant disorder: Relative significance of attachment and behavioral variables. *Journal of Abnormal Child Psychology, 23,* 487–507.

Sroufe, L. A. (1979). The coherence of individual development. *American Psychologist, 34,* 834–841.

Sroufe, L. A. (1983). Infant-caregiver attachment and patterns of adaptation in preschool: The roots of maladaptation and competence. In M. Perlmutter (Ed.), *Minnesota Symposium on Child Psychology* (Vol. 16, pp. 41–79). Hillsdale, NJ: Erlbaum.

Sroufe, L. A. (1985). Attachment classification from the perspective of infant–caregiver relationships and infant temperament. *Child Development, 56,* 1–14.

Sroufe, L. A. (1990). Considering normal and abnormal together: The essence of developmental psychopathology. *Development and Psychopathology, 2,* 335–347.

Sroufe, L. A. (1997). Psychopathology as an outcome of development. *Development and Psychopathology, 9,* 251–268.

Sroufe, L. A., Cooper, R. G., & De Hart, G. B. (1992). *Child development: Its nature and course* (2nd ed.). New York: McGraw-Hill.

Sroufe, L. A., & Fleeson, J. (1986). Attachment and the construction of relationships. In W. Hartup & Z. Rubin (Eds.), *The nature and development of relationships* (pp. 51–71). Hillsdale, NJ: Erlbaum.

Sroufe, L. A., & Rutter, M. (1984). The domain of developmental psychopathology. *Child Development, 55,* 17–24.

Stern, D. (1985). *The interpersonal world of the infant*. New York: Basic Books.

Stewart, R. B., & Marvin, R. S. (1984). Sibling relations: The role of conceptual perspective-taking in the ontogeny of sibling caregiving. *Child Development, 55,* 1322–1332.

Stewart, R. B., Mobley, L. A., Van Tuyl, S. S., & Salvador, M. A. (1987). The firstborn's adjustment to the birth of a sibling: A longitudinal assessment. *Child Development, 58,* 341–355.

Stoneman, Z., Brody, G. H., & MacKinnon, C. (1984). Naturalistic observations of children's activities and roles while playing with their siblings and friends. *Child Development, 55,* 617–627.

Strassberg, Z., Dodge, K. A., Pettit, G. S., & Bates, J. E. (1994). Spanking in the home and children's subsequent aggression toward kindergarten peers. *Development and Psychopathology, 6,* 445–461.

Sullivan, H. S. (1953). *The interpersonal theory of psychiatry.* New York: Norton.

Swanson, J. M., McBurnett, K., Christian, D. L., & Wigal, T. (1995). Stimulant medication and treatment of children with ADHD. In T. Ollendick & R. Prinz (Eds.), *Advances in clinical child psychology* (Vol. 17, 265–322). New York: Plenum Press.

Teti, D. M., & Ablard, K. E. (1989). Security of attachment and infant–sibling relationships: A laboratory study. *Child Development, 60,* 1519–1528.

Teti, D. M., Gelfand, D. M., Messinger, D. S., & Isabella, R. (1995). Maternal depression and the quality of early attachment: An examination of infants, preschoolers, and their mothers. *Developmental Psychology, 31,* 364–376.

Teti, D. M., Sakin, J. W., Kucera, E., Korns, K. M., & Das Eiden, R. (1996). And baby makes four: Predictors of attachment security among preschool-age firstborns during the transition to siblinghood. *Child Development, 67,* 579–596.

Thomas, A., Chess, S., & Birch, H. (1968). *Temperament and behavior disorders in children.* New York: New York University Press.

Thomas, A., Chess, S., & Korn, S. J. (1982). The reality of difficult temperament. *Merrill–Palmer Quarterly, 28,* 1–20.

Thompson, R. A. (1994). Emotion regulation: A theme in search of a definition. In N. A. Fox (Ed.), The development of emotion regulation. *Monographs of the Society for Research in Child Development, 59*(2–3, Serial No. 240), 25–52.

Thompson, R. A. (1998). Early socio-personality development. In W. Damon (Series Ed.) & N. Eisenberg (Vol. Ed.), *Handbook of child psychology: Vol. 3. Social, emotional, and personality development* (5th ed., pp. 25–104). New York: Wiley.

Thompson, R. A., & Nelson, C. A. (2001). Developmental science and the media: Early brain development. *American Psychologist, 56,* 5–15.

Tremblay, R. E., Pagani-Kurtz, L., Masse, L. C., Vitaro, F., & Pihl, R. O. (1995). A bimodal preventive intervention for disruptive kindergarten boys: Its impact through adolescence. *Journal of Consulting and Clinical Psychology, 63,* 560–568.

Tuma, J. M. (1989). Traditional therapies with children. In T. Ollendick & M. Hersen (Eds.), *Handbook of child psychopathology* (2nd ed., pp. 419–437). New York: Plenum Press.

van den Boom, D. C. (1994). The influence of temperament and mothering on attachment and exploration: An experimental manipulation of sensitive responsiveness among lower-class mothers with irritable infants. *Child Development, 65,* 1457–1477.

van den Boom, D. C. (1995). Do first year intervention effects endure? Follow-up during toddlerhood of a sample of Dutch irritable infants. *Child Development, 66,* 1798–1816.

van IJzendoorn, M. H., Juffer, F., & Duyvesteyn, M. G. (1995). Breaking the intergenerational cycle of insecure attachment: A review of the effects of attachment-based interventions on maternal sensitivity and infant security. *Journal of Child Psychology and Psychiatry, 36,* 225–248.

Vaughn, B. E., Egeland, B., Sroufe, L. A., & Waters, E. (1979). Individual differences in infant–mother attachment at 12 and 18 months: Stability and change in families under stress. *Child Development, 50,* 971–975.

Verhulst, F. C., & van der Ende, J. (1997). Factors associated with child mental health service use in the community. *Journal of the American Academy of Child and Adolescent Psychiatry, 36,* 901–909.

Vitaro, F., Brendgen, M., & Tremblay, R. E. (1999). Prevention of school dropout through the reduction of disruptive behaviors and school failure in elementary school. *Journal of School Psychology, 37*, 205–226.

Vitaro, F., Gendreau, P. L., Tremblay, R. E., & Oligny, P. (1998). Reactive and proactive aggression differentially predict later conduct problems. *Journal of Child Psychology and Psychiatry, 39*, 377–385.

Vitaro, F., & Tremblay, R. E. (1994). Impact of a prevention program on aggressive children's friendships and social adjustment. *Journal of Abnormal Child Psychology, 22*, 457–476.

Volling, B. L., & Belsky, J. (1992). The contribution of mother–child and father–child relationships to the quality of sibling interaction: A longitudinal study. *Child Development, 63*, 1209–1222.

Wahler R. G. (1980). The insular mother: Her problems in parent–child treatment. *Journal of Applied Behavior Analysis, 13*, 207–219.

Wallerstein, J. S., & Kelly, J. B. (1980). *Surviving the break-up: How children and parents cope with divorce.* New York: Basic Books.

Waters, E., Weinfield, N. S., & Hamilton, C. E. (2000). The stability of attachment security from infancy to adolescence and early adulthood: General discussion. *Child Development, 71*, 703–706.

Webster-Stratton, C. (1984). Randomized trial of two parent-training programs for families with conduct disordered children. *Journal of Consulting and Clinical Psychology, 52*, 666–678.

Webster-Stratton, C. (1985). The effects of father involvement in parent training for conduct problem children. *Journal of Child Psychology and Psychiatry, 26*, 801–810.

Webster-Stratton, C., & Hammond, M. (1999). Marital conflict management skills, parenting style, and early-onset conduct problems: Processes and pathways. *Journal of Child Psychology and Psychiatry, 40*, 917–927.

Weinfield, N. S., Sroufe, L. A., & Egeland, B. (2000). Attachment from infancy to early adulthood in a high risk sample: Continuity, discontinuity, and their correlates. *Child Development, 71*, 695–702.

Weiss, G., & Hechtman, L. T. (1993). *Hyperactive children grown up* (2nd ed.). New York: Guilford Press.

Weisz, J. R., & Hawley, K. M. (1998). Finding, evaluating, refining, and applying empirically supported treatments for children and adolescents. *Journal of Clinical Child Psychology, 27*, 206–216.

Weisz, J. R., & Weiss, B. (1993). *Effects of psychotherapy with children and adolescents.* Newbury Park, CA: Sage.

Weisz, J. R., Weiss, B., Alicke, M. D., & Klotz, M. L. (1987). Effectiveness of psychotherapy with children and adolescents: A meta-analysis for clinicians. *Journal of Consulting and Clinical Psychology, 55*, 542–549.

Weizman, Z. O., & Snow, C. E. (2001). Lexical input as related to children's vocabulary acquisition: Effects of sophisticated exposure and support for meaning. *Developmental Psychology, 37*, 265–279.

Wellman, H. M., Ritter, R., & Flavell, J. H. (1975). Deliberate memory behavior in the delayed reactions of very young children. *Developmental Psychology, 11*, 780–787.

Wenar, C. (1982). Developmental psychopathology: Its nature and models. *Journal of Clinical Child Psychology, 11*, 192–201.

Werner, E., Bierman, J. H., & French, F. E. (1971). *The children of Kauai.* Honolulu: University of Hawaii Press.

Werner, E., & Smith, S. (1977). *Kauai's children come of age.* Honolulu: University of Hawaii Press.

White, R. W. (1959). Motivation reconsidered: The concept of competence. *Psychological Review, 66,* 297–233.

White, S. H. (1996). The relationship of developmental psychology to social policy. In E. F. Zigler, S. L. Kagan, & N. W. Hall (Eds.), *Children, families, and government: Preparing for the twenty-first century* (pp. 409–426). New York: Cambridge University Press.

Whitebook, M. C., Howes, C., & Phillips, D. A. (1990). *Who cares? Child care teachers and the quality of care in America: Final report of the National Child Care Staffing Study.* Oakland, CA: Child Care Employee Project.

Whitebook, M. C., Sakai, L., & Howes, C. (1997). *NAEYC accreditation as a strategy for improving child care quality.* Washington, DC: National Center for the Early Childhood Work Force.

Winett, R. A. (1998). Prevention: A proactive–developmental–ecological perspective. In T. Ollendick & M. Hersen (Eds.), *Handbook of child psychopathology* (3rd ed., pp. 637–671). New York: Plenum Press.

Wolkind, S. (1985). Mothers' depression and their children's attendance at medical facilities. *Journal of Psychosomatic Research, 29,* 579–582.

Woodhead, M. (1988). When psychology informs public policy: The case of early childhood intervention. *American Psychologist, 43,* 443–454.

Yarrow, L. J., McQuiston, S., MacTurk, R. H., McCarthy, M. E., Klein, R. P., & Vietze, P. M. (1983). Assessment of mastery motivation during the first year of life: Contemporaneous and cross-age relationships. *Developmental Psychology, 19,* 159–171.

Young, K. T., & Zigler, E. (1986). Infant and toddler day care: Regulations and policy implications. *American Journal of Orthopsychiatry, 56,* 43–54.

Youngblade, L. M., & Dunn, J. (1995). Individual differences in young children's pretend play with mother and with sibling: Links to relationships and understanding of other people's feelings and beliefs. *Child Development, 66,* 1472–1492.

Zahn-Waxler, C., Cummings, E. M., McKnew, D. H., & Radke-Yarrow, M. (1984). Altruism, aggression, and social interactions in young children with a manic–depressive parent. *Child Development, 55,* 112–122.

Zahn-Waxler, C., Iannotti, R. J., Cummings, E. M., & Denham, S. (1990). Antecedents of problem behaviors in children of depressed mothers. *Development and Psychopathology, 2,* 271–291.

Zahn-Waxler, C., Radke-Yarrow, M., & King, R. A. (1979). Childrearing and children's prosocial initiations toward victims of distress. *Child Development, 50,* 319–330.

Zaslow, M., Tout, K., Smith, S., & Moore, K. (1998) Implications of the 1996 welfare legislation for children: A research perspective. *SRCD Social Policy Report, 12*(3).

Zigler, E. (1987). Formal schooling for four-year-olds? No. *American Psychologist, 42,* 254–260.

Zigler, E. F., & Gilman, E. (1996). Not just any care: Shaping a coherent child care policy. In E. F. Zigler, S. L. Kagan, & N. W. Hall (Eds.), *Children, families, and government: Preparing for the twenty-first century* (pp. 94–116). New York: Cambridge University Press.

Zigler, E., & Styfco, S. (1993). Using research and theory to justify and inform Head Start expansion. *SRCD Social Policy Report, 7*(2).

Zigler, E., & Styfco, S. (1996). Head Start and early childhood intervention: The changing course of social science and social policy. In E. F. Zigler, S. L. Kagan, & N. W.

Hall (Eds.), *Children, families, and government: Preparing for the twenty-first century* (pp. 132–155). New York: Cambridge University Press.

Zigler, E., & Valentine, J. (1979). *Project Head Start: A legacy of the War on Poverty.* New York: Free Press.

Zito, J. M., Safer, D. J., dosReis, S., Gardner, J. F., Boles, M., & Lynch, F. (2000). Trends in the prescribing of psychotropic medications to preschoolers. *Journal of the American Medical Association, 283,* 1025–1030.

Zubin, J., & Spring, B. (1977). Vulnerability: A new view of schizophrenia. *Journal of Abnormal Psychology, 86,* 103–126.

Index

325